Manual of Emergency and Critica

Second Edition

Manual of Emergency and Critical Care Ultrasound

Second Edition

Vicki E. Noble MD, RDMS, FACEP
Director, Division of Emergency Ultrasound, Department of Emergency Medicine, Massachusetts General Hospital, and Assistant Professor, Harvard Medical School, Boston, MA, USA

Bret P. Nelson MD, RDMS, FACEP
Director of Emergency Ultrasound and Associate Professor of Emergency Medicine, Mount Sinai School of Medicine, New York, NY, USA

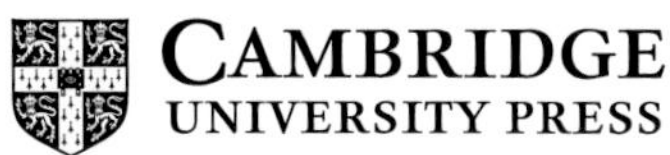

CAMBRIDGE
UNIVERSITY PRESS

University Printing House, Cambridge CB2 8BS, United Kingdom

Cambridge University Press is part of the University of Cambridge.

It furthers the University's mission by disseminating knowledge in the pursuit of education, learning and research at the highest international levels of excellence.

www.cambridge.org
Information on this title: www.cambridge.org/9780521170918

First edition published 2007
Second edition published 2011
7th printing 2015

Printed in the United Kingdom by Bell and Bain Ltd, Glasgow

A catalog record for this publication is available from the British Library

Library of Congress Cataloging in Publication data

Noble, Vicki E., 1969– author.
Manual of emergency and critical care ultrasound / Vicki E. Noble, Bret P. Nelson. – 2nd Edition.
p. ; cm.
Includes bibliographical references and index.
ISBN 978-0-521-17091-8 (Paperback)
1. Diagnostic ultrasonic imaging–Handbooks, manuals, etc. 2. Ultrasonic imaging–Handbooks, manuals, etc. 3. Emergency medicine–Diagnosis–Handbooks, manuals, etc. I. Nelson, Bret, 1973– II. Title.
[DNLM: 1. Ultrasonography–methods. 2. Critical Care–methods. 3. Emergencies. 4. Emergency Medical Services–methods. 5. Emergency Treatment–methods. WN 208]
RC78.7.U4N63 2011
616.07′543–dc22 2010046476

ISBN 978-0-521-17091-8 Paperback

Contents

Acknowledgments

Many many thanks to the nurses, doctors, residents, and support staff in the emergency department at Massachusetts General Hospital. They make me a better doctor, keep me honest, and make it fun to come to work on most days. Thanks as well to Bret for his patience with both editions of this book and for being such a strong advocate for the field of point-of-care ultrasound. He never says no even if he probaby should – and thanks to Susan for letting him say yes. Finally a million thanks to Dr. Andrew Liteplo for being such a fabulous colleague – his enthusiasm for ultrasound knows no bounds, and many of the images in the book are from his collection. It is invaluable to have a colleague who shares my enthusiasm for the potential in point-of-care ultrasound and who works tirelessly supporting the education, research, and administrative efforts behind the advancement of the field. I am very lucky and grateful.

VEN

My wife Susan and son Holden give me the strength to work and the reason to come home. This book could not have been completed without their love and support. I am also grateful for Vicki's tireless dedication to this book and the advancement of point-of-care ultrasound. Over the years I have been inspired by my colleagues, residents, and students to improve. Someday I just might.

BPN

1 Fundamentals

Introduction

To become versed in the language of ultrasonography, it is necessary to review some of the basic principles of physics. The wave physics principles of ordinary (i.e., audible) sound apply to ultrasound (US) and its applications as well. Thus, to create a foundation for further discussions, a number of definitions and basic concepts are presented here.

Basic definitions and physics principles

Amplitude is the peak pressure of a wave (Figure 1.1). Measured in decibels (dB), this can describe the volume (or "loudness") of audible sound or the strength of the echo in ultrasound.

Ultrasound machines can measure the intensity (amplitude) of the returning echo; analysis of this information affects the brightness of the echo displayed on the screen. Strong returning echoes translate into bright or white areas on the screen (known as *hyperechoic*). Weak returning echoes translate into dark gray or black areas on the screen (known as *hypoechoic* or *anechoic*, respectively). The "gray scale" of diagnostic ultrasonography is the range of echo strength as it correlates to colors on a black–white continuum (Figure 1.2).

Velocity is defined as the speed of the wave. It is constant in a given medium and is calculated to be 1540 m/s in soft tissue (i.e., the *propagation speed* of soft tissue is 1540 m/s). Using this principle, an ultrasound machine can calculate the distance/depth of a structure by measuring the time it takes for an emitted ultrasound beam to be reflected back to the source (Figure 1.3). Sonar, as used on submarines, is based on this same principle.

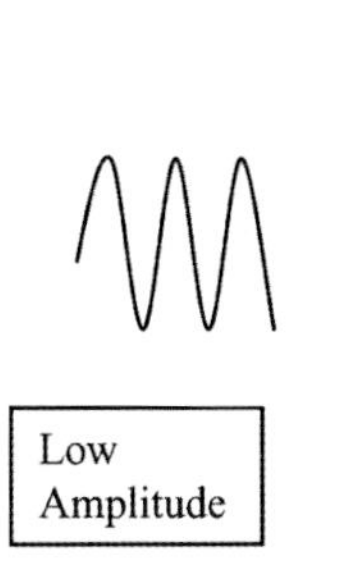

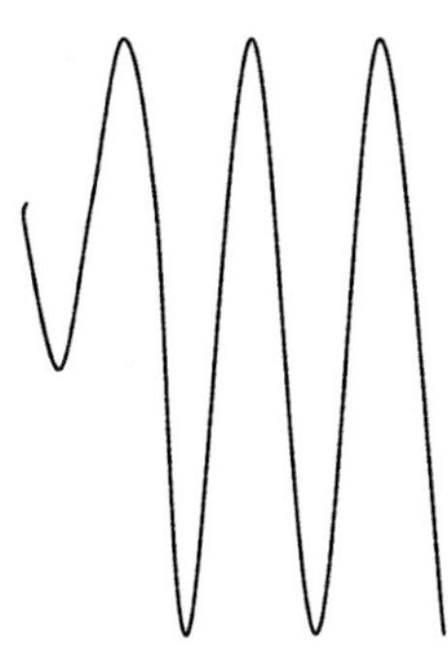

Figure 1.1 Low- and high-amplitude sound waves.

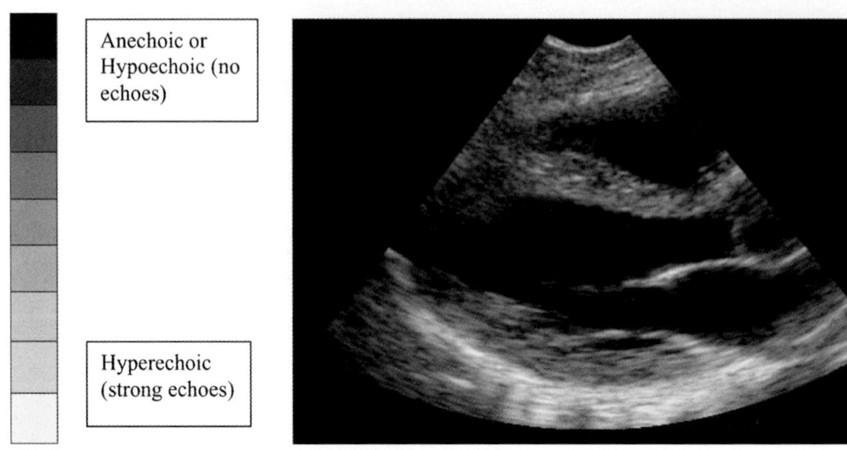

Figure 1.2
Most ultrasound machines have 256 shades of gray, corresponding to the returning amplitude of a given ultrasound wave.

Frequency is the number of times per second the wave is repeated. One hertz (Hz) is equal to one wave cycle per second. Audible sound has frequencies from 20 to 20 000 Hz. By definition, any frequencies above this range are referred to as ultrasound. The frequencies used in diagnostic ultrasound typically range from 2 to 12 MHz (1 MHz = 1 million Hz).

High-frequency sound waves generate high-resolution pictures. High-frequency sound waves use more energy because they generate more waves, which send back more echoes over short distances to the machine, creating detailed pictures of shallow depth (Figure 1.4). However, because they lose energy more rapidly, high-frequency ultrasound waves do not penetrate long distances. Conversely, lower-resolution waves conserve energy. Although they do not create pictures of equally high resolution, they are able to penetrate deeper into tissue. Imagine sitting near a high-fidelity stereo system. Your ears will note great detail in the high-frequency (treble) range, and less detail in the low-frequency (bass) range. This is why "tweeters" should be aimed at the listener while the subwoofer can be placed anywhere. Downstairs from the speakers, the treble drops off entirely and only the bass remains. Thus, frequency correlates directly to resolution and inversely to penetration in audible sound as well as ultrasound.

Wavelength is the distance the wave travels in a single cycle. Because velocity must remain constant in a given medium, wavelength is inversely related to frequency (velocity = frequency × wavelength). Therefore, high frequency decreases wavelength (and thus penetration), and lower frequency increases wavelength (and thus penetration).

Attenuation is the progressive weakening of a sound wave as it travels through a medium. The attenuation coefficients for different tissue densities in the body are shown in Table 1.1.

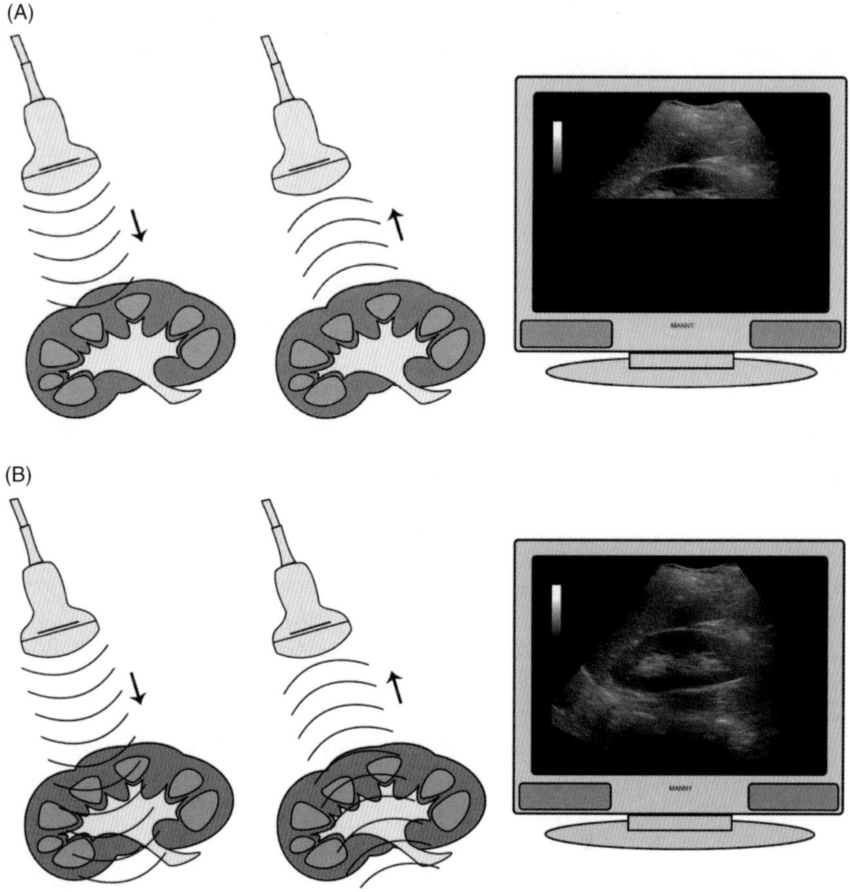

Figure 1.3

(*A*) The near field of the screen shows objects closest to the probe. (*B*) The far field of the screen shows images further from the probe. Courtesy of Dr. Manuel Colon, University of Puerto Rico Medical Center, Carolina, PR.

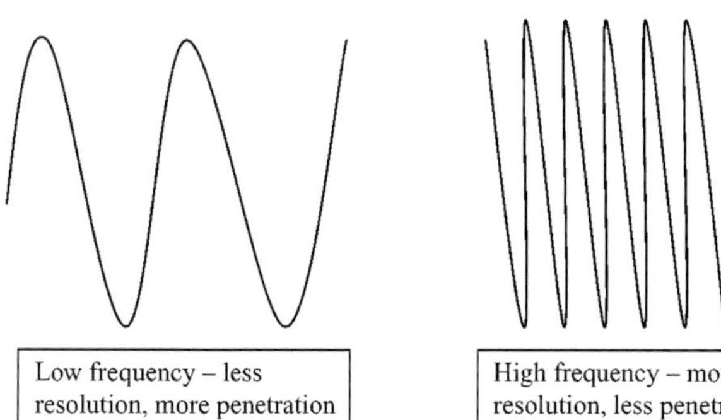

Figure 1.4

Low- and high-frequency sound waves.

Table 1.1 Attenuation coefficients for body tissues

Tissue	Attenuation coefficient	Ultrasound characterisitics
Air	4500	Poor propagation, sound waves often scattered
Bone	870	Very echogenic (reflects most back, high attenuation)
Muscle	350	Echogenic (bright echo)
Liver/kidney	90	Echogenic (less bright)
Fat	60	Hypoechoic (dark echo)
Blood	9	Hypoechoic (very dark echo)
Fluid	6	Hypoechoic (very dark echo, low attenuation)

Several factors contribute to attenuation: the density of the medium, the number of interfaces encountered, and the wavelength of the sound. Diagnostic ultrasound does not transmit well through air and bone because of scatter and reflection. However, ultrasound travels well through fluid-containing structures such as the bladder. Attenuation also occurs as sound encounters interfaces between different types of media. If a tissue is homogeneous and dense, then the number of interfaces is reduced and less attenuation occurs. If a tissue is heterogeneous and less dense, then more attenuation occurs.

Reflection is the redirection of part of the sound wave back to its source. *Refraction* is the redirection of part of the sound wave as it crosses a boundary between different media (or crosses tissues of different propagation speeds such as from muscle to bone). *Scattering* occurs when the sound beam encounters an interface that is relatively small or irregular in shape (e.g., what happens when sound waves travel through air or gas). *Absorption* occurs when the acoustic energy of the sound wave is contained within the medium.

Resolution refers to an ultrasound machine's ability to discriminate between two closely spaced objects. Figure 1.5 shows two points that are resolved as distinct by a machine with higher resolution (the paired dots) and the same structures visualized by a machine with lower resolution (the two dots are seen as a single indistinct blob). *Axial resolution* refers to the ultrasound machine's ability to differentiate two closely spaced echoes that lie in a plane parallel to the direction of the traveling sound wave. Increasing the frequency of the sound wave will increase the axial resolution of the ultrasound image. *Lateral resolution* refers to the ultrasound machine's ability to differentiate two closely spaced echoes that lie in a plane perpendicular to the direction of the traveling sound wave. In some portable ultrasound machines, the focal zone (or narrowest part of the ultrasound beam)

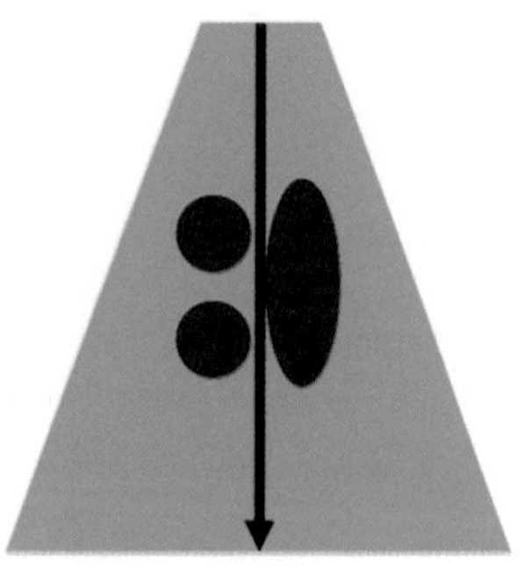

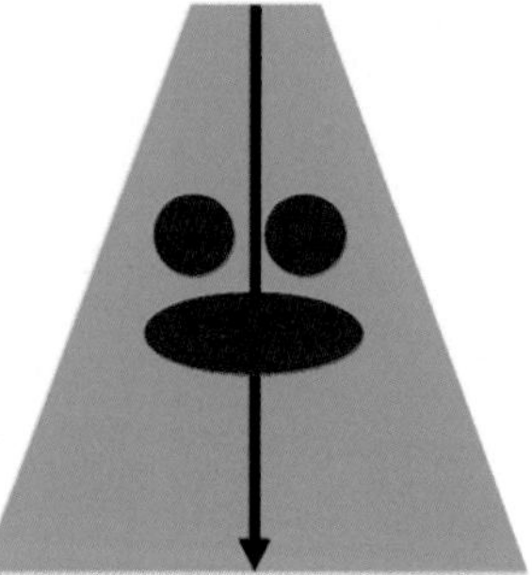

Figure 1.5
Axial resolution (*left*) improves with higher frequency. Lateral resolution (*right*) improves with narrow bandwidth (focal zone).

is automatically set over the mid-range of the screen. However, some machines have a button that allows you to shift that narrow part of the beam up and down.

Finally, *acoustic power* refers to the amount of energy leaving the transducer. It is set to a default in most diagnostic ultrasound machines to prevent adverse biologic effects, such as tissue heating or cell destruction. This is to adhere to the ALARA or "as low as reasonably acceptable" principle – meaning the lowest amount of energy is used to obtain the information clinically needed to care for the patient. Therapeutic ultrasound operates differently from the diagnostic ultrasound discussed so far in that it purposely uses the heating properties of ultrasound to affect tissue. Often, therapeutic ultrasound is used in physical therapy or rehabilitation after orthopedic injuries to help mobilize tissue that has been scarred.

Basic instrumentation

Ultrasound devices all use the same basic principle for generating ultrasound waves and receiving the reflected echoes. This principle is made possible by a property that quartz and some other compounds, both natural and synthetic, possess called the *piezoelectric effect*. The piezoelectric effect refers to the production of a pressure wave when an applied voltage deforms a crystal element. Moreover, the crystal can also be deformed by returning pressure waves reflected from within tissue. This reflected deformation generates an electric current that the machine translates into a pixel. As mentioned, this pixel's gray shade depends on the strength or amplitude of the returning echo and thus the strength of the electric current it generates.

Many different arrangements of this basic piezoelectric transducer/probe have been developed (Figure 1.6). For example, a convex probe has crystals embedded in a curved, convex array. The further the beams have to travel, the more the ultrasound beams fan out. This reduces lateral resolution in deeper tissue. It also produces a sector- or pie-shaped image. A linear array probe (Figure 1.7) has crystals embedded in a flat head. As a result, the

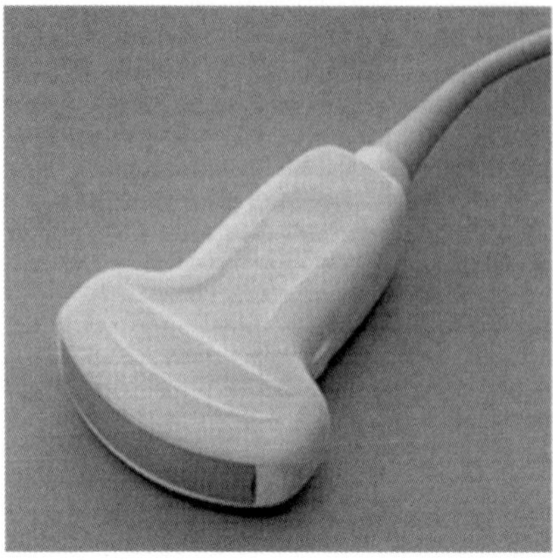

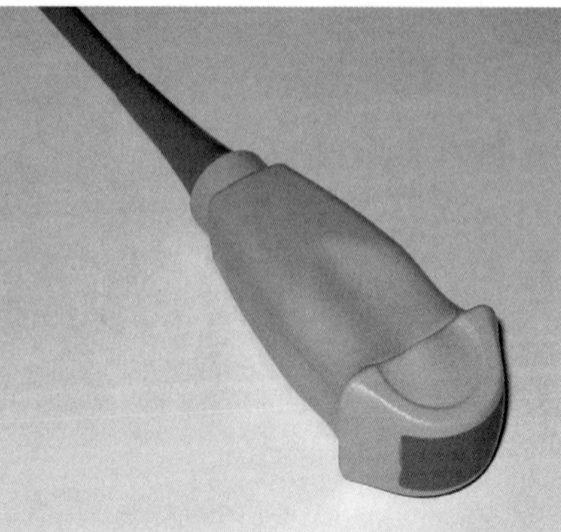

Figure 1.6
Curvilinear probe on left, microconvex probe on right.

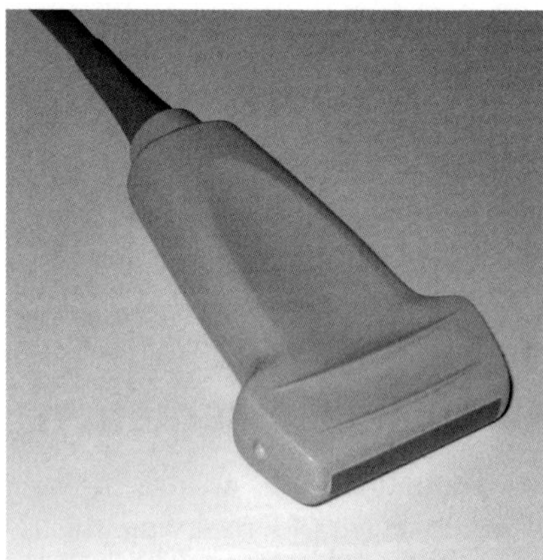

Figure 1.7
Linear probe.

ultrasound beams travel in a straight line. Because the ultrasound beams are directed straight ahead, a rectangular image is produced. Probes come in different sizes or "footprints" because sometimes smaller probes are needed to sneak through ribs or other structures that are not ultrasound-friendly. The phased-array probe (Figure 1.8) serves this purpose well and is often employed for cardiac and abdominal scanning.

Finally, each probe has a range of frequencies it is capable of generating. Usually, linear probes have higher frequency ranges and curved probes have lower frequency ranges. One exception to this is the intercavitary probe used in obstetric and gynecologic ultrasound (Figure 1.9). Although it has a curved footprint, it also uses higher-frequency ultrasound to obtain high-resolution pictures of smaller structures close to the probe.

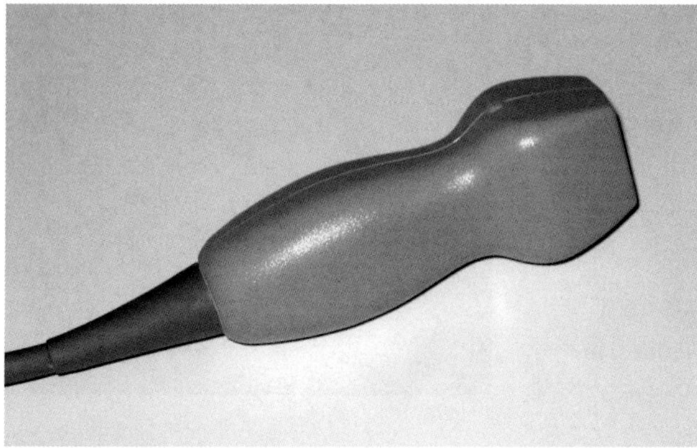

Figure 1.8
Phased-array probe.

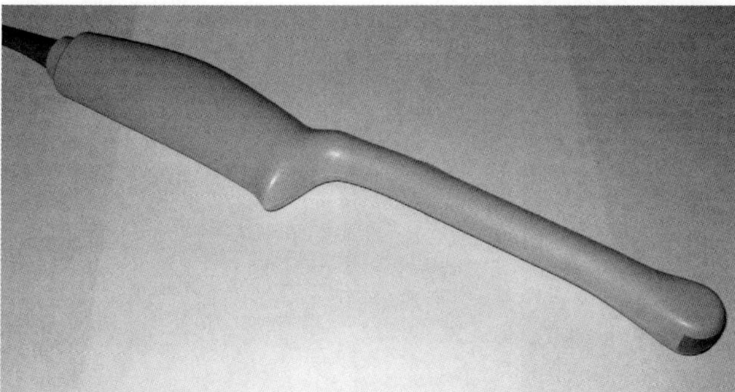

Figure 1.9
Intracavitary probe.

Using the transducer/probe

When scanning with the transducer, use adequate amounts of ultrasound gel to facilitate maneuvering the transducer and to optimize the quality of images obtained. Any air between the probe and the surface of the skin will cause sound waves traveling through that space to scatter, and the strength of the returning echoes will decrease.

It is important to hold the probe such that it does not slip from your grasp or slide around on the patient's gel-covered skin. Holding the probe with the first three to four fingers of your hand allows the fourth or fifth finger and heel of the hand to provide a stable platform for scanning. Thus, less pressure needs to be applied to maintain position on the skin surface without slipping. Holding the probe as you would a pencil is a good first pass at comfortable probe handling (Figure 1.10).

Finally, several scanning planes should be used whenever imaging any anatomic structure. It is always important to image structures in at least two planes (e.g., transverse and longitudinal), because we are looking at three-dimensional structures with two-dimensional images.

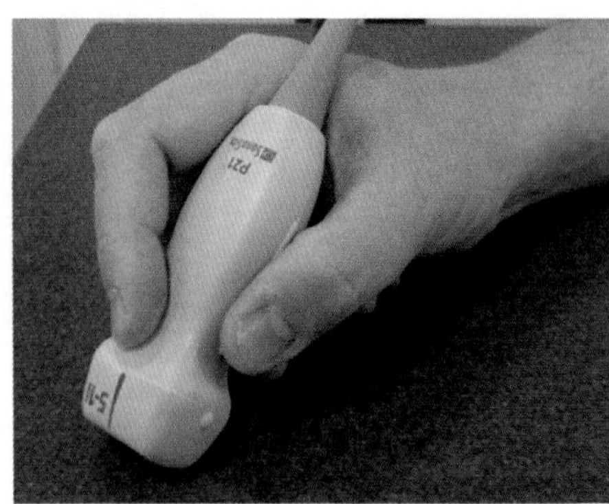

Figure 1.10
Holding the probe.

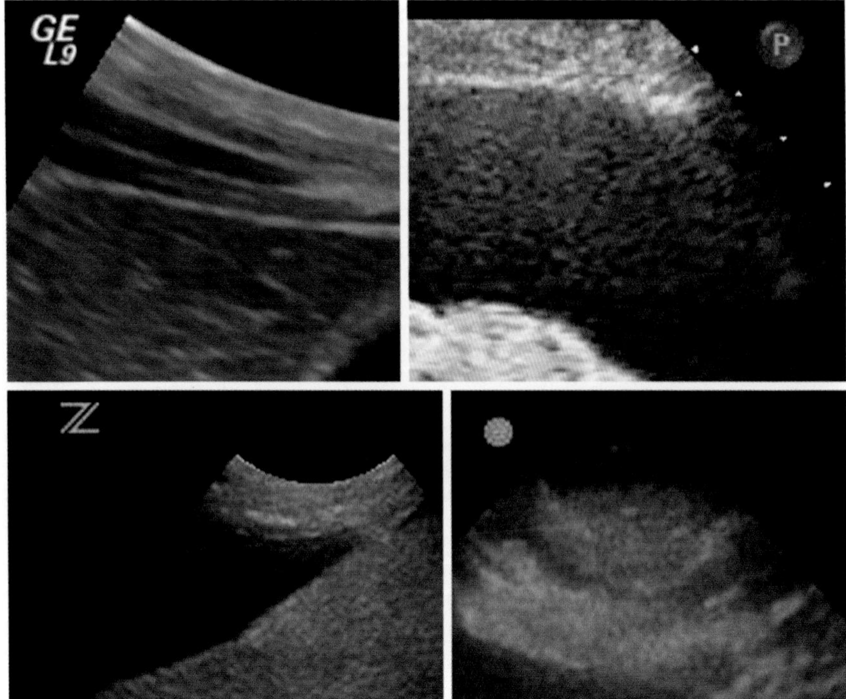

Figure 1.11
Screen markers are found on the top of the screen, usually on the left for emergency ultrasound applications. Different vendors use different symbols as markers. Clockwise from top left: GE, Philips, SonoSite, Zonare.

Probe and screen markers

One of the first principles to remember is that every probe has a raised marker or indentation on it that correlates to the side of the screen with a dot, the ultrasound manufacturer's logo, or some other identifier (Figure 1.11). Objects

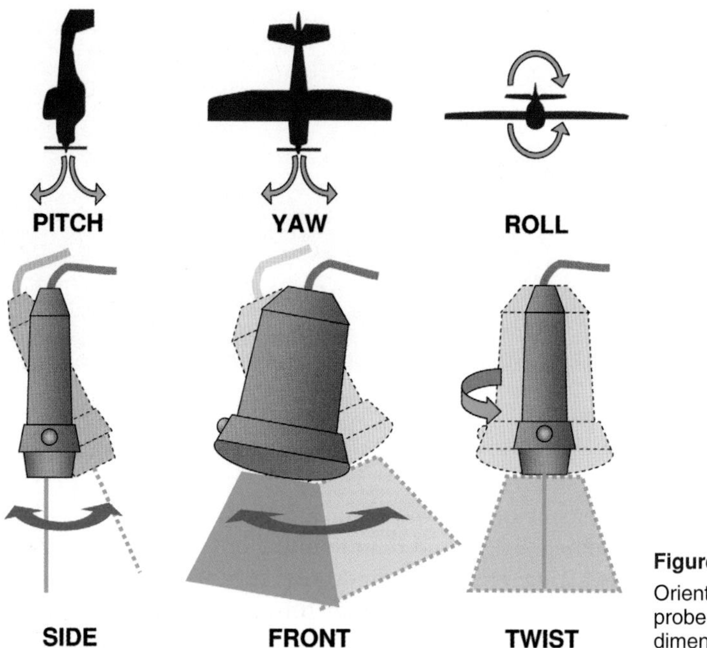

Figure 1.12
Orientation of the probe in three dimensions.

located near the probe marker on the transducer will appear near the screen marker on the screen. Objects opposite the probe marker will appear on the other side from the screen marker.

For the most part, bedside ultrasound keeps the screen marker on the left-hand side of the screen. However, formal echocardiography is performed with the marker on the right-hand side of the screen, so most machines have a button that lets you flip the screen marker back and forth. This manual describes all images with the marker on the left to keep machine settings constant. It is important to know this fact, because echocardiographers often employ different probe positions (180 degrees rotated from the descriptions in this book) based on their different screen settings.

Proprioception

As one grows more comfortable with scanning, the probe and ultrasound beam become an extension of the arm. It becomes natural to understand that moving your hand a certain way yields predictable changes in the image orientation. For novice users, it is helpful to review the standard orientation of the probe. Like any object working in three dimensions, the probe (and therefore the ultrasound beam) can be oriented in an *x*, *y*, or *z* axis. A simple analogy would be the orientation of an airplane. An ultrasound transducer is pictured in Figure 1.12 in three different orientations (short side, long side, and facing out of the page), with its beam colored green to illustrate the concept.

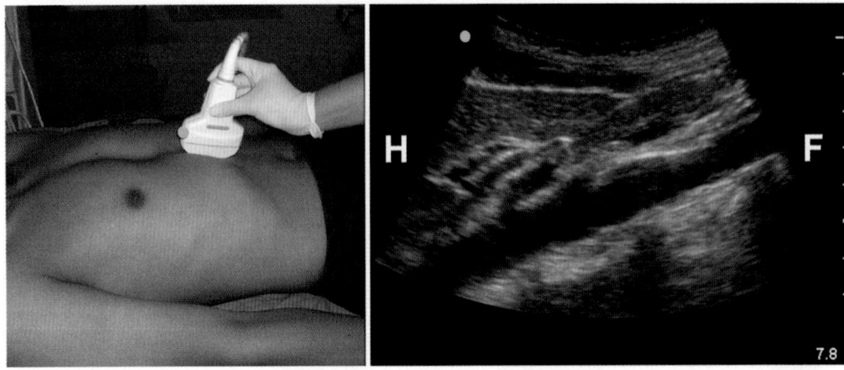

Figure 1.13
Longitudinal probe position. The probe marker and screen marker are highlighted in green.

Pitch refers to movement up or down. For a transducer in a transverse orientation on the abdomen, this would refer to tilting or "fanning" the probe toward the head or feet. *Yaw* refers to a side-to-side turn. This would correspond to angling the same probe left or right toward the patient's flanks. Finally, *roll* refers to spinning on a central long axis. If this motion is done with the aforementioned probe, the transverse orientation would become sagittal. At first, focus on moving the probe in one plane at a time, and note the impact on the image. Novice users often become disoriented when they believe that they are moving in one plane but are truly twisting through multiple axes at once.

Probe positioning when scanning

When obtaining a longitudinal or sagittal view (Figure 1.13), the transducer is oriented along the long axis of the patient's body (i.e., the probe marker is pointed toward the patient's head). This means that you will see the cephalad structures on the side of the screen with the marker (here, on the left side).

The transverse or axial view (Figure 1.14) is obtained by orienting the transducer 90 degrees from the long axis of the patient's body, producing a cross-sectional display. For the vast majority of indications, the probe marker should be oriented toward the patient's right. Again, if the marker is pointed to the right, the structures on the right side of the body will appear on the side of the screen with the marker.

The coronal view (Figure 1.15) is obtained by positioning the transducer laterally. The probe marker is still pointed to the patient's head so the cephalad structures are on the left side of the screen (marker side). The structures closest to the probe are shown at the top of the screen, and as the beam penetrates, the tissues furthest from the probe are at the bottom of the screen.

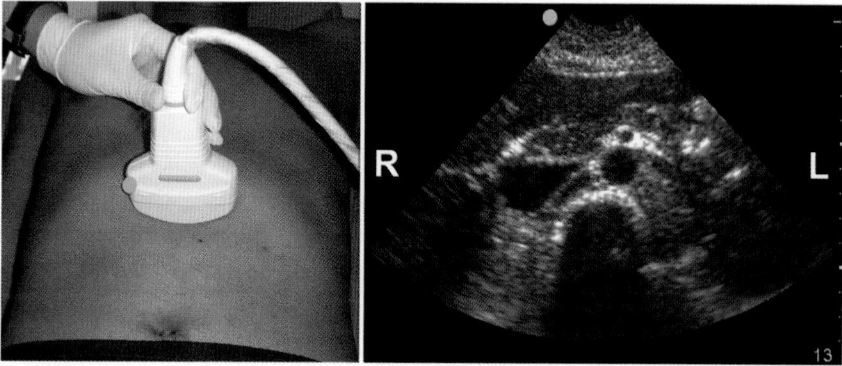

Figure 1.14
Transverse probe position. The probe marker and screen marker are highlighted in green.

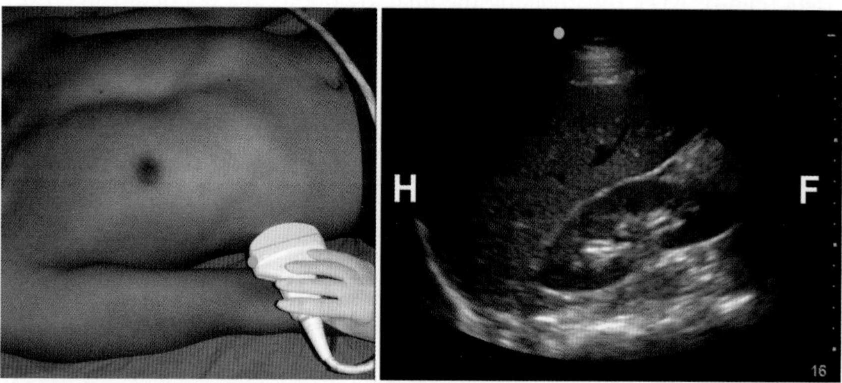

Figure 1.15
Coronal probe position. The probe marker and screen marker are highlighted in green.

Understanding the formed image

To review, a number of conventions have been almost universally adopted for translating the electrical information generated by the transducer into an image on a display screen. We say "almost" because, as mentioned previously, cardiologists have reversed their screen marker; instead of placing it on the left side of the screen, they place it on the right. Because bedside emergency ultrasound includes abdominal and other imaging, we leave the marker on the left side and describe a probe position 180 degrees reversed from the cardiology standard when doing bedside cardiac imaging. By doing this, the images will appear the same as the cardiologists' on the screen.

Again, to obtain these conventional views, you must know the orientation of the transducer's beam. The convention is that the probe indicator or marker should be to the patient's right or the patient's head. The screen marker should be on the left of the screen (Figures 1.13–1.15).

Adjusting the image

Some ultrasound machines allow the operator to choose where to focus the narrowest part of the ultrasound beam. By adjusting the *focal zone* (Figure 1.16), you can optimize lateral resolution. Focus is usually adjusted by means of a knob or an up/down button on the control panel.

Focal depth is usually indicated on the side of the display screen as a pointer. By moving the pointer to the area of interest, the beam is narrowed at that depth to improve the image quality. Not all machines allow this function to be set manually, however; some perform this function automatically at the midpoint of the screen.

Another parameter that can be adjusted by the ultrasound operator is the *depth* (Figure 1.17). By adjusting the imaging depth, the operator can ensure that the entire tissue or structure of interest is included on the screen. Depth is

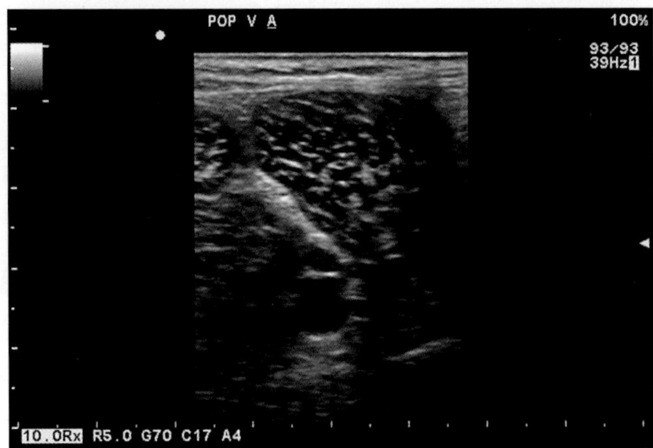

Figure 1.16
Focal zone, marked by the small white triangle at the middle right of the screen.

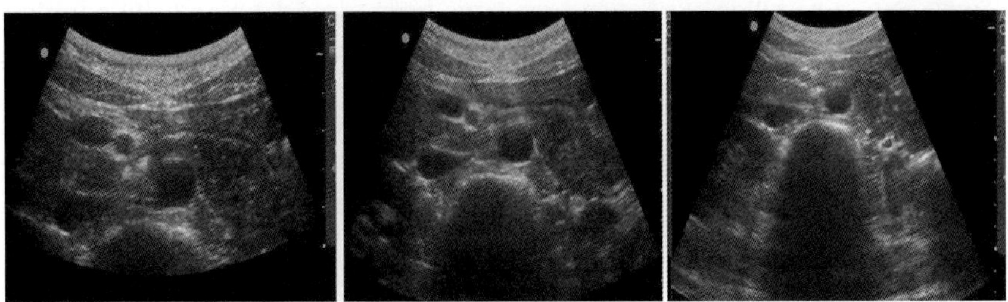

Figure 1.17
Depth. Increasing depth from the left to right panels.

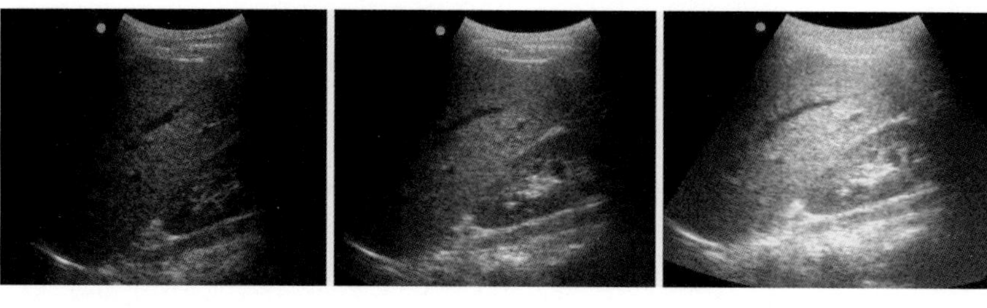

Figure 1.18
Gain. Increasing gain from the left to right panels.

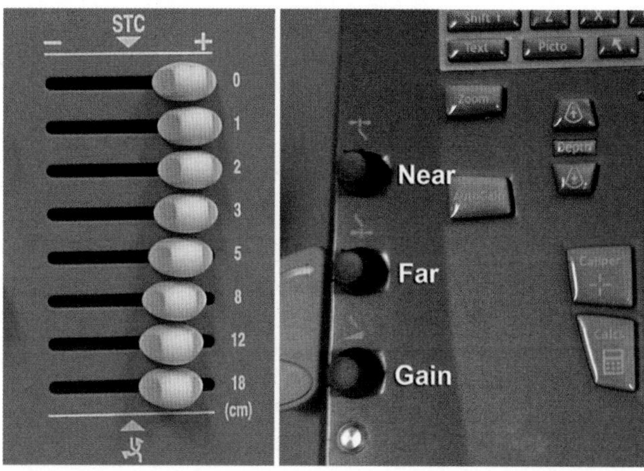

Figure 1.19
Time gain compensation (TGC) may be controlled with sliders (*left*) or knobs (*right*), and machines vary in the number of regions which may be controlled individually.

usually adjusted by means of a knob or an up/down button on the control panel. A centimeter scale is usually located on the side of the display screen to indicate the depth of the tissue being scanned.

The *gain* control offers an additional parameter for adjusting the intensity of returned echoes shown on the display screen (Figure 1.18). In other words, by increasing the gain, the entire ultrasound field (i.e., the entire display) brightens. When the gain decreases, the ultrasound field darkens. The gain function is somewhat akin to adjusting the volume on your stereo – it increases the overall volume but does not improve the quality of the sound. In the case of diagnostic imaging, it increases the brightness but does not increase the number of pixels per image. A knob or up/down button on the control panel allows the operator to adjust gain. The gain function has *no* effect on the acoustic power.

Time gain compensation (TGC) controls on an ultrasound machine allow the operator to adjust the gain *at varying depths* (Figure 1.19). Echoes returning from deeper structures are more attenuated simply because they have to travel through more tissue. Without TGC, the far field (bottom of the screen, deeper tissue) would always appear darker than the near field (top of the screen, tissue

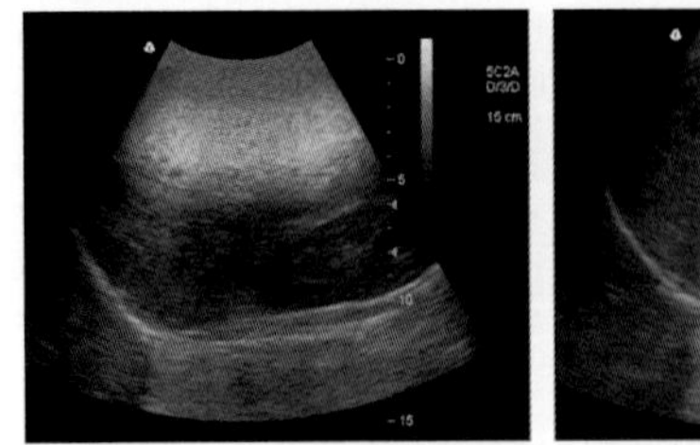
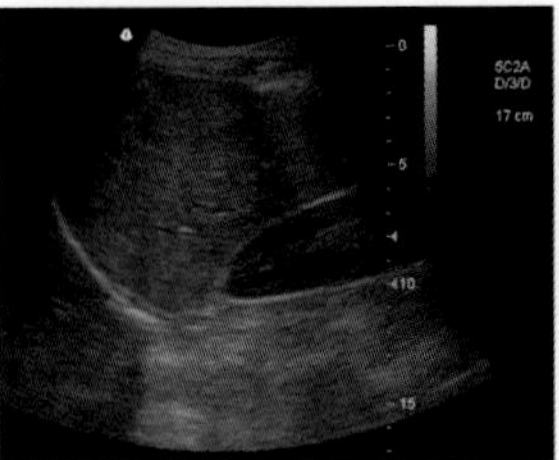
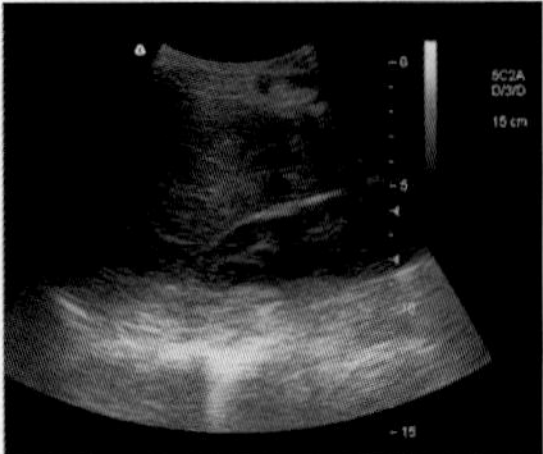

Figure 1.20
Near-field gain too high (*left*), far-field gain too high (*right*), and a well-gained image in the center.

closest to probe). TGC can boost the gain on the echoes returning from the far fields. Some machines have one button that allows you to adjust the near field relative to the far field. Other machines have multiple slider levers that allow gain control throughout the entire scanning depth. Figure 1.20 demonstrates the impact of near- and far-field gain on image quality.

Scanning modes

There are a variety of imaging modalities used in diagnostic ultrasound.

A, or *amplitude*, mode is an imaging modality largely of historical interest, although it is used in ophthalmologic applications today (Figure 1.21). It uses an oscilloscope display for returning amplitude information on the vertical axis and the reflector distance information on the horizontal axis. There is no picture; distance and amplitude are represented by a graph. In Figure 1.21 the vertical axis *A* represents the amplitude of the signal returned to the transducer, and the depth *D* is calculated based on the round-trip time of the ultrasound beam signal.

B, or *brightness*, mode is the modality which has been described up to this point; it is what we use for diagnostic imaging. B-mode scanning converts these amplitude waveforms into an image by using the gray-scale converter discussed previously. Most scanners now display images with up to 256 shades of gray, allowing for visualization of subtle differences within tissues/structures. As mentioned, the gray-scale assignment of each pixel is based on the signal amplitude or strength of the returning wave from a given point.

M, or *motion*, mode plots a waveform that depicts the motion of the tissue/structure of interest relative to the transducer's image plane (line through the

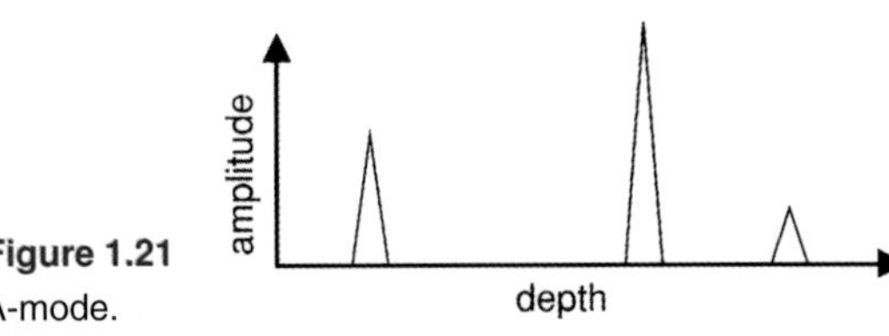

Figure 1.21
A-mode.

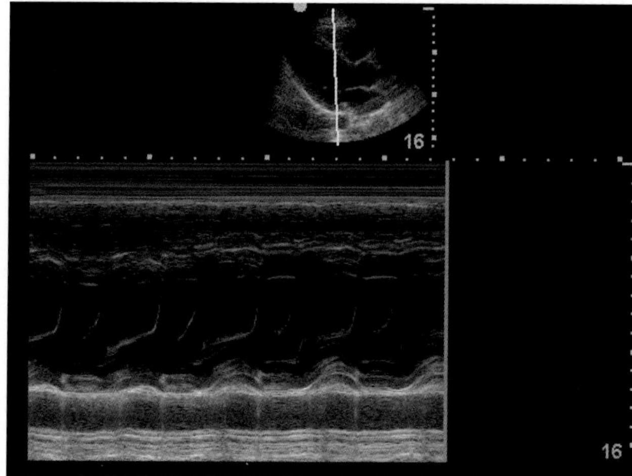

Figure 1.22
M-mode.

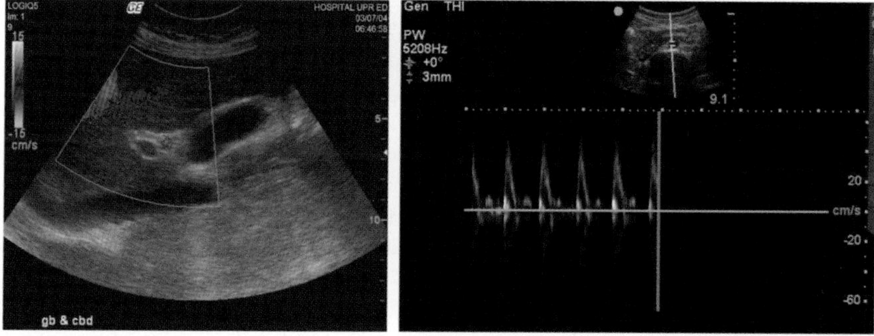

Figure 1.23
Color Doppler (*left*) and spectral Doppler (*right*).

structure) on the vertical axis, and time on the horizontal axis (Figure 1.22). This is often used simultaneously with B-mode scanning to study the motion of valves or to measure/document fetal cardiac activity. Many new bedside ultrasound machines are capable of performing this function.

D, or *Doppler*, mode is an imaging modality that relies on the principle of Doppler/frequency shift. Consider the example of a moving train: a pedestrian at a crossing will hear an increase in the pitch of the train whistle as it approaches and a decrease in pitch as it moves away. However, the train engineer will not hear this change in pitch – this audible shift in frequency – because he or she is traveling with the sound. Doppler ultrasound can differentiate movement of the reflected ultrasound waves toward and away from the probe. This is represented either by color changes (color Doppler) or by audible or graphical peaks (spectral Doppler).

The left image in Figure 1.23 shows color Doppler. The blue and red do not identify venous and arterial flow – rather, they describe whether flow is

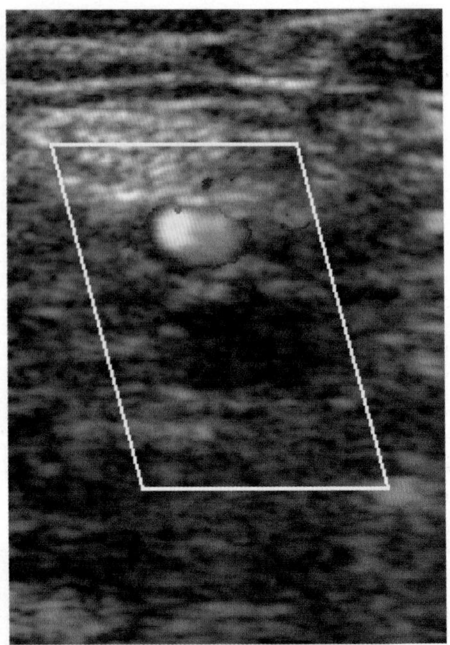

Figure 1.24
Power Doppler.

toward or away from the probe and depend on probe orientation. The legend on the left of the screen defines the directional color assignment. In this example, red flow is toward the transducer (toward the top of the screen), and blue flow is away from the transducer (toward the bottom of the screen). The right image in Figure 1.23 is an example of pulsed-wave or spectral Doppler. Spectral Doppler waveforms can be helpful in identifying and distinguishing venous from arterial waveforms.

Power Doppler is a form of color Doppler that uses a slightly different component of returned signal and seems to be more sensitive in low-flow states (Figure 1.24). This mode sacrifices the ability to demonstrate the direction of flow to gain sensitivity in detecting lower levels of flow.

We review when D- and M-mode functions are useful in the diagnostic and procedural applications sections of the chapters that follow.

Effects and artifacts

Understanding image artifacts and their formation is of the utmost importance. Unrecognized artifacts can lead to misinterpretation and can undermine the utility of the bedside ultrasound exam.

Acoustic shadowing is a characteristic ultrasound effect that can aid in the diagnosis of certain conditions (e.g., cholelithiasis) and act as a hindrance to the visualization of distal structures (e.g., deep-to-rib shadows) (Figure 1.25). When sound travels from a medium of one density to another, some energy

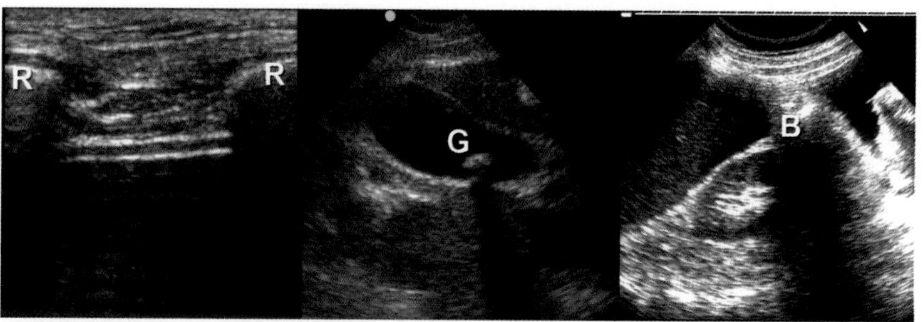

Figure 1.25

Shadowing caused by rib (R, *left*), gallstone (G, *middle*), and air (bowel gas, B, *right*). Note the dark shadows cast from the object toward the far end of the screen.

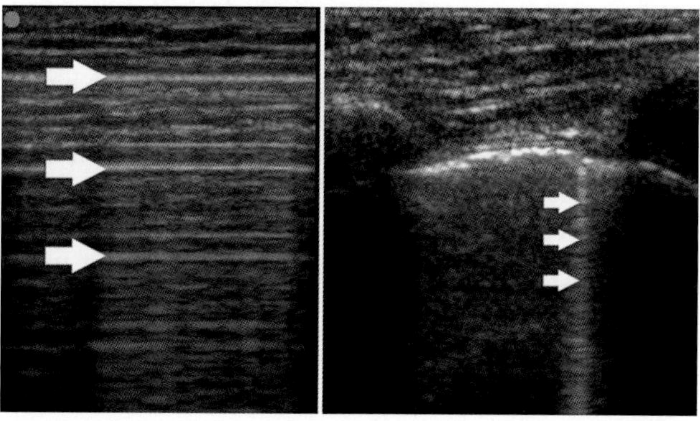

Figure 1.26

Reverberation artifact (arrows, *left*) and comet tail artifact or B-lines (arrows, *right*).

is reflected, some refracted. The greater the density difference, the more acoustic energy is reflected. Ultrasound transducers and coupling gel have roughly the density of liquid. Thus, we always begin with liquid density when performing diagnostic sonography. When the beam encounters skin, soft tissue, muscle, organs, or other roughly liquid-dense structures, a small degree of refraction and reflection take place: most acoustic energy travels deeper into the tissue. When the beam encounters structures much denser than liquid (such as bone or calcifications) or much less dense than liquid (air), a great deal of scatter and reflection occur. This leads to a loss of signal penetration distal to the air or bone. Thus, structures with a density much different than liquid are often referred to as strong reflectors.

Acoustic shadowing extends from the strong reflector to the edge of the screen, much as the shadow from someone standing up during a movie extends all the way from that person to the movie screen.

Reverberation occurs when the sound beam "bounces" between two highly reflective structures (Figure 1.26). It can appear as recurrent bright arcs that are displayed at equidistant intervals from the transducer. These arcs – called A-lines when visualized on imaging the lung – represent reflections between the skin/transducer interface and the pleura or other bright reflectors in the

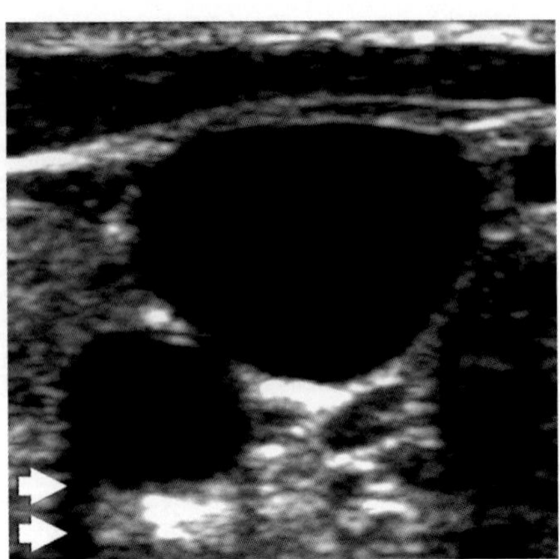

Figure 1.27
Refraction artifact (arrows).

body. Thus, artifactual "pleura" lines appear on the screen at depths which are multiples of the true distance from skin to pleura. A second clinically important variation on this is when sound gets trapped between two highly reflective structures that are closely opposed, such as visceral and parietal pleura. The fibrous tissue traps the sound beam, and it "bounces" infinitely back and forth such that the reflected echo is interpreted as a straight bright white echo also known as a *comet tail*. This concept is reviewed again in subsequent chapters because these artifacts are clinically important when evaluating the lung.

Reverberation can also refer to the property of some materials to vibrate in response to the energy of the ultrasound beam. Metallic objects such as needles create bright white lines distal as they vibrate and create additional signal interpreted by the ultrasound machine as additional iterations of the same object, deeper than the true object. This phenomenon has also been described as a *ring-down* artifact.

Refraction occurs when a sound beam obliquely crosses a boundary between tissues with different propagation speeds (Figure 1.27). It appears as an acoustic shadow, originating from the point where the sound beam changes direction. This is often seen at the edge of a blood vessel in transverse orientation.

Mirror images occur when an ultrasound beam undergoes multiple reflections and an incorrect interpretation results (Figure 1.28). When the beam encounters a bright reflector (*R*), some of the acoustic energy is reflected backward. When this beam path encounters an object (*A*), information about its relative brightness is relayed back to the transducer. However, its depth is miscalculated because the machine assumes the ultrasound beam took a straight path toward the target object. Because the reflected path (solid arrows) has a longer round-trip time than a path directly to and from the target, the machine calculates that the structure is deeper than it is. This yields a false object (*B*), calculated by the machine to lie along a linear path from the initial ultrasound beam. Mirroring appears as a duplication of structures, with the mirror image always appearing deeper than the real structure.

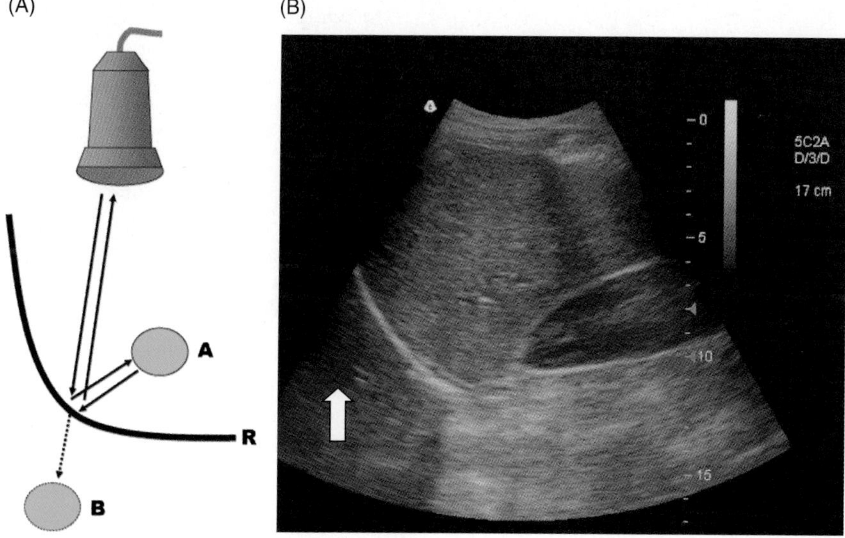

Figure 1.28

Mirror image artifact. (*A*) The path of the ultrasound beam as it encounters an acoustic reflector. (*B*) The arrow indicates the mirror image of liver tissue cephalad to the diaphragm.

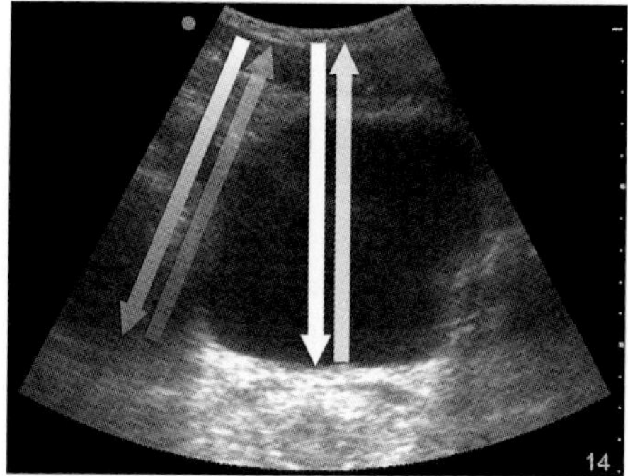

Figure 1.29

Posterior acoustic enhancement posterior to the bladder. The same acoustic energy (represented by the brightness of the arrows) enters the tissue. After significant attenuation (left pair) or no attenuation (right pair) the beams return with different amounts of energy. These are assigned different brightness values by the ultrasound machine.

The mirror image will disappear with subtle changes in position of the transducer, whereas the real image should be visible in multiple planes. This artifact is useful during the FAST exam, where it is present as a normal artifact in the right and left upper quadrants above the diaphragm. When liquid (effusion of hemothorax) replaces air (lung) above the diaphragm, this artifact disappears.

Enhancement (or *posterior acoustic enhancement*) is artifactual brightness deep to an anechoic structure, commonly a cystic structure or blood vessel. It occurs when sound crosses an area of low signal attenuation. There is an increase in echogenicity posterior to the low-attenuation structures because the sound returns to the transducer with greater intensity than from adjacent areas. For example, in Figure 1.29 the beams on the left are uniformly attenuated as they pass through the body. They return to the transducer with

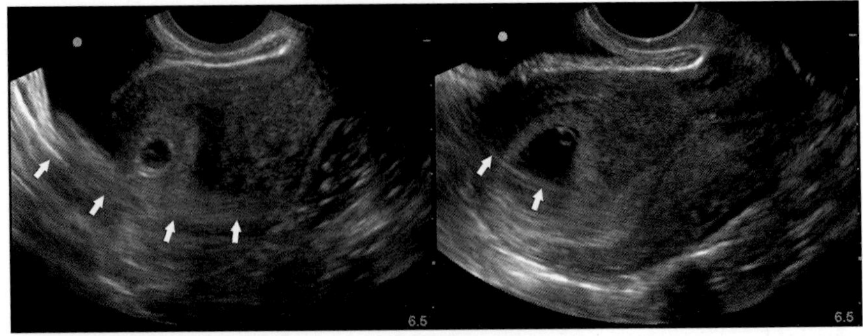

Figure 1.30
Two examples of the side lobe artifact seen originating deep to the bladder and obscuring the view of the uterus. Note that in both examples the artifact sweeps across anatomic planes and parallel to the sweep of the ultrasound beam. This appearance helps distinguish artifact from true anatomy.

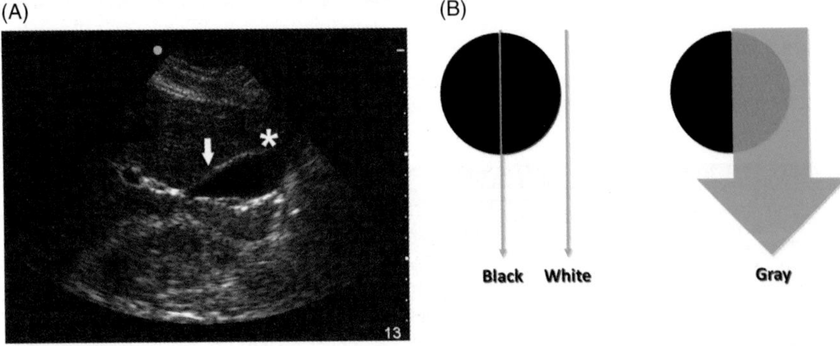

Figure 1.31
Beam width artifact. (*A*) The gallbladder is filled with bile of a consistent density, yet it appears more anechoic near the neck (arrow) than the fundus (*). At this angle, the ultrasound beam averages signal received near the edge from inside and outside the gallbladder, yielding a mid-range result. (*B*) Very thin slices near the edge of the black structure (*left*) travel through mostly black or mostly white areas. A thick beam (*right*) will cover both simultaneously, and thus return data that averages to gray.

far less energy (darker arrow) than they started with. The beam in the center loses no energy as it passes through the bladder, and thus it has much more energy (brighter white) as it returns to the transducer.

The *side lobe* (or *grating lobe*) artifact occurs when ultrasound energy which is emitted outside of the central axis of the ultrasound beam is reflected back to the transducer. It is interpreted as signal originating from within the central axis of the beam, and therefore creates a false image. This is frequently encountered during pelvic ultrasound when side lobes reflecting strong signal distal to the bladder are interpreted as originating from within the uterus (Figure 1.30).

Beam width artifact is encountered because the ultrasound beam is several millimeters thick, although it is generally described as if it had no thickness at all. It is similar in concept to volume averaging, which impacts computed tomography. When the beam encounters an interface between two structures of different echogenicity (such as gallbladder and liver), parts of the beam sample through brighter and some through less bright reflectors. This information is averaged as it returns to the transducer, producing a mid-range echogenicity value. Areas near the edge of the anechoic gallbladder will appear gray, for example, and may mimic sludge (Figure 1.31).

Section 1

Diagnostic ultrasound

When we wrote the introduction in the first edition of this book in 2007, this picture of an early ultrasound machine was a favorite. We wrote, "In the 1950s, when medical diagnostic ultrasonography was in its infancy, it was hard to imagine that the average physician would find it helpful. The technology required that patients be immersed in a tub of water and be hemodynamically stable enough to spend long periods of time in the tub. Ultrasound waves generated a graph representing the strength of returning echoes from the patient and were challenging to translate into anatomic images. Not only was the whole process cumbersome (and likely chilly and uncomfortable), it also required much training and skill to interpret the data generated."

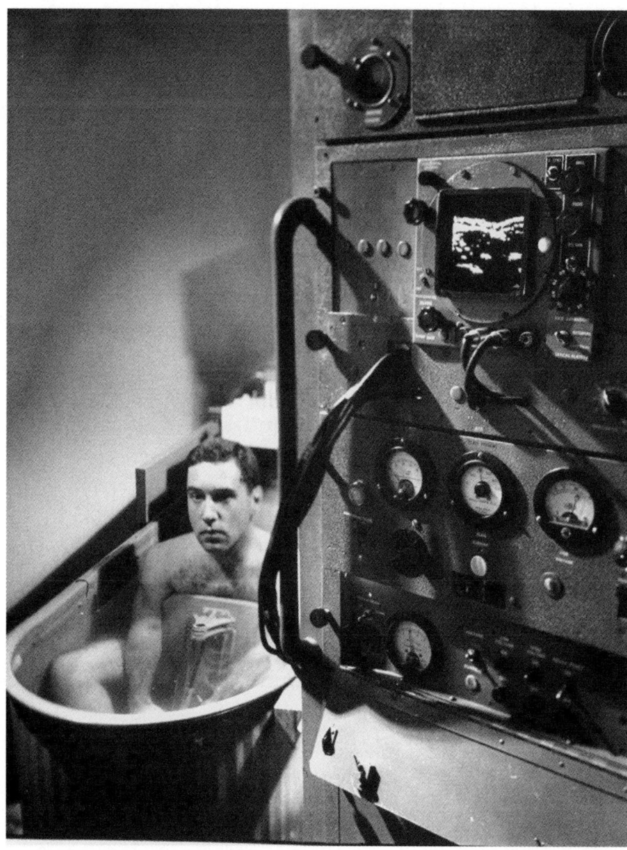

Reproduced with permission from Carl Iwasaki/Life Magazine/Getty Images.

We commented then that the technology revolution and advances in ultrasound technology were similar to the incredible developments taking place in other digital media arenas. Cellphones, video games, personal computers, and ultrasound machines are all faster, easier to use, more powerful and more capable than ever before. What we weren't sure about in 2007 was whether medicine would recognize and embrace the potential that we saw in ultrasound technology.

This is now happening, and quickly. Ultrasound education is now part of emergency medicine, critical care, and surgical training programs. Several medical schools in the United States are longitudinally integrating ultrasound into their curriculum – both in the preclinical (anatomy, pathophysiology) and clinical years. Internationally, the opportunity that even one ultrasound machine offers in terms of diagnostic and procedural capability has also been recognized by clinicians. Organizations such as the World Interactive Network Focused on Critical Ultrasound (WINFOCUS) have taught courses in over 40 different countries over the last five years. The demand is greater than the ability of organizations like WINFOCUS to keep up. Moreover, in the United States there is a growing awareness of the risks of repeated radiation exposure from computed tomography and a new appreciation of rising healthcare costs. This has focused attention toward point-of-care diagnostic testing such as ultrasound, and has sparked a reassessment of diagnostic imaging strategies. There has never been a greater opportunity for ultrasound, and our challenge now is to pursue a research agenda that evaluates how to incorporate point-of-care ultrasound into patient care safely, efficiently, and effectively.

The benefits of ultrasound as outlined in our previous introduction are the same: "Not only can it assist the physician at the bedside in making diagnoses, it can do so without exposing the patient to harmful radiation and it can be repeated infinitely without requiring transportation as clinical situations change. It can assist in performing invasive procedures under direct visualization. It can help guide the physician in mobilizing further resources or consultations, direct which testing should be done next, or provide the proof needed to undertake more invasive procedures to stabilize patients. Most importantly, it enables physicians to understand and diagnose pathophysiology directly with moving images in real time."

Today, the groundswell of interest is greater and so we must strive even harder to find the best way to use this powerful tool. Our goal in this edition is the same as it was in 2007. We want to introduce physicians to the way the machine works, and to give an overview of the basic principles needed to operate a bedside ultrasound machine. We have expanded the list of applications to incorporate new research and development since the last edition. And most importantly, we want to continue to communicate the potential of ultrasound and to inspire physicians to use it more widely. Ultrasound is not just another innovation – it can play a key role in advancing our diagnostic capability, and therefore in providing safe and efficient treatment for our patients.

2 Focused assessment with sonography in trauma (FAST)

Introduction

Ultrasound (US) was first used in the evaluation of trauma patients in Europe in the 1970s. The German surgery board has required certification in ultrasound skills since 1988. Since the mid 1980s in the United States, the use of ultrasound in trauma has become more widespread and has all but replaced diagnostic peritoneal lavage (DPL) in most trauma centers. The FAST exam has been included as part of the advanced trauma life support course since 1997 [1]. In addition, the American College of Surgeons has included ultrasound as one of several "new technologies" that surgical residents must be exposed to in their curriculum. Both the American College of Emergency Physicians and the Society for Academic Emergency Medicine support the use of ultrasound to evaluate blunt abdominal trauma as well. Since 2001, training in emergency ultrasound has been required for all emergency medicine residents [2–4]. Therefore, all physicians who will be evaluating trauma patients must become proficient in the use of trauma ultrasound.

The objective of the FAST exam is to detect free intraperitoneal, intrathoracic, and pericardial fluid in the setting of trauma. The cardiac windows are especially critical in penetrating trauma and are reviewed in this section and in Chapter 3. Not only can the physician identify free intraperitoneal fluid with the FAST exam, but pleural fluid and other signs of thoracic injury can be assessed as well. Although computed tomography (CT) provides excellent and more detailed solid-organ evaluation, it often requires transportation of the patient to a less monitored setting (thus the trauma adage, "death begins in radiology"). In addition, CT requires exposure to radiation and is more expensive. DPL is more sensitive for detecting intraperitoneal blood than ultrasound. It is considered positive with 100 000 red blood cells (RBCs)/mm^3, which is 20 mL of blood per liter of lavage fluid. However, DPL is an invasive test that can be complicated by pregnancy, previous surgery, and operator inexperience. In addition, DPL's high sensitivity leads to false positives (in the form of non-therapeutic laparotomies) at reported rates of 6–26% [5]. The evolution from surgical treatment of many splenic and liver injuries to non-operative management means that the high sensitivity and invasive nature of the DPL has become less useful [5–8]. Ultrasound can reliably detect as little as 250 mL of free fluid in Morison's pouch [9]. It is also inexpensive, rapid, and easily repeated. In addition, ultrasound has a higher specificity for therapeutic laparotomy than DPL [10].

To take advantage of the strengths and weaknesses of all three diagnostic options for trauma (CT, US, and DPL), a combination approach is best. There is an overwhelming amount of data supporting the use of the FAST exam as the initial screening tool for evaluation of the abdomen and thorax in trauma [10–21]. In addition, in an era of cost consciousness, there is even evidence that shows that using FAST as a screening tool helps reduce testing, hospital stays, and intensive care unit requirements and thus can also significantly decrease cost [11,12]. Therefore, it is important to remember the strengths and weaknesses of all three diagnostic options for trauma. In this chapter, we discuss the FAST scanning technique, review positive and negative images, and present potential clinical algorithms for FAST use.

Focused questions for the FAST exam

The focused questions for the FAST exam are as follows:

1. Is there free fluid/blood in the abdomen?
2. Is there fluid/blood in the pericardium?

There have also been a number of studies demonstrating the utility of ultrasound in evaluating the thorax as part of the FAST examination to detect pneumothorax and hemothorax [22–24]. This has been called the extended FAST (eFAST), and most trauma centers are now using this technique. We discuss ultrasound diagnosis of pneumothorax at the end of this chapter and show how the eFAST can diagnose blood in the thorax during the following discussion. For the eFAST, there are two additional focused questions:

3. Is there fluid/blood in the thorax?
4. Is there a pneumothorax?

Anatomy

The shape of the peritoneal cavity provides several dependent areas when a patient is in the supine position. The site of accumulation of fluid depends on the source of bleeding and the position of the patient. Because most trauma patients are transported supine on a backboard, we use this as the starting position.

The right paracolic gutter runs from Morison's pouch to the pelvis. The left paracolic gutter is not as deep as the right paracolic gutter. In addition, the phrenocolic ligament blocks fluid movement to the left paracolic gutter. As a result, fluid flows more freely toward the right paracolic gutter.

The hepatorenal recess (Morison's pouch) is the potential space located in the right upper quadrant (RUQ) between Glisson's capsule of the liver and Gerota's fascia of the right kidney (Figures 2.1–2.3). In a normal exam, there is no fluid between these two organs, and the fascia appears as a bright hyperechoic line separating the liver from the kidney.

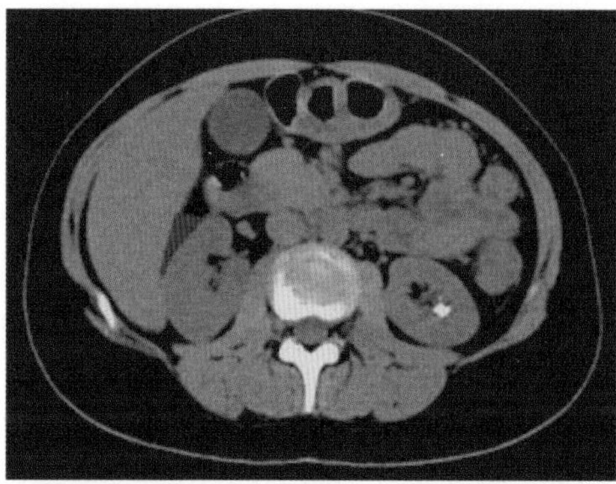

Figure 2.1

Computed tomography view of Morison's pouch (*red*). Courtesy of Dr. Lauren Post, Mount Sinai School of Medicine, New York, NY.

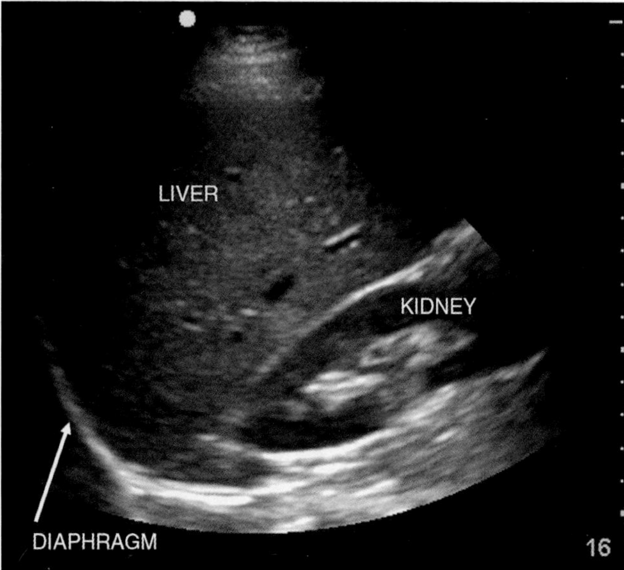

Figure 2.2

Ultrasound view of Morison's pouch.

The splenorenal recess is the potential space located in the left upper quadrant (LUQ) between the spleen and Gerota's fascia of the left kidney (Figures 2.4 and 2.5). Again, in the normal ultrasound exam of this quadrant, there is no fluid or hypoechoic area separating the spleen from the kidney, and the fascia appears as a bright hyperechoic line separating the two organs. However, because of the position of the splenocolic ligament and the shearing effect on the splenic hilum in blunt trauma, blood usually collects in the subdiaphragmatic space in the LUQ, and looking at the space between the spleen and the diaphragm is much more likely to yield results than the splenorenal recess. This is an important difference between the essential views of the RUQ and LUQ.

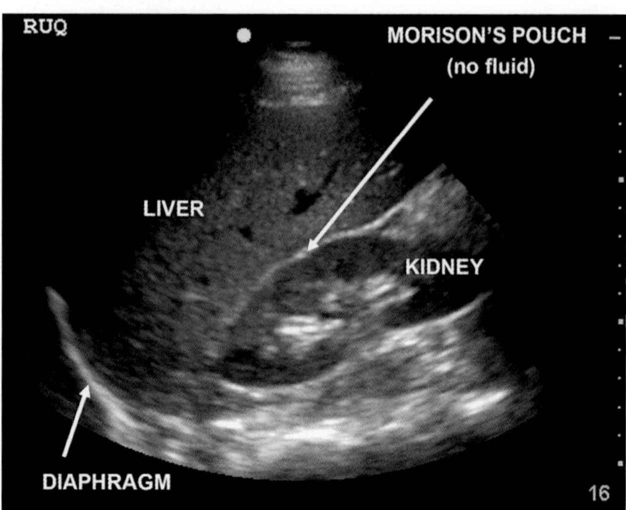

Figure 2.3
Labeled view of Morison's pouch.

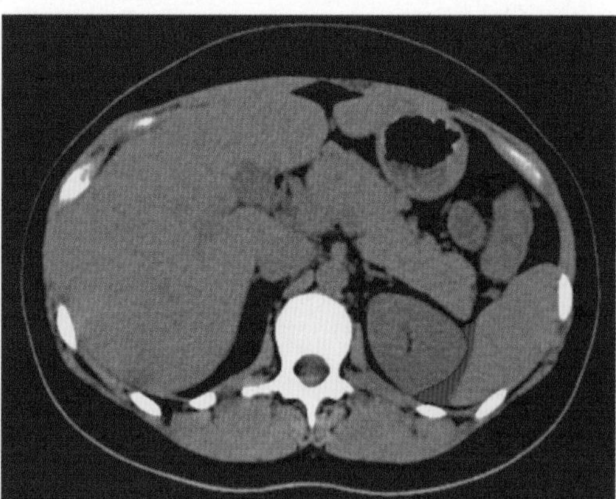

Figure 2.4
Computed tomography view of splenorenal recess (*red*). Courtesy of Dr. Lauren Post, Mount Sinai School of Medicine, New York, NY.

The rectovesical pouch (Figure 2.6A) is the pocket formed by the reflection of the peritoneum from the rectum to the male bladder. It is the most dependent area of the supine male.

The rectouterine pouch (pouch of Douglas) (Figures 2.6B and 2.7) is the pocket formed by the reflection of the peritoneum from the rectum and the back wall of the uterus. It is the most dependent area of the supine female.

Figure 2.8 shows movement patterns of free intraperitoneal fluid. In the supine patient, fluid in the RUQ will collect first in Morison's pouch. Overflow will travel down the right paracolic gutter into the pelvis. Free fluid in the LUQ will collect first between the spleen and the left hemidiaphragm. Fluid will then move into the splenorenal recess, toward the left paracolic

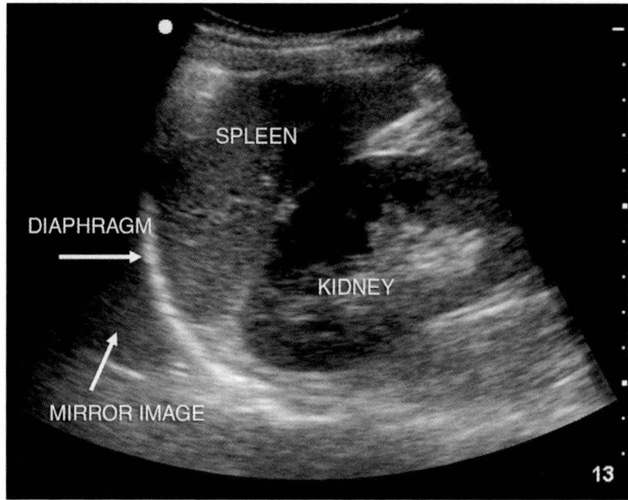

Figure 2.5
Labeled view of a normal splenorenal recess.

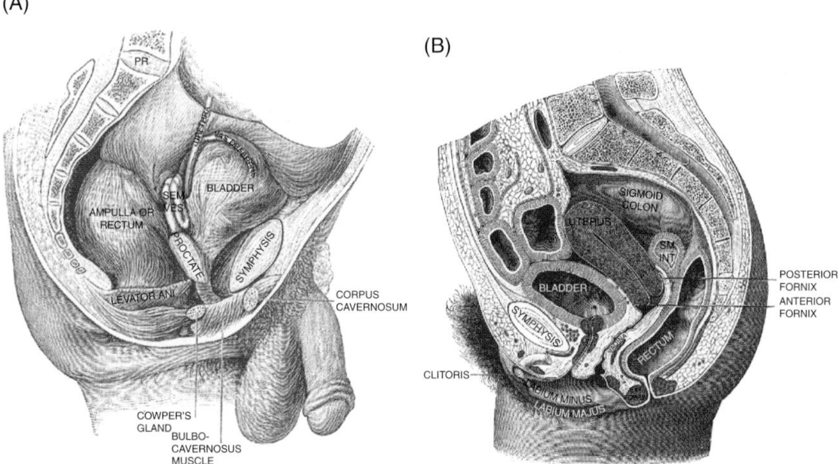

Figure 2.6
(*A*) Male and (*B*) female pelvic anatomy. Images reproduced from *Gray's Anatomy*, 1918 (image out of copyright).

gutter into the pelvis. As mentioned, the phrenocolic ligament often shunts fluid to Morison's pouch before filling the left paracolic gutter. Free fluid in the pelvis will first collect either in the rectovesical pouch or in the pouch of Douglas and then start to flow cephalad toward the paracolic gutters. Of course this depends largely on where the bleeding is coming from. If there is pelvic bleeding only, a large amount of accumulation is necessary

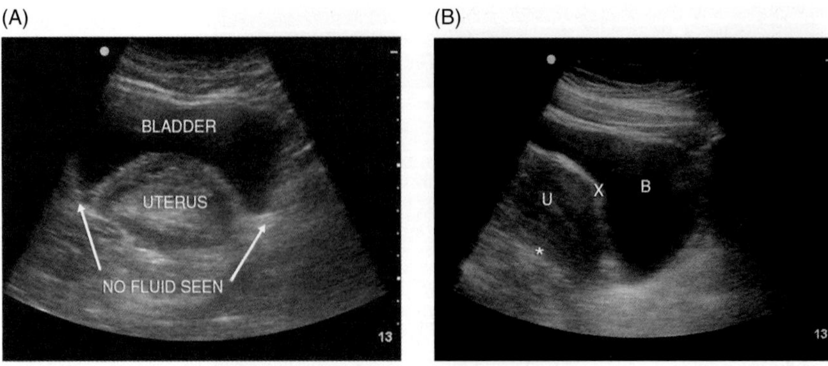

Figure 2.7

(*A*) Labeled transverse suprapubic view in female. (*B*) Longitudinal suprabic view in female. B, bladder, U, uterus; X, vesiculouterine space; *, pouch of Douglas.

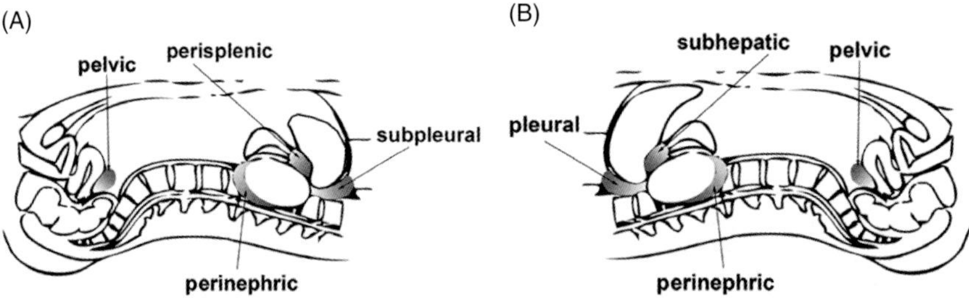

Figure 2.8

The areas of greatest dependence in the supine patient. Fluid will collect in the areas marked in blue, as seen when investigating (*A*) the left side and (*B*) the right side of the peritoneal and thoracic cavities. Images used with permission from Hoffmann B (ed.). *Ultrasound Guide for Emergency Physicians*, www.sonoguide.com, courtesy of Dr. Beatrice Hoffmann.

before there is blood in Morison's pouch, and the pelvic view will be positive much earlier. The converse would be true for bleeding originating from the RUQ.

Technique

Probe selection

A phased-array or curvilinear 2.5–5.0 MHz probe is most commonly used for the FAST exam. The views and windows used in the exam may all be obtained with a single probe. Some sonographers prefer larger-footprint probes that provide greater resolution of deep structures, while others prefer narrower-footprint microconvex or phased-array probes to obtain images between the ribs more readily.

Views

The FAST exam is performed using four views (Figure 2.9):

1. Hepatorenal recess or Morison's pouch (RUQ)
2. Splenorenal or perisplenic view (LUQ)
3. Pelvic view
4. Pericardial or subxiphoid view

With the eFAST exam, the probe slides superiorly from the standard RUQ and LUQ views to visualize the costophrenic angle and assess for blood in the thorax pooling in the costophrenic space and for normal sliding of the lung pleura with respiration (discussed below).

Morison's pouch

The starting probe position when looking for Morison's pouch should be the anterior axillary line in the seventh to ninth intercostal space (Figure 2.10). The probe marker (green dot on the probe in Figure 2.10) should be pointing toward the patient's head. To get a good view of the entire recess, the probe can be moved toward the head and then back toward the feet along this plane. If rib shadows obscure the image, the probe's orientation may be rotated from a pure sagittal plane to a slightly oblique plane parallel to the ribs (usually 10–20 degrees). Thus, the probe will sit within a rib space, and the plane of the ultrasound beam will cut across fewer ribs.

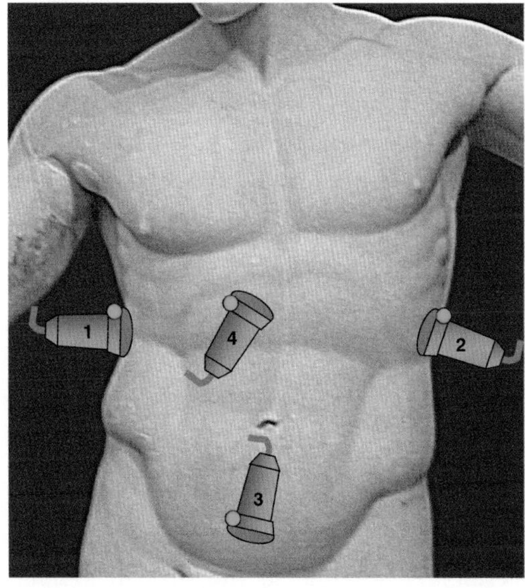

Figure 2.9
The four views that comprise the FAST exam.

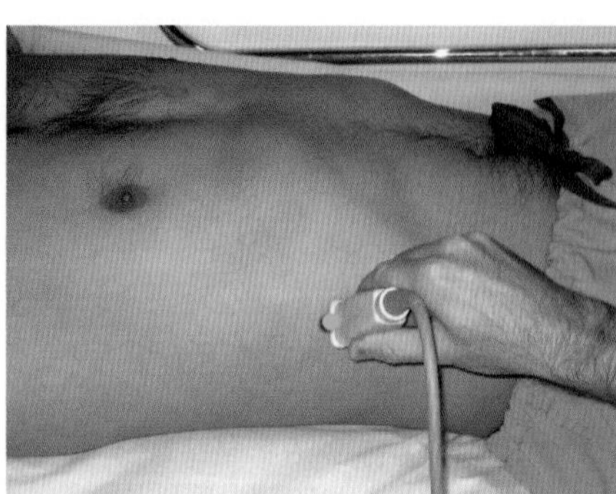

Figure 2.10
Probe positioning in the right upper quadrant.

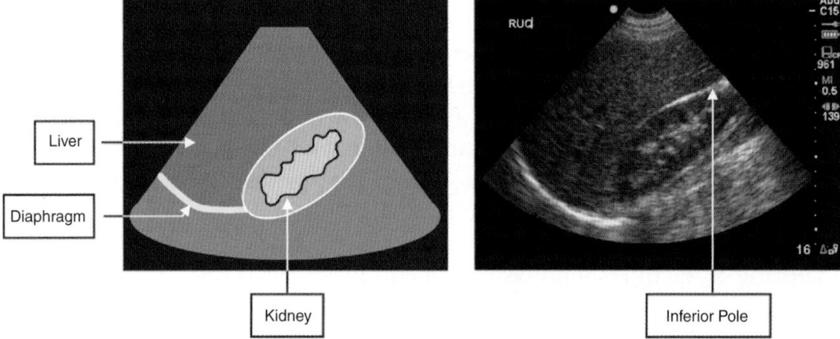

Figure 2.11
Normal ultrasound view of right upper quadrant/Morison's pouch. Hyperechoic Gerota's fascia seen here surrounding the kidney.

Do not forget to visualize the inferior pole! In a supine patient, the inferior pole of the kidney on both right and left upper quadrant views is the most posterior or dependent part of the peritoneal cavity (Figure 2.11). It is seen by sliding the probe more inferiorly or toward the feet along the axillary line. It is also important to fan anterior and posterior with the probe at each level to make sure the entire area is interrogated.

Figure 2.12 shows how it is possible to miss the more subtle stripe of free fluid between the liver and the kidney more inferiorly if you do not image the inferior pole.

Perisplenic space

The spleen is smaller than the liver, so the left kidney is more posterior and superior than the right kidney. Therefore, the starting probe position on the left should be in the posterior axillary line in the fifth to seventh

(A)

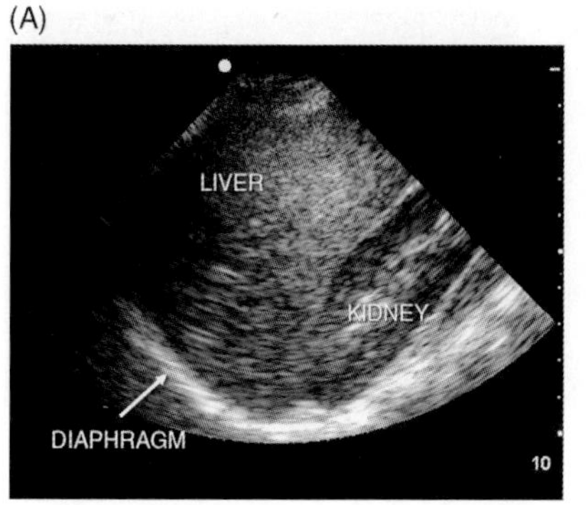

(B)

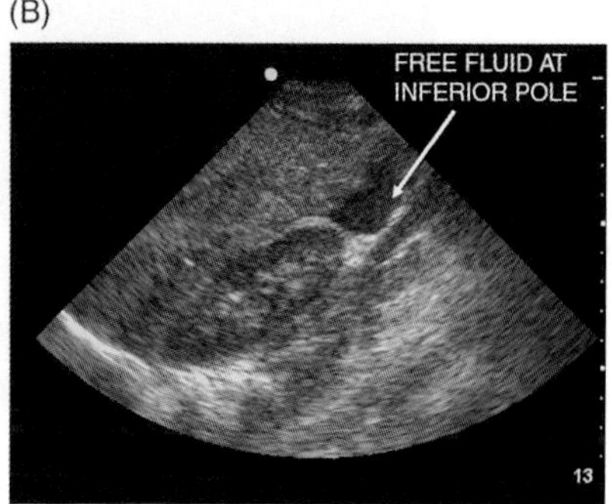

Figure 2.12

Positive FAST. (*A* and *B*) Views of Morison's pouch showing fluid along the inferior pole of the right kidney (only visible in *B*).

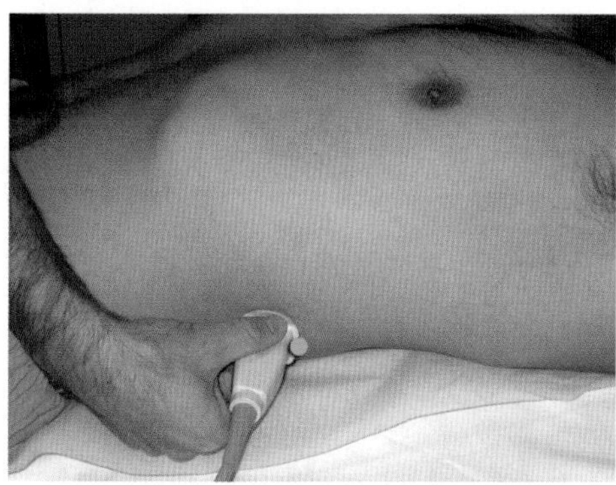

Figure 2.13

Probe positioning in the left upper quadrant.

intercostal space (Figure 2.13). Again, the marker should be pointed toward the patient's head. As with the RUQ view, the probe's orientation may be rotated to a slightly oblique plane parallel to the ribs (usually 10–20 degrees more posterior). Thus, the probe will sit within a rib space, and the plane of the ultrasound beam will cut across fewer ribs (Figure 2.14). It is important to slide the probe superior to fully investigate the space between the diaphragm and the spleen as this is usually the first space where fluid will collect. Again, fan the probe anterior to posterior at each probe position as the probe is moved from superior to inferior, to get a three-dimensional view of the entire space.

Pelvis

If this part of the exam can be done before the bladder is emptied (i.e., before a Foley catheter is placed), it is much easier. If a bladder catheter has

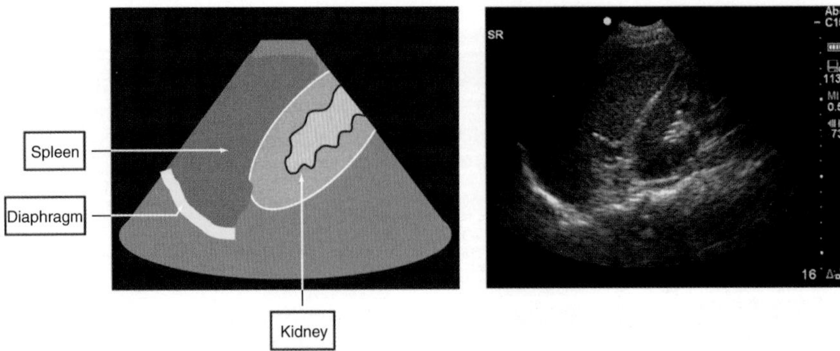

Figure 2.14

In the RUQ, it is critical to visualize the inferior pole of the right kidney, since fluid tracks here first and the large liver maintains an interface with the kidney through most of the kidney's length. In contrast, the LUQ has a much smaller interface between the smaller spleen and the kidney. Early fluid tracking tends to be close to this interface or even between the spleen and the diaphragm as a result of the splenocolic ligament, and therefore it is not as critical to visualize the inferior pole of the left kidney.

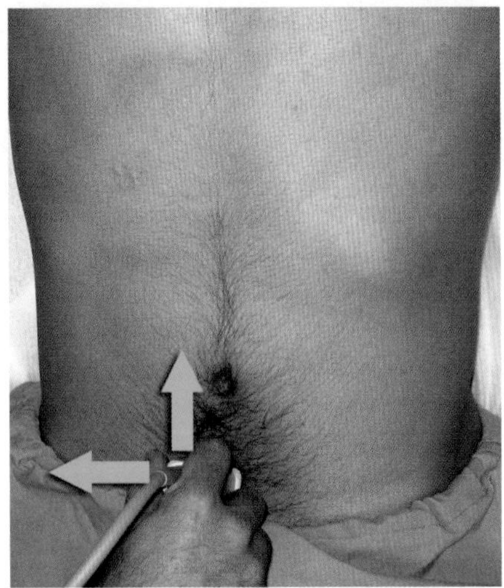

Figure 2.15

Probe positioning for the transverse suprapubic view (green arrow pointing to patient's right) and longitudinal suprapubic view (green arrow pointing to patient's head).

already been placed, accuracy of the study can be increased by instilling saline into the bladder until it is easily visualized using ultrasound, but this is not mandatory – always take a look first, and if the view is positive for fluid no further maneuvers are necessary. Place the probe in the transverse position (probe marker to the patient's right) on the symphysis pubis and angle toward the patient's feet (Figure 2.15). The bladder is not always perfectly midline, so sometimes sliding to the right and left above the symphysis pubis will bring the bladder into view (Figure 2.16). The most common reason for

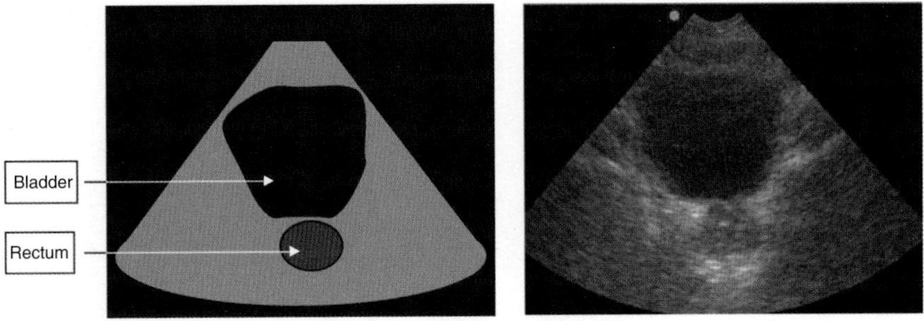

Figure 2.16
Normal transverse view of the pelvis.

difficulty visualizing the bladder is a probe position that is too superior. Remember that the bladder is a pelvic organ and only emerges from above the symphysis pubis as it becomes distended. Examine for fluid posterior to the bladder, posterior to the uterus, and between loops of bowel. It is important to look in both transverse and longitudinal planes for fluid behind the bladder, as the sagittal or longitudinal view is more sensitive for small amounts of fluid. Once the bladder is identified transversely, rotate the probe 90 degrees for the longitudinal view. The longitudinal view is more sensitive for free fluid, because free fluid outside the posterior bladder wall is easier to identify in this plane. Moreover, occasionally if the bladder is very full the transverse view is obtained higher in the peritoneal cavity and so the most dependent part of the pelvis (the rectovesicular space) is missed. Finally, it is important to fan anterior to posterior in the transverse view and side to side in the longitudinal view in order to fully interrogate this space.

Subxiphoid

Cardiac views are reviewed in more detail in Chapter 3. For the FAST subxiphoid view, position the probe almost flat on the abdomen with the marker to the patient's right and angle the probe to the patient's left shoulder (Figure 2.17). If the patient can bend his or her knees, sometimes this helps relax the abdominal wall muscles. It is also important to remember to bring the depth out to its maximal level for this view, because often the distance from the subxiphoid to the heart is at least 6 cm. With shallow depth settings, the heart will not be visualized. In addition, sometimes a stomach full of air can scatter the ultrasound beams before they reach the heart in the left chest. If this is a problem, slide the probe to the patient's right and shoot through the left lobe of the liver (as detailed in Chapter 3). The liver will act as a better acoustic window than the stomach, and the heart will be easier to visualize (Figure 2.18).

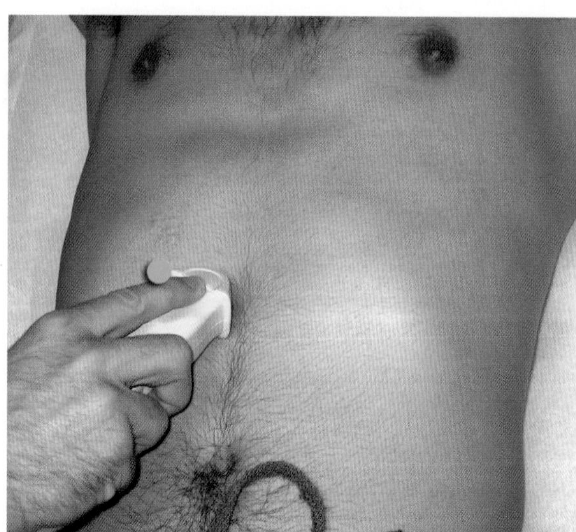

Figure 2.17
Probe positioning for subxiphoid view.

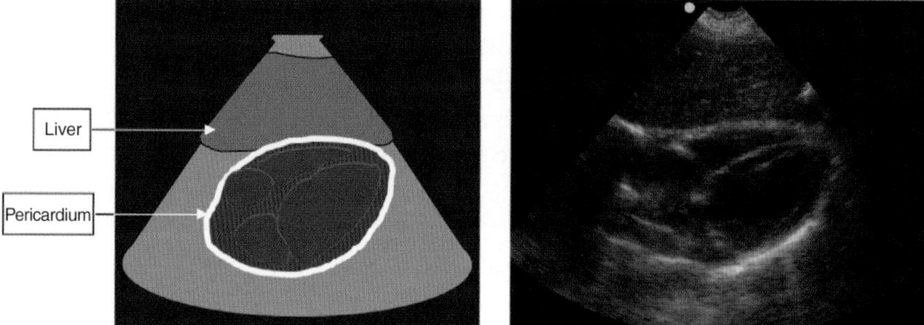

Figure 2.18
Normal subxiphoid view.

Scanning tips

Trouble with the RUQ view

Rib shadow in the way?

- Try angling the probe obliquely to sneak in between the ribs.
- Have the patient take a deep breath to lower the diaphragm and bring Morison's pouch lower in the abdomen below the ribs.

Can't see the diaphragm?

- Try bringing the probe lower on the abdominal wall (toward the stretcher in a more posterior coronal plane).

- Try sliding the probe on the same coronal plane toward the head or toward the feet to see if something familiar pops into view.

Trouble with the LUQ view

Rib shadow in the way?

- Try the same techniques as listed previously.
- Sometimes, because the spleen is so much smaller than the liver, it is actually easier to visualize the splenorenal recess from a more anterior plane. Slide the probe over the spleen anteriorly and angle the probe through the spleen to the kidney from anterior to posterior.

Trouble with the pelvic view

Can't find the bladder?

- This is most often because the probe is too cephalad. Bring the probe almost on top of the symphysis pubis, angling toward the feet.
- The bladder is sometimes off midline. Position the probe transverse (marker to the patient's right) and slide from right to left.
- Has the Foley catheter already been placed or the bladder decompressed? Try again after some fluid is given.

Trouble with the cardiac view

Can't find the heart?

- This is most often because the angle of the probe is too steep when looking subcostally. Position the probe almost flat on the abdomen in the subxiphoid position.
- The second most common problem is that the depth on the machine is set too shallow. Bring the depth out as deep as the machine allows and look for the moving organ. The depth can be readjusted to a more shallow view once the heart is found.
- Often, because a trauma patient has swallowed a lot of air, the stomach is distended. When looking subcostally, the beam is trying to reach the heart through an air-filled stomach. Slide the probe more to the right, and try looking for the heart through the liver, not the stomach. Occasionally this just won't work, and a second cardiac view should be tried (see Chapter 3).

Normal images

Figures 2.19–2.25 are examples of normal FAST ultrasound scans.

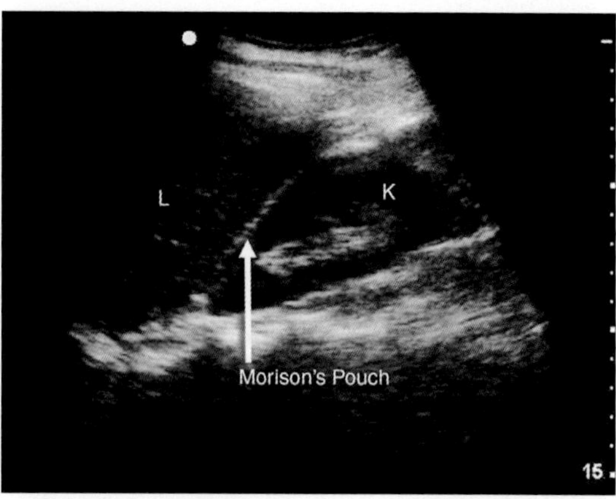

Figure 2.19
Normal RUQ. K, kidney; L, liver.

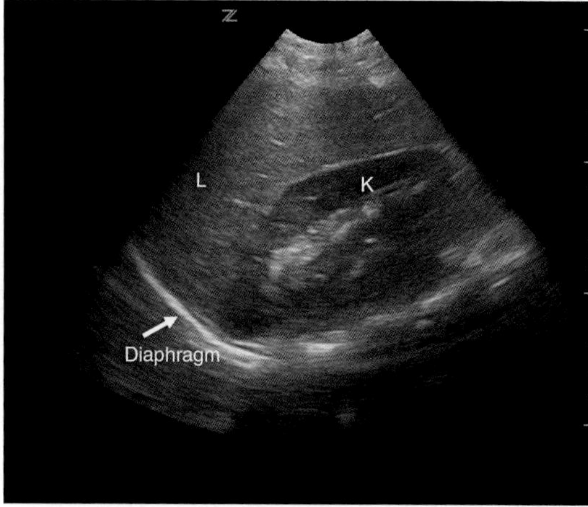

Figure 2.20
Negative view of RUQ with no fluid in Morison's pouch. K, kidney; L, liver.

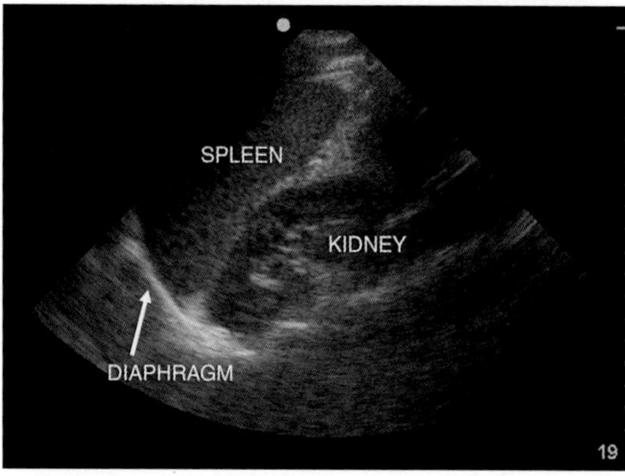

Figure 2.21
Normal LUQ.

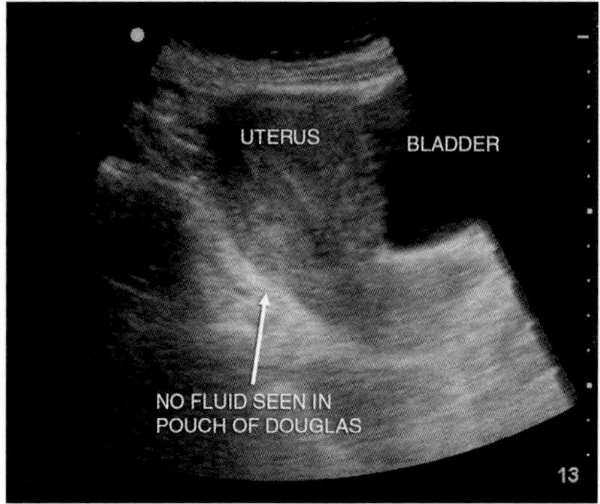

Figure 2.22
Normal female suprapubic view. This is a longitudinal view, because you see the uterus in its longitudinal orientation and the probe marker is toward the patient's head.

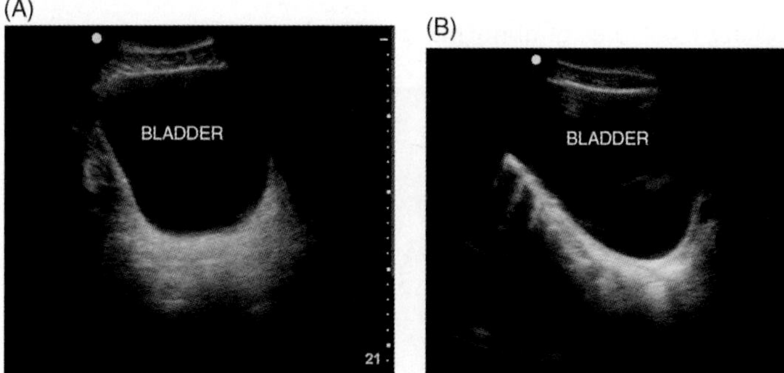

Figure 2.23
Normal (*A*) transverse and (*B*) longitudinal views of the male pelvis.

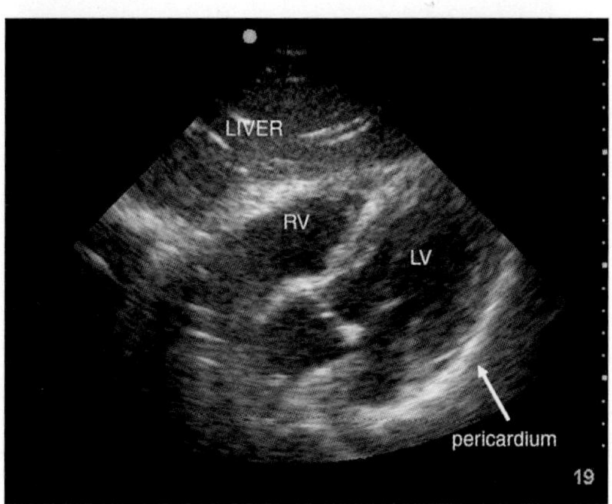

Figure 2.24
Normal subxiphoid view. LV, left ventricle; RV, right ventricle.

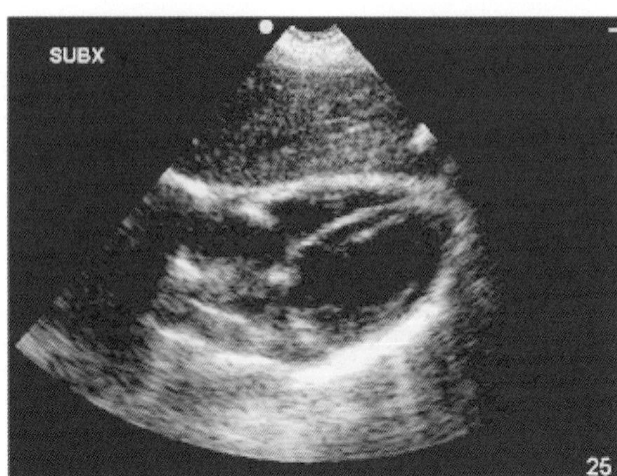

Figure 2.25
Normal subxiphoid view.

Abnormal images

Figures 2.26–2.39 are examples of abnormal FAST ultrasound scans.

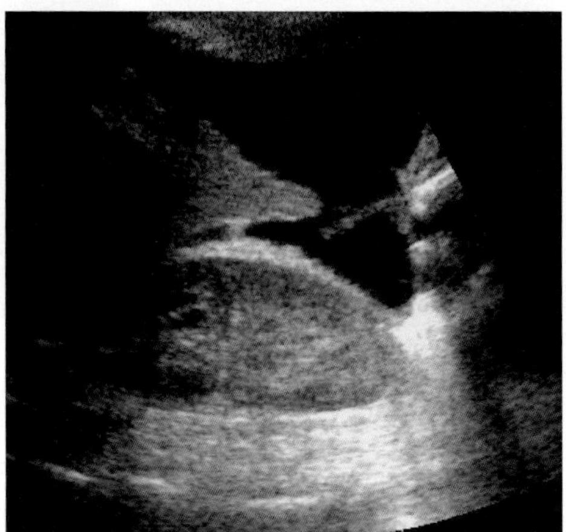

Figure 2.26
A large pocket of free fluid seen around the liver edge.

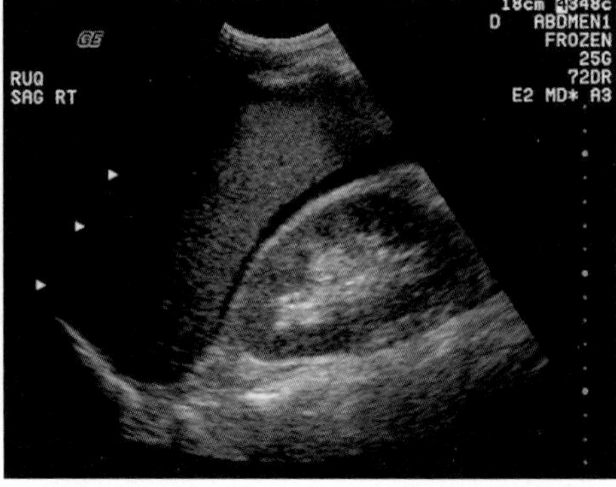

Figure 2.27
A stripe of fluid is seen in Morison's pouch. Diaphragm and Gerota's fascia well visualized as hyperechoic bright lines.

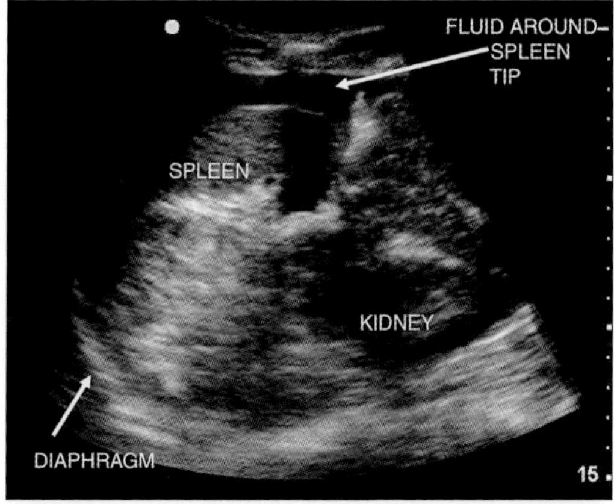

Figure 2.28

Fluid is seen at the spleen tip and in the subdiaphragmatic space, stressing the importance of these views.

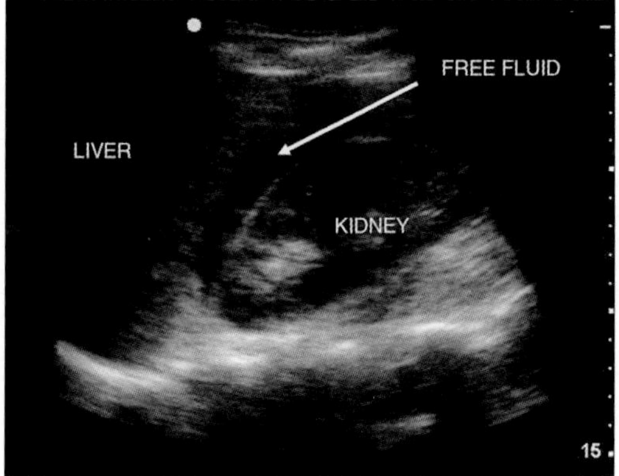

Figure 2.29

Fluid in Morison's pouch.

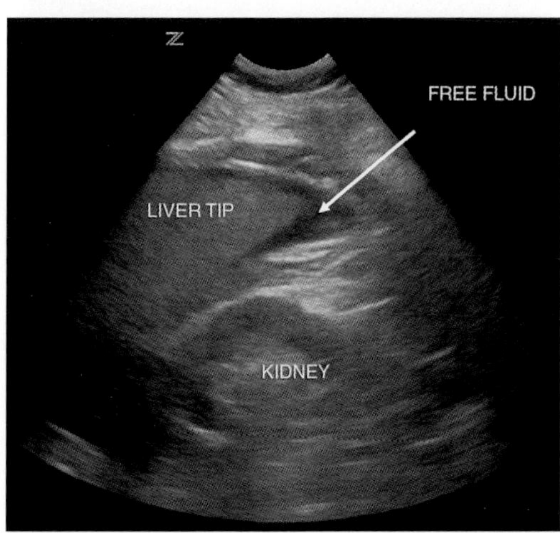

Figure 2.30

Fluid around tip of liver and heterogeneous material outside Gerota's fascia in the free fluid pocket suggests clot.

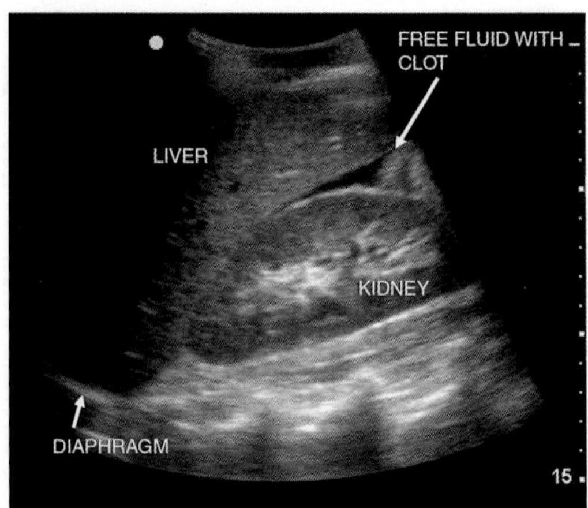

Figure 2.31

Fluid stripe in Morison's pouch. The heterogeneous echogenic material at the inferior pole of the kidney suggests clot.

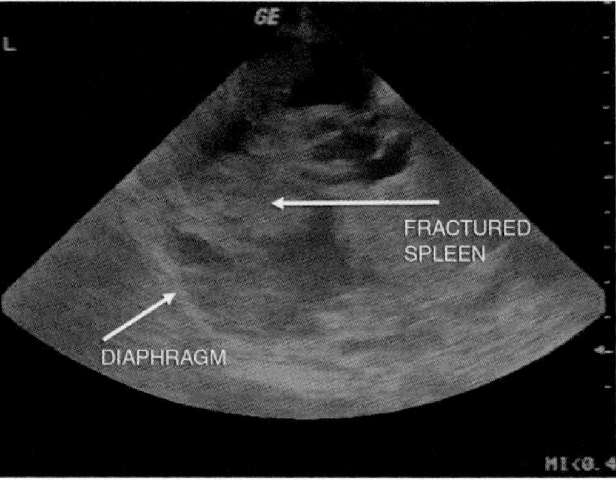

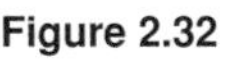

Figure 2.32

This is an unusual image in that the fracture of the spleen can be well visualized. In any case, large amounts of free fluid around the spleen are seen. Courtesy of Emergency Ultrasound Division, St. Luke's–Roosevelt Hospital Center, New York, NY.

(A)

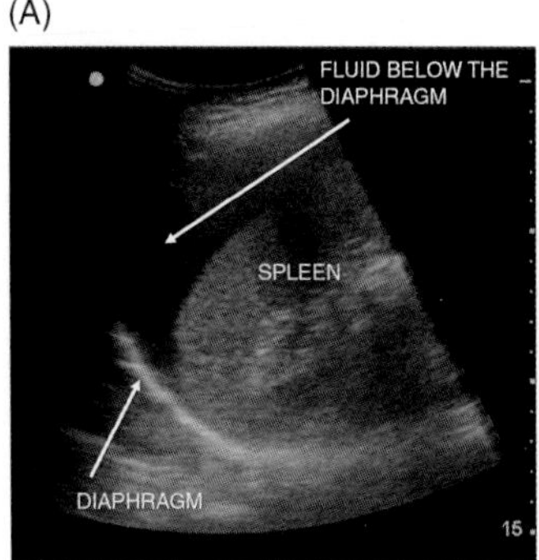

(B)

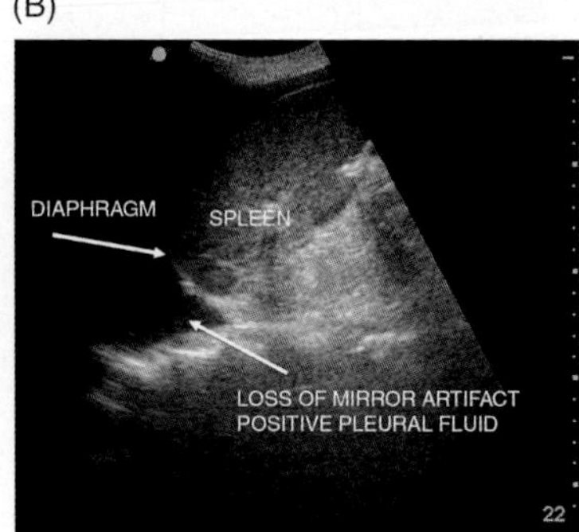

Figure 2.33

These images show how important it is to use the diaphragm as a landmark to identify whether fluid is intrathoracic or intraperitoneal. (*A*) Fluid collecting above the spleen in the subphrenic space below the bright diaphragm before filling the splenorenal recess. (*B*) Fluid above the bright hyperechoic diaphragm indicates that this is a pleural effusion.

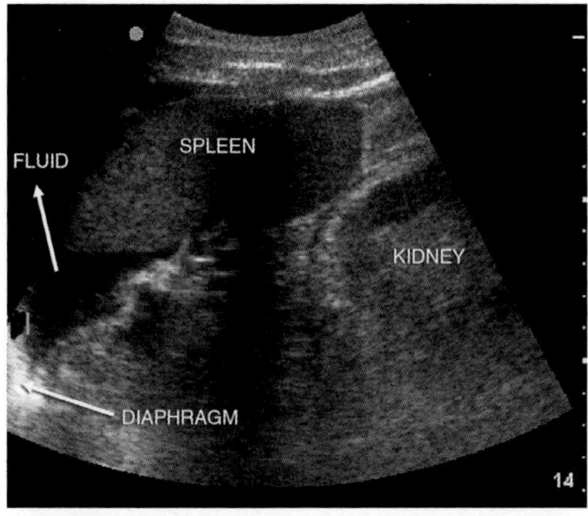

Figure 2.34

There is free fluid between the spleen and the left hemidiaphragm.

(A)

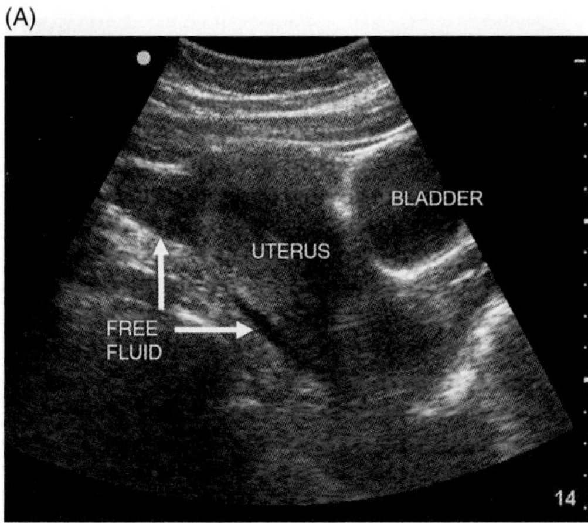

(B)

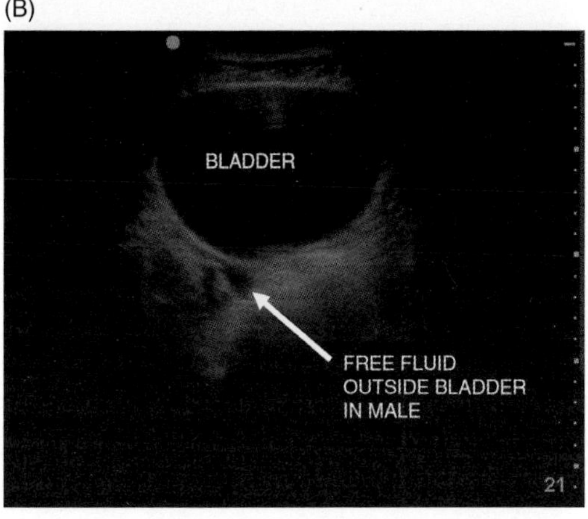

Figure 2.35

(*A*) Fluid is seen behind the uterus and tracking above the fundus. (*B*) Fluid can be seen outside the bladder wall and tracking into the rectovesicular space.

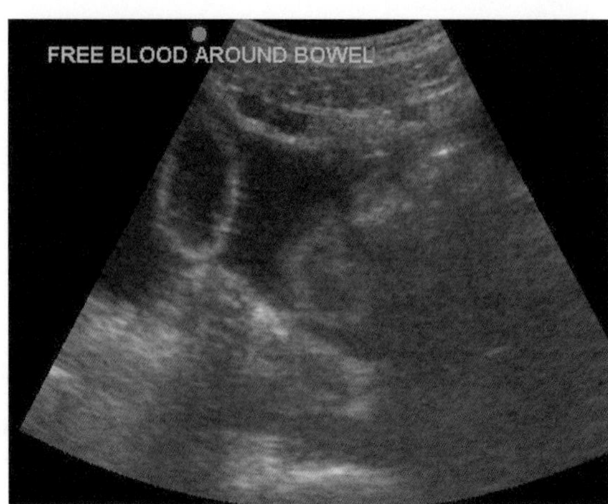

Figure 2.36
Bowel loops floating in free fluid in the pelvis.

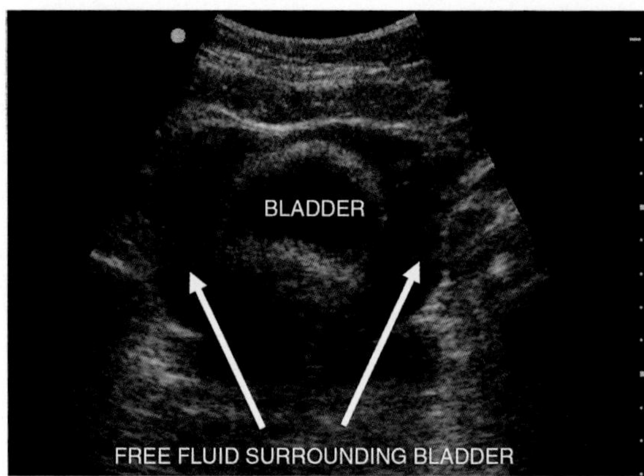

Figure 2.37
Free fluid in the pelvis surrounding the bladder.

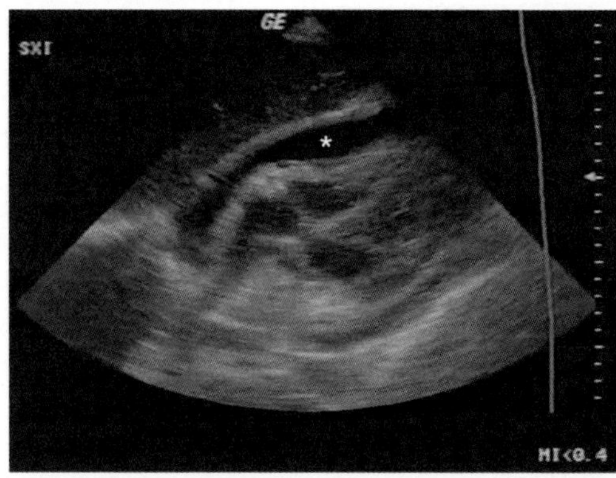

Figure 2.38
Fluid (*) is seen here both anteriorly and posteriorly separating the pericardium (bright white line) from myocardium. The right ventricle is also bowed inward, which is concerning for tamponade physiology (see Chapter 3). Courtesy of Emergency Ultrasound Division, St. Luke's–Roosevelt Hospital Center, New York, NY.

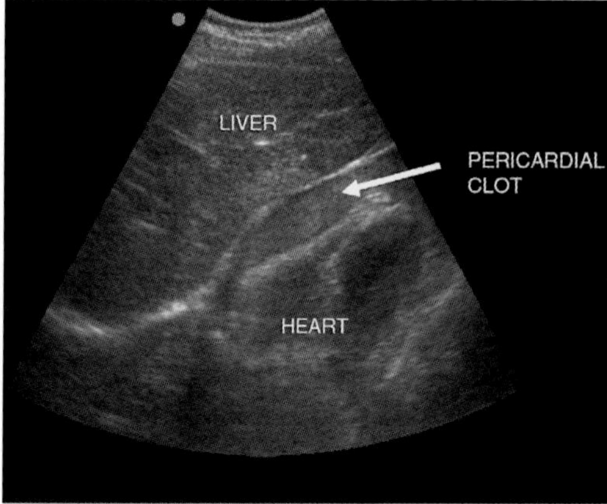

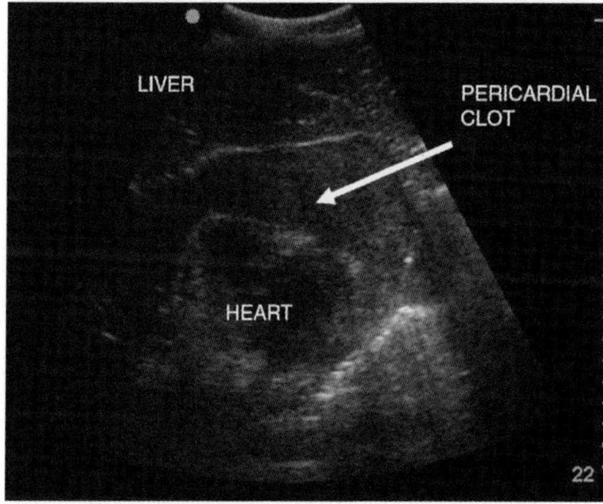

Figure 2.39

In these two pictures, clot is seen in the pericardial space. The importance of recognizing this can be lifesaving, as not all fluid is anechoic.

Extended FAST or eFAST

In the normal right upper quadrant and left upper quadrant views of the FAST exam, the diaphragm acts as a strong reflector of ultrasound beams. Therefore, if you remember the description of the mirror image from Chapter 1, the diaphragm reflects the normal splenic or liver tissue, so an additional "mirror image" is present above the diaphragm (Figure 2.40). The ability of the eFAST to rapidly and accurately diagnose traumatic hemothoraces has been well documented [22,23]. If there is fluid in either the right or the left chest, the mirror image is lost above the diaphragm and black fluid is seen instead (Figure 2.41). In addition, the vertebral shadow that is visible when there is no fluid in the thoracic cavity stops at the diaphragm, since the air in the thoracic cavity scatters the sound waves and prevents further penetration. However, when there is fluid in the thoracic cavity sound waves can travel to the thoracic spine and so the vertebral shadow is visible above the diaphragm (Figure 2.41).

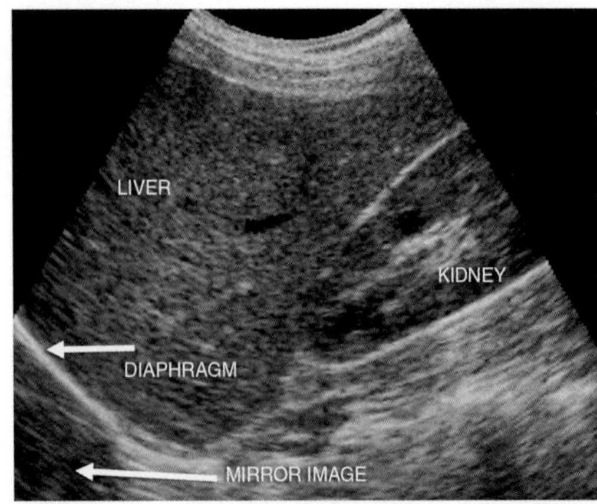

Figure 2.40

Mirror image. Liver-tissue artifact seen above the diaphragm.

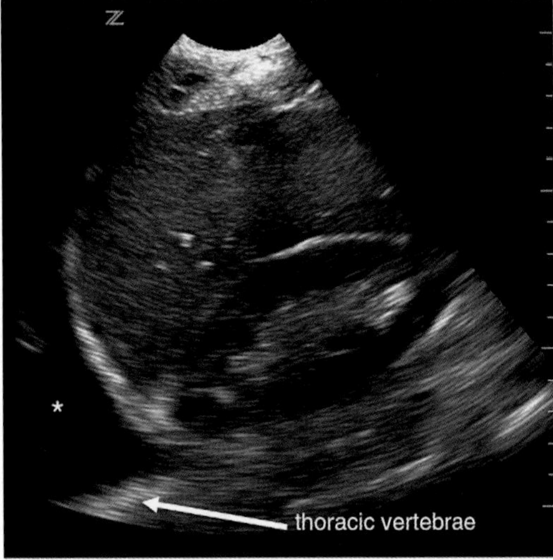

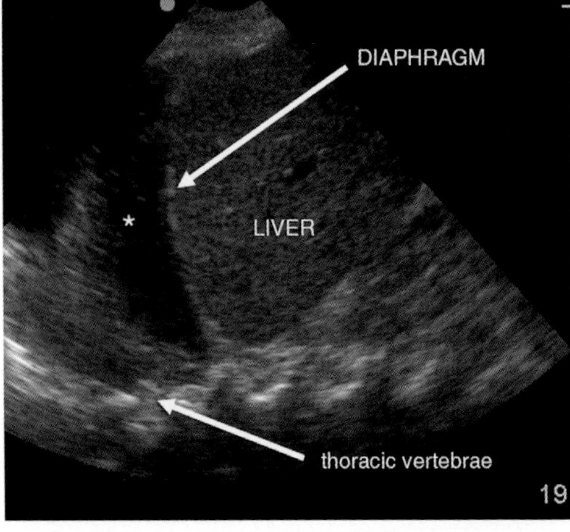

Figure 2.41

Loss of mirror image in both images because of fluid in the thoracic cavity. In addition, when fluid is present in the thorax, ultrasound can penetrate and reach the thoracic vertebrae, so the presence of thoracic vertebral shadows above the diaphragm is pathognomonic for pleural fluid.

Sample clinical protocol

While it is important to remember that the FAST exam was introduced as a way to evaluate blunt trauma, it can also be performed on patients with penetrating trauma. It is particularly useful and lifesaving when evaluating penetrating thoracic or cardiac trauma to look for hemopericardium [25,26] (see Chapter 3), but it can also be used in evaluating penetrating abdominal trauma if there is clinical concern for abdominal hemorrhage. If the FAST exam is positive in penetrating trauma, similar clinical algorithms to blunt trauma can be followed (see below). It should be remembered, however, that ultrasound is not sensitive in diagnosing specific solid-organ injuries. Most penetrating trauma patients, including those with concern for bowel or diaphragmatic injuries, will require CT or exploratory laparotomy to evaluate their injuries further. In addition, FAST can be used in non-trauma patients with concern for abdominal hemorrhage. In the case of a young woman presenting with atraumatic acute peritonitis, or a patient with clinical suscpicion for spontaneous splenic rupture (mononucleosis, hematologic malignancies), a quick look for intra-abdominal hemorrhage can be lifesaving.

Figure 2.42 illustrates the International Consensus Conference recommendations [27].

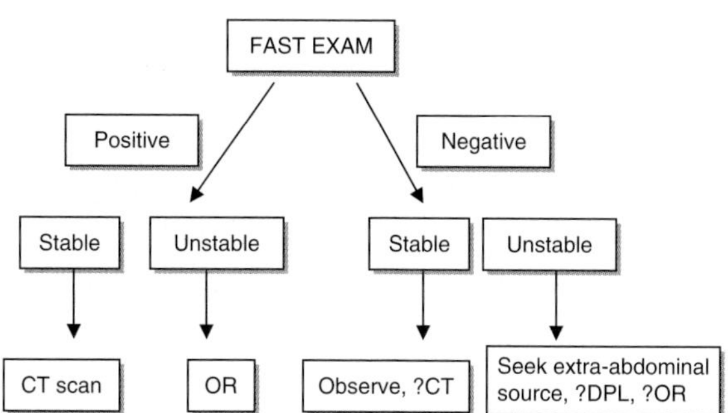

Figure 2.42 Consensus FAST protocol [27].

The decision of what to do with negative FAST patients is still somewhat dependent on the trauma center. In some centers, patients with stable vital signs and a negative FAST exam are observed for 4 hours, undergo repeat FAST exam, and are then discharged home if the FAST remains negative. In unstable patients with a negative FAST exam, extra-abdominal sources of hypotension (intrathoracic trauma, blood loss from extremity or pelvic trauma, spinal shock, head injuries) must be carefully ruled out. DPL can also be performed if FAST images are not clear or difficult to obtain for technical reasons (e.g., subcutaneous air, bowel gas).

Literature review

Reference	Methods	Results	Notes
Melniker *et al.* 2006 [12]	Randomized trauma patients to US-based pathway vs. trauma evaluations without FAST.	FAST led to more rapid time to operating room (OR), fewer CT scans, fewer complications, reduced length of stay, and lower charges.	Outcomes-based study on use of FAST exam. FAST improved outcomes in almost every clinical parameter evaluated.
Plummer *et al.* 1992 [25]	Penetrating trauma patients randomized to emergency department (ED) echo vs. "standard of care" evaluation (echo called in).	Not only diagnosis and disposition expedited in ED echo group, but there was a survival benefit if patients had ED cardiac ultrasound.	Mortality benefit of ED cardiac ultrasound in penetrating cardiac injury.
Branney, *et al.* 1997 [11]	Randomized trauma patients to US-based pathway vs. "standard of care" trauma evaluations (no FAST).	In US-based pathway, DPL use decreased 13%, and CT use decreased 30%. No "significant" injuries missed. Cost savings estimated at $450 000.	First study to note cost savings with implementation of FAST. Also first to document decrease in DPL and CT use.
McKenney *et al.* 2001 [10]	Developed and tested FAST score to help predict need for therapeutic laparotomy. Measured depth of fluid in deepest pocket, and 1 point was added for fluid in each of the other areas (4 maximum).	85% of patients with score > 3 required therapeutic laparotomy, whereas 15% of patients with a score ≤ 2 required surgery.	Further defined characteristics of positive FAST that indicate need for therapeutic laparotomy. More evidence of US benefit over DPL because US predictive value more clinically useful.
Moylan *et al.* 2007 [28]	Looked at the rate of therapeutic laparotomy for normotensive blunt-trauma patients who have a positive FAST exam.	Retrospective cohort study. Unadjusted odds ratio for a positive FAST and laparotomy was OR 116 (95% CI 49.5–273). 37% of patients with a positive FAST required therapeutic laparotomy. Only 0.5% of patients with a negative FAST went to the OR.	Even in normotensive patients, the FAST exam is highly predictive of the need for an operation and is very helpful in risk stratification and prioritization for CT scanning.

Reference	Methods	Results	Notes
Scalea *et al.* 1999 [27]	First consensus statement on how to use FAST in clinical algorithm.	NA	Has not been prospectively validated to date.
Sisley, *et al.* 1998 [22]	Results from initial chest x-ray (CXR) and chest US compared in 360 trauma patients.	US more sensitive (97.5% vs. 92.5% in 360 patients with 40 effusions) and faster (1.3 vs. 14.2 min) in diagnosing traumatic hemothoraces.	Comparison with gold standard showed US to be superior for hemothorax diagnosis.
Rowan *et al.* 2002 [24]	Results from chest US compared to CXR and CT scan test results.	11 pneumothoraces in 70 patients. Thoracic US detected 11/11, CXR 4/11.	US as sensitive as CT, significantly more sensitive than CXR for pneumothorax diagnosis in trauma patients.
Ma *et al.* 2008 [29]	First longitudinal study looking at novice sonographer learning curve over 18 months with respect to test accuracy.	Evaluated image interpretation accuracy at 6-month intervals in an emergency medicine (EM) residency training program.	At 12 months (or after performing 35 examinations) novice EM residents achieved accuracy numbers consistent with published data for FAST exams.

Detection of pneumothorax

Traditionally, the standard test for the initial evaluation of the thorax in trauma patients is the supine chest x-ray. However, supine chest x-rays are notoriously inaccurate when looking for pneumothoraces because air layering anteriorly will be difficult to see. In this context, the sensitivity of ultrasound for diagnosing pneumothorax is an improvement on the current standard practice [24] and one of the most practice-changing diagnostic imaging developments to occur in medicine. This improvement is true not only for trauma but also for many critical care fields of medicine.

A review of the literature describes a technique that first identifies the pleural line. A normal ultrasound examination of the lung includes both lung sliding and comet tail artifacts. *Lung sliding* is the back-and-forth movement of the visceral pleura synchronized with respiration, as seen in real-time scanning. Comet tail artifacts occur when the ultrasound beam bounces back and forth between two closely spaced interfaces, causing multiple reverberations to merge and form a *comet tail pattern* or bright line (see Chapter 1). If a pneumothorax is present, air within the pleural space hinders the propagation of ultrasound waves, thereby preventing the formation of comet tail artifacts and obscuring lung sliding as the visceral pleura is no longer visualized. Therefore, an ultrasound is positive for pneumothorax when lung sliding and comet tail artifacts are absent. One advantage of bedside ultrasound is that each patient will have his or her own control, because comparing left to right thorax will often help make the diagnosis easier. A second technique uses M-mode to visually demonstrate lung sliding or absence of lung sliding (as described in the following section).

Technique

Using a high-frequency linear transducer (5.0–10.0 MHz), longitudinal scans of the anterior chest wall are obtained with the patient in the supine position (Figure 2.43). Place the transducer over the third or fourth intercostal space anteriorly and in the third to fifth intercostal space in the anterior axillary line. The respiratory expansion of the lung (and thus the amount of sliding) may be greater in the anterior axillary-line view. It is also possible to use the same lower-frequency probe (2.5–5 MHz) that is used for FAST exams. Although the image detail may be somewhat less with the lower-frequency probe, sliding or its absence is still readily detectable.

First, identify the rib shadow. This allows you to locate the intercostal plane. Next, identify the pleural line. This is the hyperechoic line located between and below two ribs. In the normal subject, this pleural line is characterized by lung sliding. You should also look for comet tail artifacts as seen in Figures 2.44 and 2.45. Normal lung sliding and the presence of the comet tail artifact rule out pneumothorax with a 100% negative predictive value (Table 2.1).

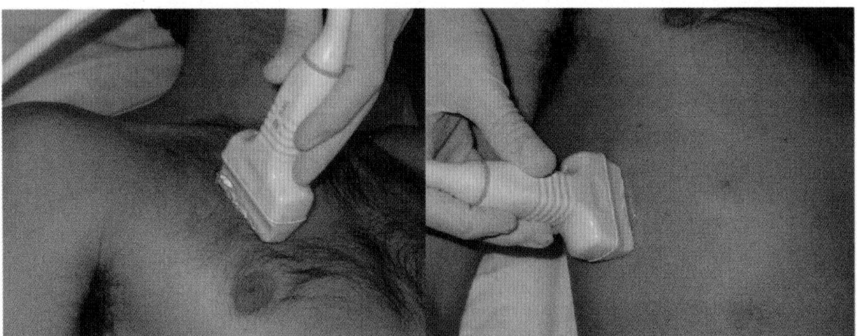

Figure 2.43

Anterior positioning of probe on chest wall (*left*), and anterior axillary-line positioning (*right*). Greater lung sliding is usually seen with axillary-line probe positioning because of greater lung excursion with respirations at this level. However, the anterior position is more sensitive in the supine patient because air layers anteriorly. Courtesy of Dr. Greg Press, University of Texas – Houston, Hermann Memorial Hospital, Houston, TX.

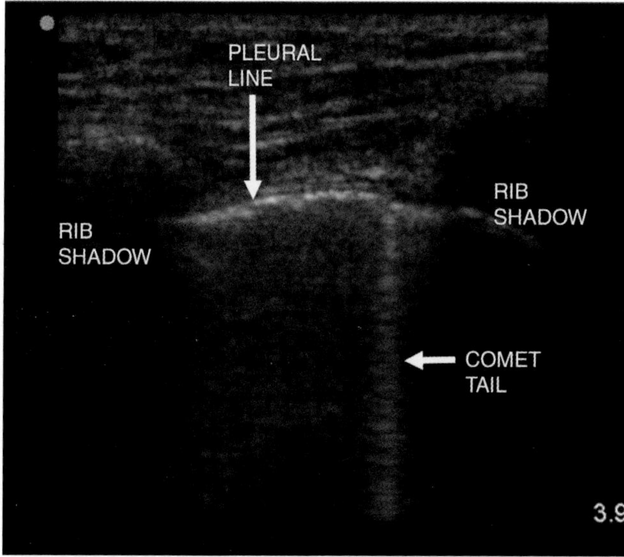

Figure 2.44
Longitudinal scan of the anterior chest wall of a normal patient. The "pleural line" and a comet tail artifact are labeled. The normal to-and-fro sliding movement of this pleural line, synchronized with the respiratory cycle, can be observed in real time.

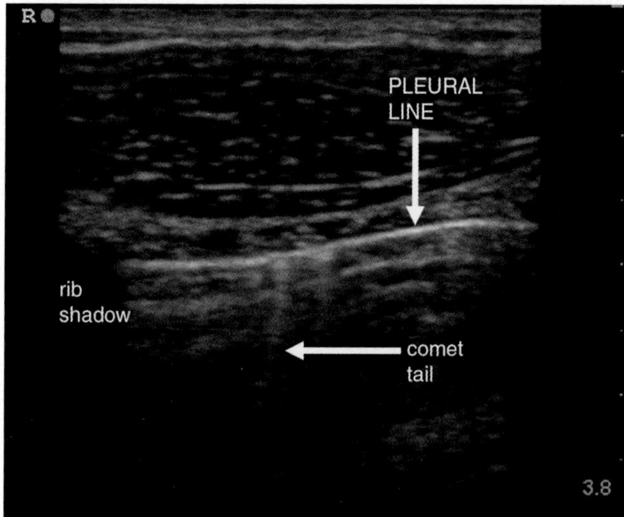

Figure 2.45
Here you can see the rib shadow, pleural line, and comet tail artifact of a normal lung image.

There are three ways to assess the presence of lung sliding using ultrasound. First, the lung slide can be directly observed in real time using two-dimensional ultrasonography, and images can be saved as video. Second, power Doppler can be used to highlight the motion of the pleura. Positive and negative Doppler images are demonstrated in Figure 2.46. Third, M-mode can be used to demonstrate lung sliding on a static image. When using M-mode for this technique, follow a line that includes subcutaneous tissue, chest wall musculature, pleura, and lung and make sure to avoid

Table 2.1 Literature support for ultrasound diagnosis of pneumothorax

Reference	Feature	Performer	Probe	Patients	Standard	Sens	Spec	NP	PP
Blaivas *et al.* 2005 [30]	LS	ED		176 blunt trauma	CT	98	99	99	98
Rowan *et al.* 2002 [24]	LS, comet tail	Radiology	7.0 MHz	27 ED trauma getting CT	CT	100	94	100	92
Dulchavsky *et al.* 2001 [31]	LS, comet tail	Surgery	4.0 Mhz	382 trauma	CXR	94	100	99.4	95
Lichtenstein *et al.* 1999 [32]	LS, comet tail	ICU	3.5 MHz	115 ICU	CXR, CT	100	96.5	100	89
Lichtenstein *et al.* 1995 [33]	LS	ICU	3.0 MHz	111 hemitho-races in ICU	CXR, CT	95.3	91.1	100	87

LS, lung sliding; ED, emergency department; ICU, intensivist; Sens, sensitivity; Spec, specificity; NP, negative predictive value; PP, positive predictive value; CT, computed tomography; CXR, chest x-ray.

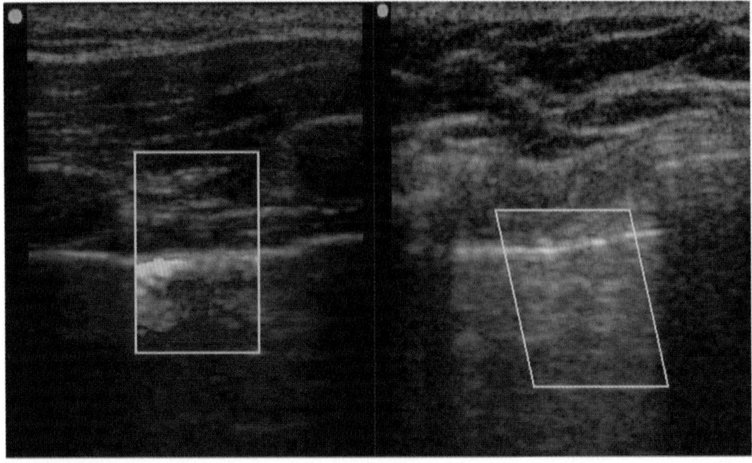

Figure 2.46

Presence of color (*left*) indicates movement or sliding and thus normal lung when using power Doppler. Its absence (*right*) indicates pneumothorax.

placing the M-mode line over a rib. In a normal lung, the image obtained using M-mode should demonstrate smooth lines superficially (because the chest wall should not move much with respiration in this view). Deep to the pleura, the sliding lung will produce enough motion artifact to create

(A)

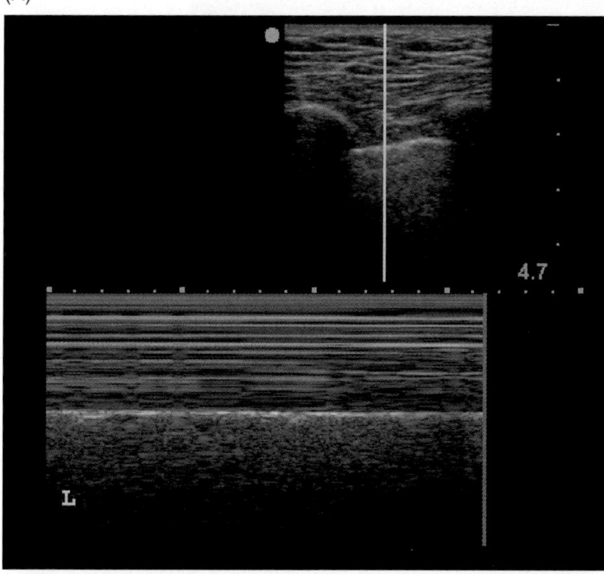

(B)

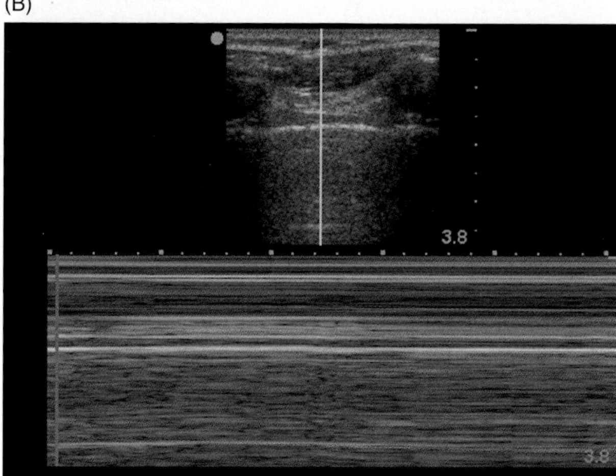

Figure 2.47

(*A*) The "seashore" or normal lung: the pleural line marks a difference in texture above and below (moving lung below the pleura). (*B*) The "barcode sign," with the same texture seen above and below the pleural line.

a rougher, grainier image. The interface between the smooth lines of the chest wall and the rough texture of the moving lung has been described as a "waves on a beach" or "seashore" image (Figure 2.47A). In the case of pneumothorax, no motion will be visible in the chest wall or lung. Thus the lines will be uniformly straight and smooth. This has been called the "barcode" sign (Figure 2.47B) [34]. One of the most specific signs for pneumothorax has been described as the "lung point" sign. This is where the area of pleural reattachment can be seen, represented on ultrasound by an image which is half no lung sliding and half lung sliding [34]. M-mode demonstrates

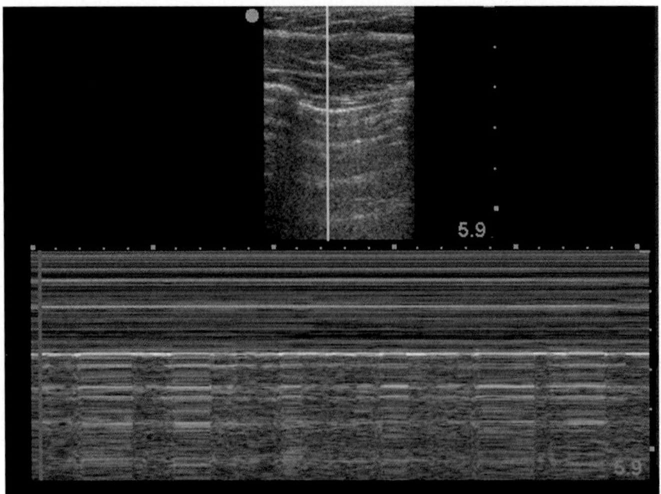

Figure 2.48
M-mode imaging demonstrating the "lung point" sign (half "seashore," half "barcode").

this in a still image by showing half the image as "seashore" and half as "barcode" (Fig 2.48).

One of the most important things to remember when evaluating the thoracic cavity for pneumothorax is that the probe can only interrogate the area of pleura directly beneath the probe footprint. Therefore, if the patient is upright, the most important place to look for a pneumothorax is the apices bilaterally. If a patient is supine, the most important place to look for a pneumothorax is the anterior chest wall. If a patient has penetrating trauma or has just had a procedure, the most important place to look for lung sliding is directly below the point of penetration. Obviously looking in more places increases the sensitivity and specificity of the exam.

New directions

As promised, most chapters will try to stimulate creative thinking about new diagnostic applications for bedside ultrasound. One interesting idea is the concept of using M-mode to diagnose diaphragmatic injury. Diaphragmatic injuries are notoriously difficult to diagnose; even CT scans can be fooled. The gold standard is usually laparoscopy or laparotomy to directly visualize the diaphragm. Blaivas *et al.* [35] describe using M-mode to show whether the diaphragm maintains its respiratory movement/contraction or whether it becomes fixed after injury. Cases where fixed M-mode images correlate with diaphragmatic injury are reported (Figure 2.49).

Another area for research is the evaluation of trauma ultrasound applications in the prehospital setting. Could identifying intraperitoneal fluid in a

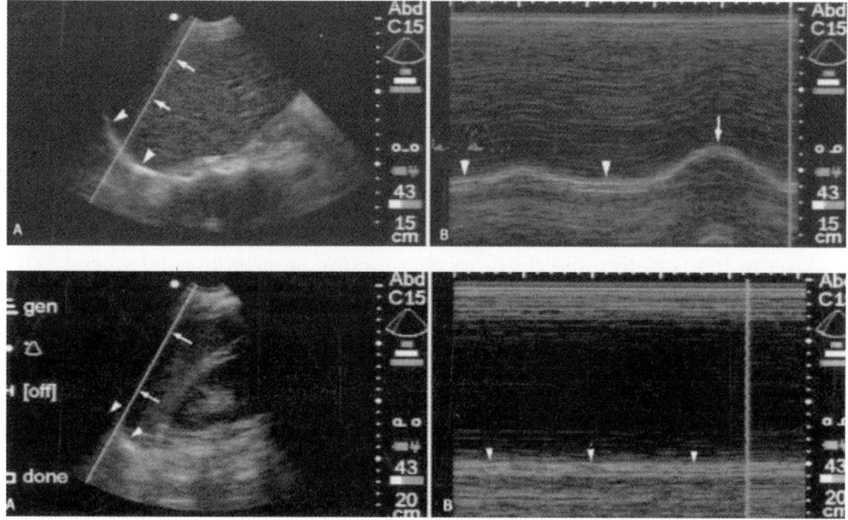

Figure 2.49

The top image demonstrates normal diaphragmatic movement in M-mode during the respiratory cycle. The bottom image illustrates the loss of movement in the setting of diaphragmatic injury. From Blaivas *et al.* [35]. Reprinted with permission from Dr. Michael Blaivas, Professor of Emergency Medicine, Northside Hospital Forsyth, Atlanta, GA.

hypotensive patient help mobilize the operating room more effectively? Could identifying lung sliding prevent unnecessary bilateral needle decompression in a hypotensive patient and thus avoid tube thorocostomy? There is increasing research looking at this, but good outcome-oriented data are needed [36].

References

1. American College of Surgeons (ACS). *Advanced Trauma Life Support for Physicians*. Chicago, IL: ACS; 1997.
2. American College of Emergency Physicians. Use of ultrasound imaging by emergency physicians. Policy 400121. www.acep.org.
3. American College of Emergency Physicians. Emergency ultrasound guidelines 2001. www.acep.org.
4. Society for Academic Emergency Medicine. Ultrasound position statement. www.saem.org.
5. Henneman PL, Marx JA, Moore EE, Cantrill SV, Ammons LA. Diagnostic peritoneal lavage: accuracy in predicting necessary laparotomy following blunt and penetrating trauma. *J Trauma* 1990; **30**: 1345–55.
6. Cogbill TH, Moore EE, Jurkovich GJ, *et al*. Nonoperative management of blunt splenic trauma: a multicenter experience. *J Trauma* 1989; **29**: 1312–17.

7. Bose SM, Mazumdar A, Gupta R, *et al*. Expectant management of haematoperitoneum. *Injury* 1999; **30**: 269–73.
8. Minarik L, Slim M, Rachlin S, Brudnicki A. Diagnostic imaging in the follow-up of nonoperative management of splenic trauma in children. *Pediatr Surg Int* 2002; **18**: 429–31.
9. Branney SW, Wolfe RE, Moore EE, *et al*. Quantitative sensitivity of ultrasound in detecting free intraperitoneal fluid. *J Trauma* 1995; **39**: 375–80.
10. McKenney KL, McKenney MG, Cohn SM, *et al*. Hemoperitoneum score helps determine need for therapeutic laparotomy. *J Trauma* 2001; **50**: 650–4.
11. Branney SW, Moore EE, Cantrill SV, Burch JM, Terry SJ. Ultrasound based key clinical pathway reduces use of hospital resources for the evaluation of blunt abdominal trauma. *J Trauma* 1997; **42**: 1086–90.
12. Melniker LA, Leibner E, McKenney MG, *et al*. Randomized controlled trial of point-of-care limited ultrasonography for trauma in the emergency department: the first sonography outcomes assessment program trial. *Ann Emerg Med* 2006; **48**: 227–35.
13. Kimura A, Otsuka T. Emergency center ultrasonography in the evaluation of hematoperitoneum: a prospective study. *J Trauma* 1991; **31**: 20–3.
14. Rothlin MA, Naf R, Amgwerd M, *et al*. Ultrasound in blunt abdominal and thoracic trauma. *J Trauma* 1993; **34**: 488–95.
15. Rozycki GS, Ochsner MG, Jaffin JH, Champion HR. Prospective evaluation of surgeons' use of ultrasound in the evaluation of the trauma patient. *J Trauma* 1993; **34**: 516–27.
16. Ma OJ, Mateer JR, Ogata M, *et al*. Prospective analysis of a rapid trauma ultrasound examination performed by emergency physicians. *J Trauma* 1995; **38**: 879–85.
17. Ma OJ, Kefer MP, Mateer JR, Thoma B. Evaluation of hemoperitoneum using a single vs multiple-view ultrasonographic examination. *Acad Emerg Med* 1995; **2**: 581–6.
18. McElveen TS, Collin GR. The role of ultrasonography in blunt abdominal trauma: a prospective study. *Am Surg* 1997; **63**: 184–8.
19. Bode PJ, Edwards MJ, Kruit MC, van Vugt AB. Sonography in a clinical algorithm for early evaluation of 1671 patients with blunt abdominal trauma. *AJR Am J Roentgenol* 1999; **172**: 905–11.
20. Thomas B, Falcone RE, Vasquez D, *et al*. Ultrasound evaluation of blunt abdominal trauma: program implementation, initial experience and learning curve. *J Trauma* 1997; **42**: 384–8.
21. Gracias VH, Frankel HL, Gupta R, *et al*. Defining the learning curve for the focused abdominal sonogram for trauma (FAST) examination: implications for credentialing. *Am Surg* 2001; **67**: 364–8.
22. Sisley AC, Rozycki GS, Ballard RB, *et al*. Rapid detection of traumatic effusion using surgeon-performed ultrasonography. *J Trauma* 1998; **44**: 291–6.
23. Ma OJ, Mateer JR. Trauma ultrasound examination vs chest radiography in the detection of hemothorax. *Ann Emerg Med* 1997; **29**: 312–15.

24. Rowan KR, Kirkpatrick AW, Liu D, *et al*. Traumatic pneumothorax detection with US: correlation with chest radiography and CT – initial experience. *Radiology* 2002; **225**: 210–14.
25. Plummer D, Brunette D, Asinger R, Ruiz E. Emergency department echocardiography improves outcome in penetrating cardiac injury. *Ann Emerg Med* 1992; **21**: 709–12.
26. Rozycki GS, Feliciano DV, Ochsner MG, *et al*. The role of ultrasound in patients with possible penetrating cardiac wounds: a prospective multicenter study. *J Trauma* 1999; **46**: 543–51.
27. Scalea TM, Rodriguez A, Chiu WC, *et al*. Focused assessment with sonography for trauma (FAST): results from an international consensus conference. *J Trauma* 1999; **46**: 466–72.
28. Moylan M, Newgard CD, Ma OJ, *et al*. Association between a positive ED FAST examination and therapeutic laparotomy in normotensive blunt trauma patients. *J Emerg Med* 2007; **33**: 265–71.
29. Ma OJ, Gaddis G, Norvell JG, Subramanian S. How fast is the focused assessment with sonography for trauma examination learning curve? *Emerg Med Australas* 2008; **20**: 32–7.
30. Blaivas M, Lyon M, Duggal S. A prospective comparison of supine chest radiography and bedside ultrasound for the diagnosis of traumatic pneumothorax. *Acad Emerg Med* 2005; **12**: 844–9.
31. Dulchavsky SA, Schwarz KL, Kirkpatrick AW, *et al*. Prospective evaluation of thoracic ultrasound in the detection of pneumothorax. *J Trauma* 2001; **50**: 201–5.
32. Lichtenstein D, Meziere G, Biderman P, Gepner A. The comet-tail artifact: an ultrasound sign ruling out pneumothorax. *Intensive Care Med* 1999; **25**: 383–8.
33. Lichtenstein DA, Menu Y. A bedside ultrasound sign ruling out pneumothorax in the critically ill. Lung sliding. *Chest* 1995; **108**: 1345–8.
34. Lichtenstein DA. Pneumothorax and introduction to ultrasound signs in the lung. In Lichtenstein DA (ed.), *General Ultrasound in the Critically Ill*. New York, NY: Springer; 2004: 105–14.
35. Blaivas M, Brannam L, Hawkins M, Lyon M, Sriram K. Bedside emergency ultrasonographic diagnosis of diaphragmatic rupture in blunt abdominal trauma. *Am J Emerg Med* 2004; **22**: 601–4.
36. Heegaard W, Hildebrandt D, Spear D, *et al*. Prehospital ultrasound by paramedics: results of field trial. *Acad Emerg Med* 2010; **17**: 624–30.

3 Cardiac ultrasound

Introduction

Cardiac ultrasound can benefit the practice of both novice and seasoned physician sonographers. Differentiating between pulseless electrical activity (PEA) and asystole in cardiac arrest, identifying pericardial effusions, and estimating volume status or global cardiac function in shock are all applications that can make a difference in patient treatment and outcome. However, it is important to note that this manual is not meant to teach a non-cardiologist to be an echocardiographer. Bedside cardiac ultrasound is a tool to be used by clinical practitioners who need rapid answers to specific questions about cardiac function in critically ill patients. Any good physician must recognize the limitations of his or her knowledge and skill; in cases where ambiguity remains after bedside ultrasonography, follow-up testing should occur in accordance with normal practice patterns [1].

This chapter also reviews how to make estimations of global cardiac function and a basic assessment of right ventricular strain. This can impact the care of patients in whom pulmonary embolism is being considered.

Cardiac ultrasound is essential in looking for wall motion abnormalities in ischemic heart disease and in evaluating valvular cardiac disease, but these applications can be complicated and require more extensive training. Again, knowing the limitations of bedside ultrasonography is essential for practicing safely.

Focused questions for cardiac ultrasound

Two distinct applications are considered primary indications for emergency department cardiac ultrasound, and they also have a role in other areas of critical care medicine:

1. Is there a pericardial effusion?
2. Is cardiac activity present?

For the novice sonographer, assessing for cardiac activity and pericardial effusion can alter management and impact patient care. These should be the foundation on which further cardiac assessment is built. As comfort with these applications grows, more advanced questions can be addressed:

3. What is the global function/contractility (hypercontractile, normal, decreased)?
4. Are signs of right ventricular strain present?

Anatomy

Because the heart lies obliquely in the chest, standard positional nomenclature (e.g., sagittal and coronal) is not useful. Instead, there are standard planes commonly used to visualize key cardiac structures, and these provide the basis for a complete exam. Basic anatomy of the heart is detailed in Figure 3.1. Commonly used planes include (1) the long axis, which "cuts" the heart along its long axis from the atria to the apex, and (2) the short axis, which cuts a cross-section from anterior to posterior.

There are common probe positions used to view these planes. These positions have been selected to avoid artifacts from rib shadows or lung:

- Parasternal position
- Subxiphoid position
- Apical position

By using these positions (or windows), one can obtain common views (or planes) of the heart that are comparable to those used by echocardiographers.

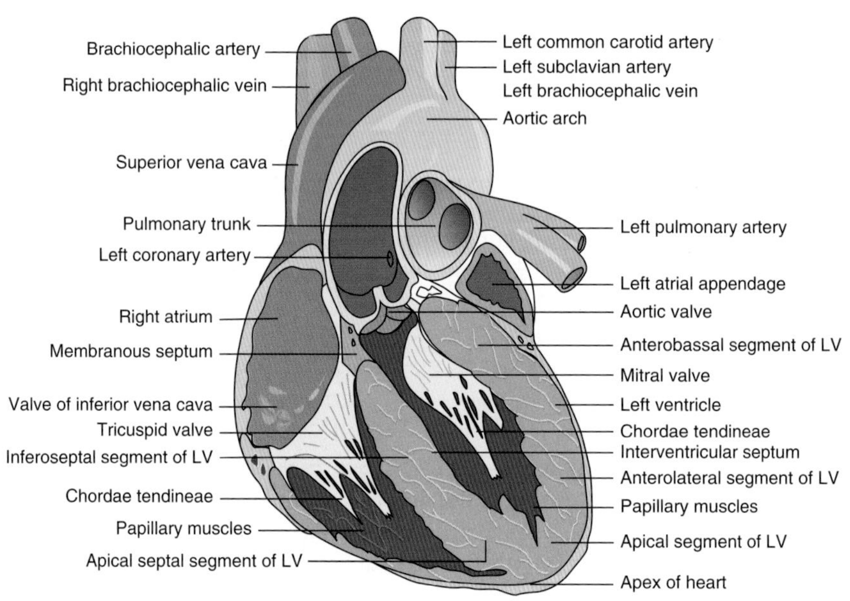

Figure 3.1

Anatomy of the heart. Courtesy of Patrick Lynch, Yale University School of Medicine, New Haven, CT.

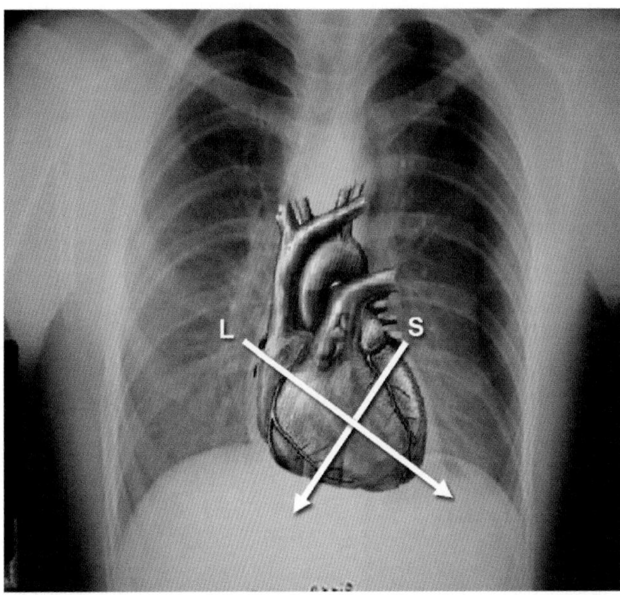

Figure 3.2
Position of the heart in the thoracic cavity with major axes (arrows). L, long axis; S, short axis. Courtesy of Dr. Manuel Colon, Hospital of the University of Puerto Rico, Carolina, PR.

Most clinical applications can be supported using four basic sonographic views of the heart:

- Subcostal or subxiphoid four-chamber view
- Parasternal long-axis view
- Parasternal short-axis view
- Apical four-chamber view

When learning bedside cardiac ultrasound the most important concept to remember is that the heart lies in the chest at somewhat of an oblique angle, with the apex pointing toward the left hip (Figure 3.2). The right ventricle in the majority of patients will be more anterior (closer to the anterior chest wall) than the left ventricle because of the normal anatomic rotation of the heart. This means that for most imaging the right ventricle will be more anterior or closer to the probe than the left ventricle. The other obvious anatomic difference between the left and right ventricle is that the left ventricle is a high-pressure system with thicker myocardium, while the right ventricle is a lower-pressure system, and thus in normal physiology the walls of the right ventricle are much thinner. Of course, this normal appearance is changed with certain types of pathophysiology, but it is a good place to begin.

Technique

Historically, cardiac ultrasound adopted standard views in which the left side of the heart was portrayed on the right side of the ultrasound screen. There are two ways in which such cardiac-oriented images may be obtained.

First, image in "cardiac mode" on the ultrasound machine, which will flip the screen image 180 degrees and will place the screen marker on the right of the image screen. Then place the probe with the marker to the patient's left or pointing to the patient's shoulders. More commonly, however, point-of-care sonographers leave the screen marker on the left as it is in abdominal imaging and place the probe marker to the patient's right or pointing to the patient's hips. Either way will generate the same image when looking at the screen.

The second technique is described here. This allows the sonographer to keep the abdominal image settings on the machine the same, to avoid confusion, but the pictures generated will look identical to those made using cardiology settings and probe positioning. However, if the first option is preferred, just invert the probe positions described here by 180 degrees.

Probe selection

The probe used for cardiac ultrasound is most often a phased-array probe – ideally with the smallest possible footprint, useful in imaging between ribs. It is usually a lower-frequency probe with ranges between 2 and 5 MHz. Some machines also have cardiac presets in their setup menus that help the machine optimize digital image processing for cardiac imaging (such as altering dynamic range and contrast to enhance wall detection, and increasing frame rate for better detection of motion).

Views

Multiple ultrasound views are used to assess the heart at the bedside. The two views most commonly used by the non-cardiologist to look for contractility and evaluate for pericardial effusion are the subxiphoid four-chamber view and the left parasternal view. We review these two positions first, and then supplement with parasternal short-axis and apical four-chamber views to give the bedside ultrasonographer multiple options for evaluating the heart. Note that only the subxiphoid and apical views allow for four-chamber visualization and comparison of right and left ventricular cavity size.

Subcostal/subxiphoid view

The subxiphoid probe position uses the liver as an acoustic window through which the heart is well visualized. The probe should be placed in the subxiphoid position (Figure 3.3). Aim toward the left shoulder and place the probe at a 15-degree angle to the chest wall. The probe indicator should be pointing toward the patient's right (Figure 3.4). Many novices place the probe at too steep an angle, and thus the ultrasound beam being generated is too steep – that is, it is not projecting toward the left chest cavity where the heart lies. In some people, the probe is almost flat against the abdominal wall. Because the beam is transmitted over a

(A)

(B)

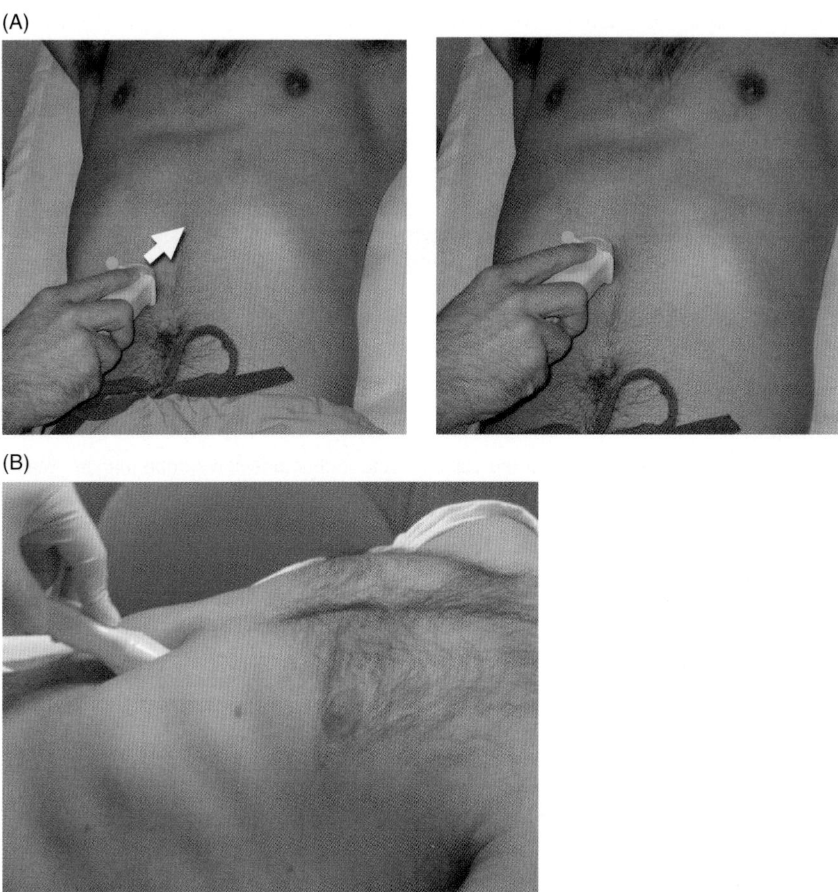

Figure 3.3

Probe positioning for subxiphoid view. (*A*) Begin with the probe several centimeters inferior to the xiphoid process and slide the probe cephalad (in direction of arrow) until (*B*) it "nestles" in the subxiphoid area. (*C*) Note the angle the transducer must make in order to visualize the heart. Probe marker (green dot) faces patient's right side.

fairly long distance (usually 7–10 cm), it is best to start with the screen at maximum depth so the longest distance is visualized on the screen. Once the heart is identified, the depth can be adjusted to enlarge the image as appropriate.

The liver and then right ventricle are closest to the probe and so will be most superior on the ultrasound screen. The bright white pericardium is seen in Figure 3.5; it is flush up against the gray myocardium, indicating no effusion is present. Often stomach or intestinal gas interferes with the subxiphoid view. When this occurs the probe should be moved toward the patient's right side to better use the liver as an acoustic window (Figure 3.6)

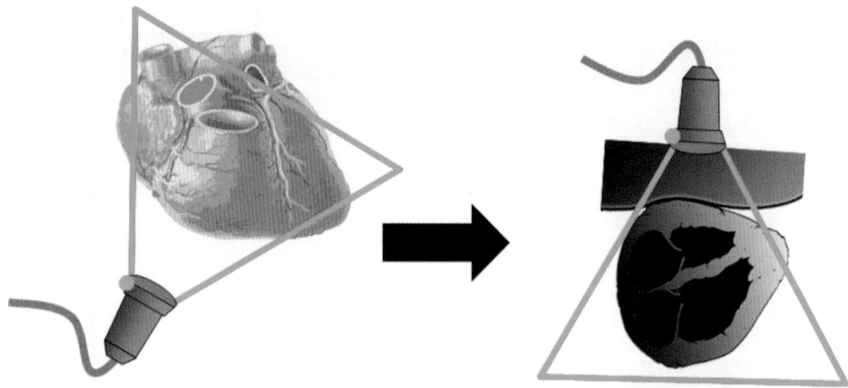

Figure 3.4
Orientation of probe and image for the subxiphoid four-chamber view (probe marker noted with a green dot).

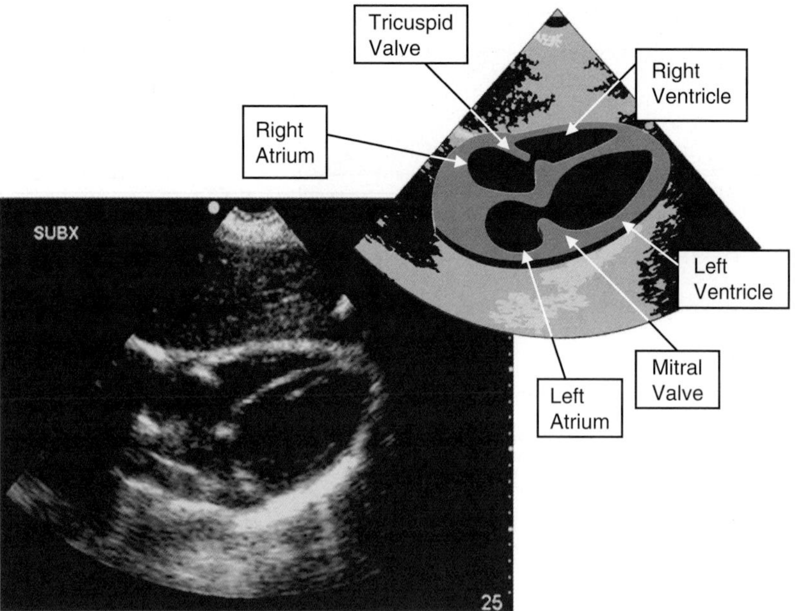

Figure 3.5
Cartoon of subxiphoid view with corresponding anatomy as visualized by ultrasound. Courtesy of Dr. Manuel Colon, Hospital of the University of Puerto Rico, Carolina, PR.

The subxiphoid four-chamber view gives a good view of the right ventricle and is often used to look for a pericardial effusion. It is also the standard view for cardiac evaluation during the FAST exam.

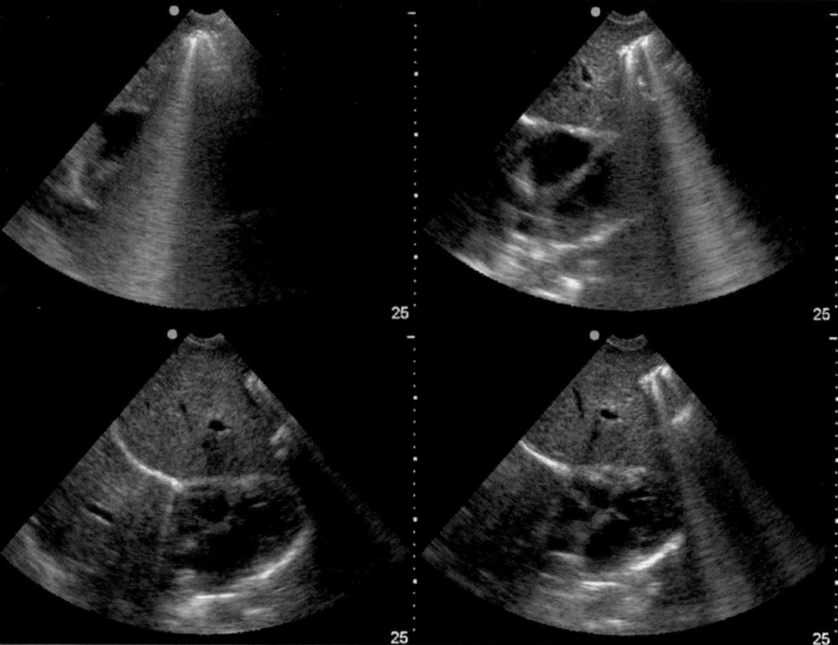

Figure 3.6

Moving the probe toward the patient's right side avoids bowel gas and optimizes the liver window in the subxiphoid view. Note significant interference from stomach gas obscuring view. This is decreased incrementally (clockwise from top left) as the probe is moved toward the patient's right side, maximizing use of the liver as a window.

Left parasternal long-axis view

Assuming the long axis of the heart to be from the patient's right shoulder to the left hip, the transducer probe should be placed in the third or fourth intercostal space, immediately left of the sternum (Figure 3.7). The probe indicator should be pointing toward the 5 o'clock position or toward the patient's left hip (Figure 3.8). In this position, the depth on the machine does not need to be as great because the structures of interest should be fairly close to the probe. The angle of the probe should be adjusted to place the beam along the electrical vector of the heart.

There are three points which define the plane of the parasternal long-axis view:

- Mitral valve
- Aortic valve
- Cardiac apex

When these three structures are visualized simultaneously, the probe is oriented correctly along the long axis of the heart. This is not only

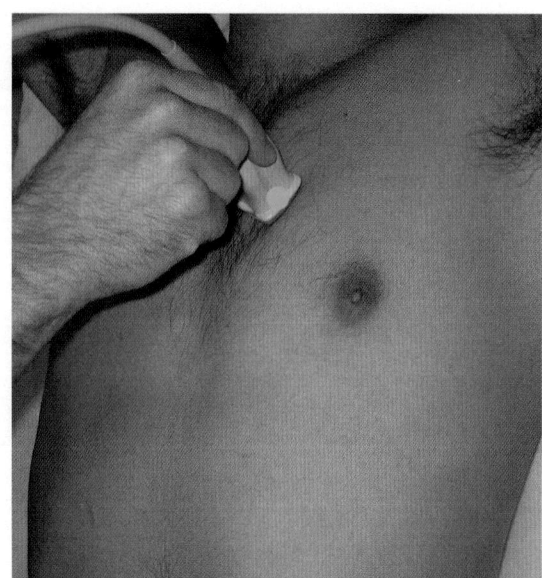

Figure 3.7

Probe positioning for parasternal long-axis view. Probe marker (green dot) faces patient's left side, pointing toward the apex.

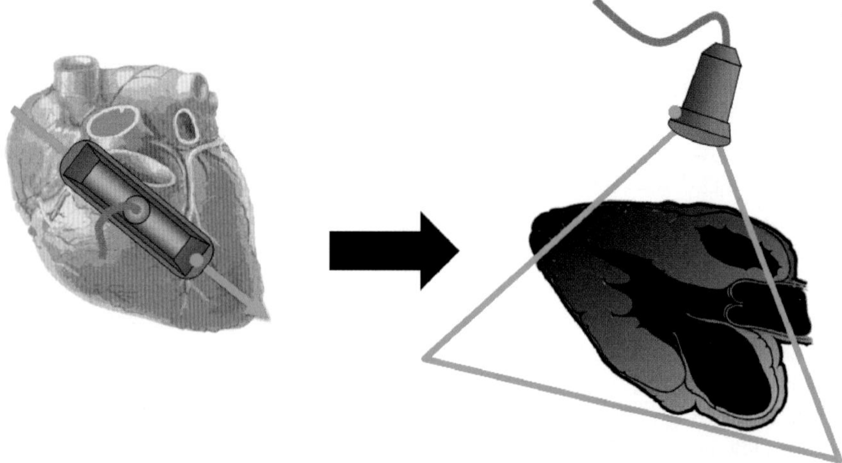

Figure 3.8

Orientation of probe (probe marker direction shown by green dot) and corresponding image orientation in parasternal long-axis view.

important for consistency of terms between clinicians. The appearance of contractility and other assessments may be altered by an incorrect or off-plane orientation.

The parasternal view is often easier in obese patients, although it can be challenging in patients with significant pulmonary disease. Again, the right

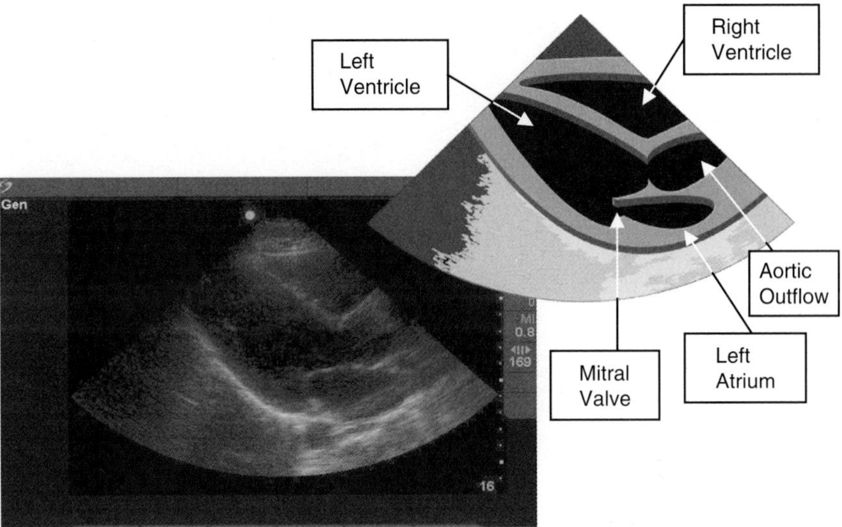

Figure 3.9

Cartoon of parasternal long-axis view with corresponding anatomy as visualized by ultrasound. Courtesy of Dr. Manuel Colon, Hospital of the University of Puerto Rico, Carolina, PR.

ventricle will be the chamber closest to the top of the screen, because it is closest to the probe (Figure 3.9).

Most important, the parasternal long-axis view can help distinguish pleural from pericardial effusions. Large pleural effusions can appear to surround the heart, but they will taper to the descending aorta, which can often be seen in the parasternal view. Pericardial effusions will cross anterior to the descending aorta. This is because the pleura will insert where the descending aorta travels through the thoracic cavity. The pericardium is a self-contained space that will cross the midline. In Figure 3.10 the pericardium is flush up against the myocardium, and there is no effusion.

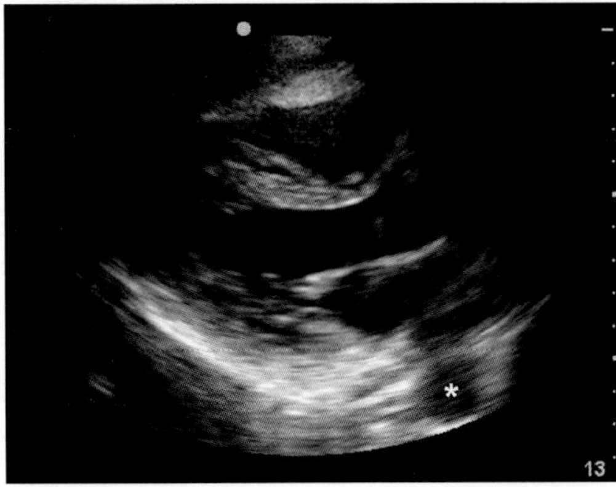

Figure 3.10

Normal parasternal long-axis view with no pericardial effusion, and descending thoracic aorta visible (*).

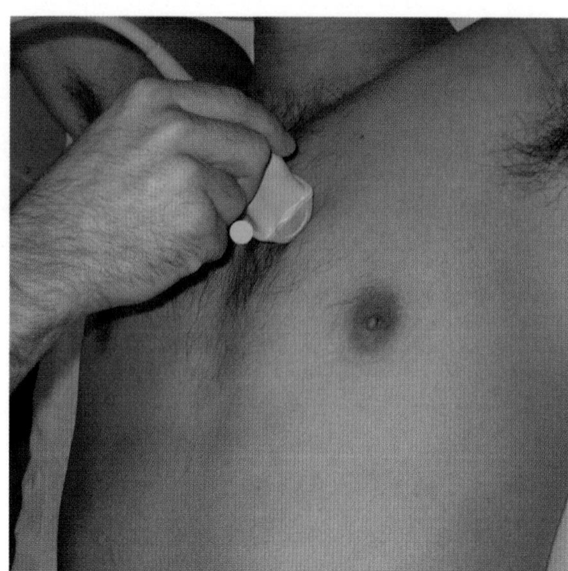

Figure 3.11
Probe position for short-axis view. Starting with a parasternal long-axis view, simply rotate the probe 90 degrees. Probe marker faces caudally (green dot).

Left parasternal short-axis view

Assuming the short axis to be from the patient's left shoulder to the right hip, the transducer probe should be placed in the third or fourth intercostal space, immediately left of the sternum (Figure 3.11). If the parasternal long-axis view has already been obtained, simply rotate the transducer 90 degrees clockwise toward the patient's right hip to find the short-axis view (Figure 3.12). By sliding the probe toward the right shoulder or toward the left hip, the ultrasonographer can slice the short axis at different cross-sections – usually this view visualizes the mitral valve in cross-section (Figure 3.13), but by sliding toward the right shoulder the aortic valve can be seen, or by sliding toward the left hip more focused images of the heart's apex can be seen. This plane gives an excellent circumferential view of the left ventricle and is often used for assessment of contractility and even regional wall motion abnormalities.

Apical four-chamber view

This window is obtained at the apex of the heart, which is usually located along the T4–5 level or nipple line. If possible, rotate the patient onto his or her left side to reduce any lung artifact and to bring the heart closer to the anterior chest wall. Position the transducer at the patient's point of maximal impulse (PMI) – or about the fifth intercostal space – aiming toward the patient's right shoulder (Figure 3.14). The probe indicator should be pointed toward the patient's right (Figure 3.15).

This is an important view, because it yields information about the relative dimensions of the left and right ventricles (Figure 3.16). An important rule

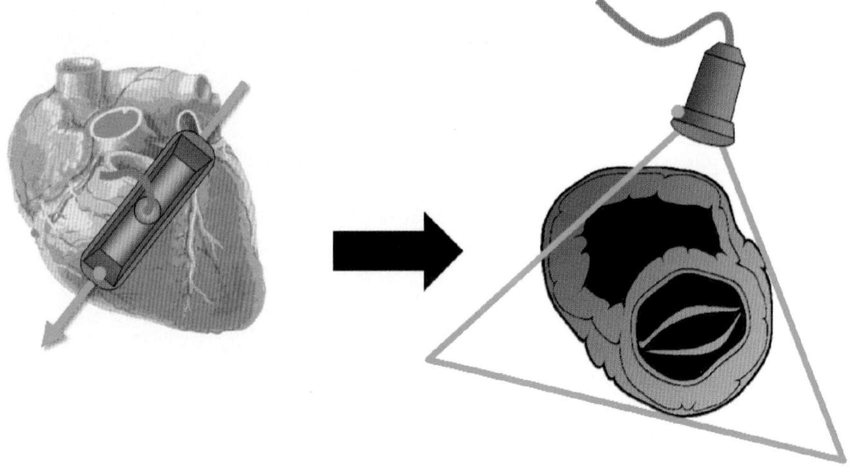

Figure 3.12
Orientation of probe (probe marker direction shown by green dot) and corresponding image orientation in parasternal short-axis view.

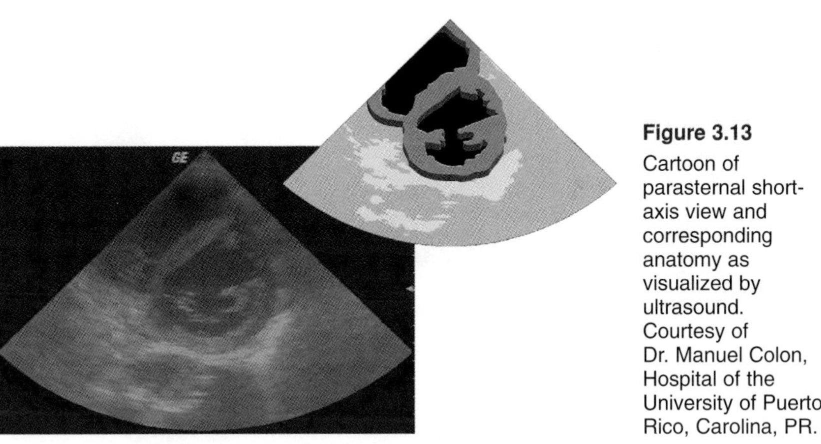

Figure 3.13
Cartoon of parasternal short-axis view and corresponding anatomy as visualized by ultrasound. Courtesy of Dr. Manuel Colon, Hospital of the University of Puerto Rico, Carolina, PR.

of thumb is that the ratio of right-ventricle to left-ventricle diameter is less than 0.7 at the level of the tricuspid and mitral valves. That is, the width from myocardial inner wall to septal inner wall of the right ventricle is about half that of the left ventricle. Although a RV/LV ratio of greater than 0.7 indicates a dilated right ventricle, many authors use a ratio of greater than 1 : 1 to indicate a pathologically dilated RV [2]. Abnormal movement of the septum away from the right ventricle during diastole indicates increased right ventricular pressures. Normally the right ventricle is a low-pressure system, and therefore relaxation would mean the septum would bow away from

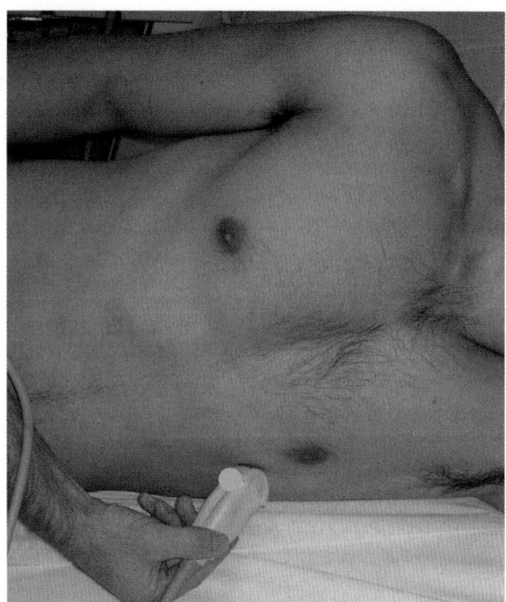

Figure 3.14

Probe positioning in apical four-chamber view (probe marker direction shown by green dot). Note that the patient is placed in the left lateral decubitus position whenever possible. This improves the quality of all cardiac views but is often the *only* position in which an adequate apical four-chamber view can be obtained.

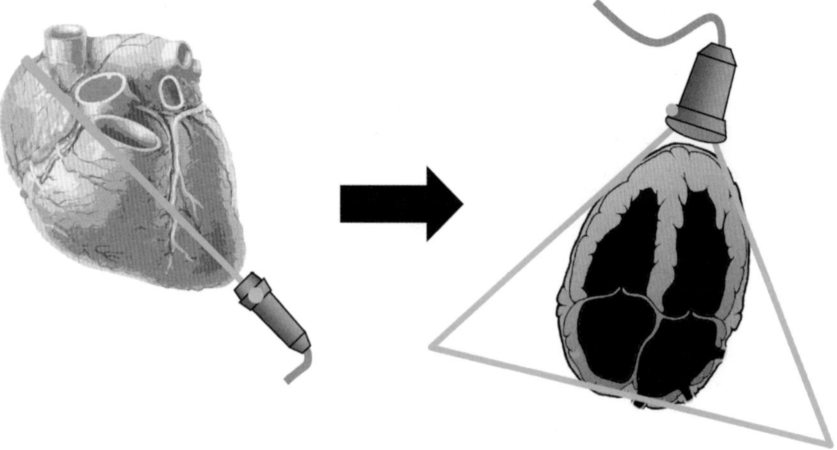

Figure 3.15

Orientation of probe (probe marker direction shown by green dot) and corresponding image orientation in apical four-chamber view. Note that the probe marker is on the same side as the right ventricle.

the higher-pressure left ventricle. Both this abnormal septal movement and increased right ventricular size are evidence of right ventricular dysfunction [2]. For the bedside echocardiographer, these findings are only helpful in the right clinical setting, i.e., critically ill patients. However, if the clinical

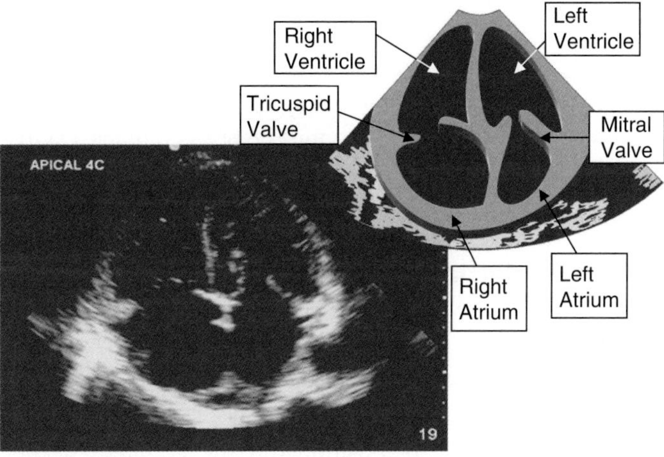

Figure 3.16

Cartoon of apical four-chamber view and corresponding anatomy as visualized by ultrasound. Courtesy of Dr. Manuel Colon, Hospital of the University of Puerto Rico, Carolina, PR.

suspicion for pulmonary embolus is high and these findings are seen, this may help support the decision for lysis in critical patients in the right clinical setting [3].

Scanning tips

Trouble with the subcostal four-chamber view

Can't see anything recognizable?

- Try increasing the depth to its maximal level to make sure the beam is reaching the part of the thoracic cavity containing the heart.
- Flatten the probe on the abdominal wall to make sure the beam is angling toward the left thoracic cavity.
- Slide the probe over to the right to use the liver as an acoustic window and to get away from the stomach, which may be scattering the sound waves.
- Have the patient bend his or her knees if possible. This helps relax the abdominal wall muscles and can sometimes make visualization easier.

Trouble with the parasternal long-axis view

Rib shadow in the way?

- Try angling the probe obliquely to sneak through the intercostal space.

Can't see a recognizable image?

- Try sliding the probe along the third or fourth intercostal space toward and away from the sternum. Occasionally, the long-axis view is not adjacent to the sternum but more in the middle of the thoracic cavity.
- Have the patient lie in the left lateral decubitus position to bring the heart closer to the chest wall and limit interference from the lung.

Trouble with the parasternal short-axis view

Can't find the heart?

- Try sliding the probe in the intercostal space toward and away from the sternum. Try angling the probe obliquely as well.
- If the patient can sit forward or be positioned in the left lateral decubitus position, the heart will be brought forward in the chest and will be closer to the probe, making for easier scanning.

Trouble with the apical four-chamber view

Can't find the heart?

- This can be the trickiest view to find, and sometimes sliding the probe around where you think the PMI might be will result in a recognizable image popping into view.
- If the patient can sit forward or be positioned in the left lateral decubitus position, the heart will be brought forward in the chest and will be closer to the probe.
- Try to start with a parasternal long-axis view, and slide the probe laterally (left) along the chest wall until the apex is centered on the screen. Then adjust the angle and direction of the transducer to create an apical window.

Normal images

Figure 3.17 demonstrates normal subxiphoid four-chamber views. Note the liver visible in the near field acting as a good acoustic window for this view.

Figure 3.18 demonstrates normal parasternal long-axis views. Note that the descending thoracic aorta is visible as a brightly outlined circle in the far field deep to the heart.

Figure 3.19 demonstrates normal parasternal short-axis views. The left ventricle appears as a circle.

Figure 3.20 demonstrates normal apical four-chamber views. The right ventricle should be on the same side as the probe marker, and the left and right ventricle sizes can be compared well in this view.

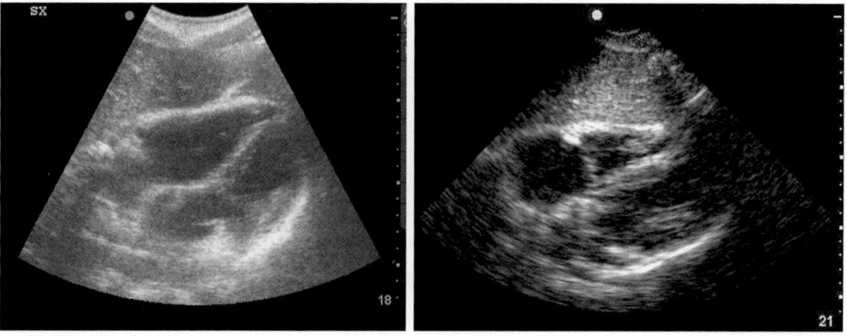

Figure 3.17
Normal subxiphoid four-chamber views.

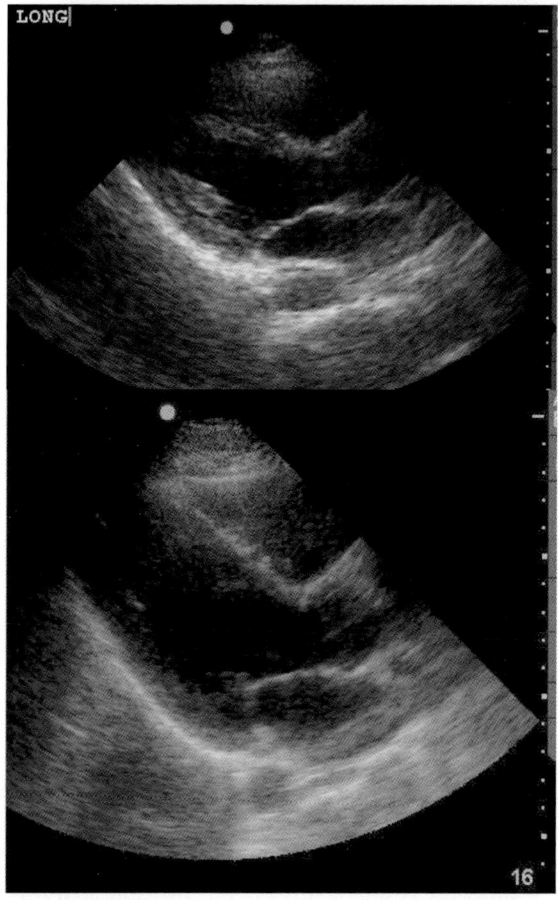

Figure 3.18
Normal parasternal long-axis views.

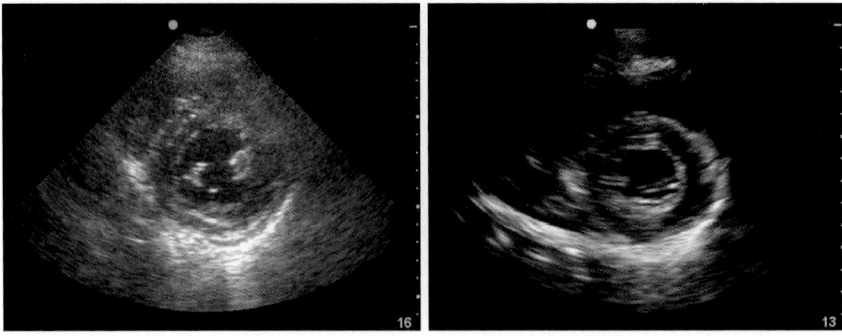

Figure 3.19
Normal parasternal short-axis views.

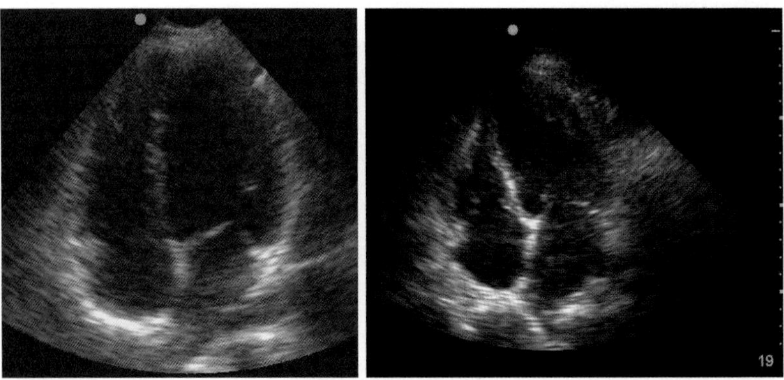

Figure 3.20
Normal apical four-chamber views. Note that the right ventricle diameter is smaller than the left.

Abnormal images

Pericardial fluid

Pericardial effusions are defined as the presence of fluid in the pericardial space. They can be caused by a variety of local and systemic disorders or trauma, or they can be idiopathic. They can be acute or chronic, and the time course of development has a great impact on the patient's symptoms.

The pericardium itself is a dense, fibrous sac that completely encircles the heart and a few centimeters of the aorta and pulmonary artery. The dense parietal pericardial tissue is highly echogenic (looks white on ultrasound) and is recognized both anteriorly and posteriorly as the sonographic border of the cardiac image. A pericardial effusion is characterized on ultrasound by an anechoic (black) fluid collection between the visceral and parietal pericardium

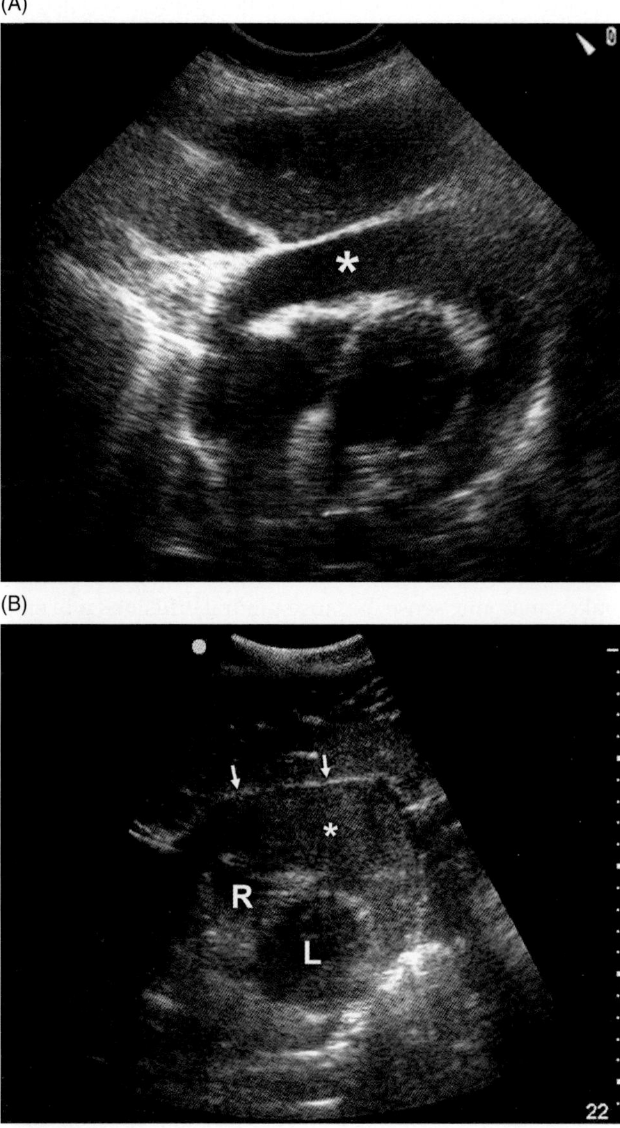

Figure 3.21

(*A*) The black stripe (*) separating the pericardium from the myocardium is the surrounding pericardial effusion. (*B*) Here, the pericardial effusion (asterisk) is grainy and gray, consistent with coagulating blood, pus, or other echogenic material. The fluid (*) separates the right (R) and left (L) ventricles from the pericardium (arrows).

(Figure 3.21A) – keeping in mind that the visceral pericardium is not usually seen by transthoracic cardiac ultrasound. Therefore, a pericardial effusion appears as a fluid collection that separates the bright white, highly reflective parietal pericardium from the heterogeneous gray myocardium.

If the fluid has pus, blood mixed with fibrin, or is malignant, it can appear echogenic or have a gray appearance (Figure 3.21B). Although this can make the diagnosis more challenging, in real time this "gray" appearance is swirling in a pocket of black fluid that separates the parietal pericardium from the myocardium.

In certain clinical scenarios, pericardial fluid volumes of up to 50 mL can be physiologic. Small effusions are usually located posterior and inferior to the left ventricle. Moderate effusions extend toward the apex of the heart, and large effusions circumscribe the heart. Most textbooks define a moderate effusion as an echo-free pericardial space (anterior plus posterior) of 10–20 mm during diastole and a large effusion as an echo-free space of more than 20 mm [4]. Figure 3.22 demonstrates pericardial effusions in three different cardiac views.

Occasionally, either intra-abdominal fluid or pleural effusions may be confused with pericardial effusions. Therefore, it is absolutely necessary to visualize the hyperechoic image of the pericardium to ensure that the anechoic fluid is indeed intrapericardial. In addition, when visualizing the descending thoracic aorta via a parasternal long-axis window, one will observe that pleural effusions do not cross the aorta, whereas pericardial effusions will. This makes anatomic sense, because pleural effusions will stop at the insertion of the pleura, whereas pericardial effusions will cross the midline (Figure 3.23).

Another pitfall can be the mistaken impression that an echo-free collection anterior to the right ventricle is fluid. Many patients have an "epicardial fat pad" that will appear as an anechoic area anterior to the heart. Because most patients have their ultrasounds in a relatively supine position you would expect fluid to collect posteriorly, and thus fluid seen *only* anteriorly should be suspect. A fat pad will not exert pressure on the right ventricle causing deformation.

Cardiac tamponade

Cardiac tamponade is the compression of the heart caused by blood or fluid accumulation in the space between the myocardium and the pericardium. It is less dependent on the amount of fluid, but rather on the rate of fluid collection within the pericardial sac. It is important to remember that although pericardial effusions are a diagnosis made by ultrasound, tamponade is a *clinical* diagnosis based on a patient's hemodynamics and clinical picture. Ultrasound may be useful in confirming the diagnosis in a patient with the classic triad of muffled heart tones, hypotension, and jugular venous distension. More importantly, ultrasound may demonstrate early warning signs of tamponade before the patient becomes hemodynamically unstable.

Several sonographic signs suggestive of tamponade physiology have been described, although appreciation of these may be subtle [4]. *The most important finding is a circumferential pericardial effusion with a hyperdynamic heart that*

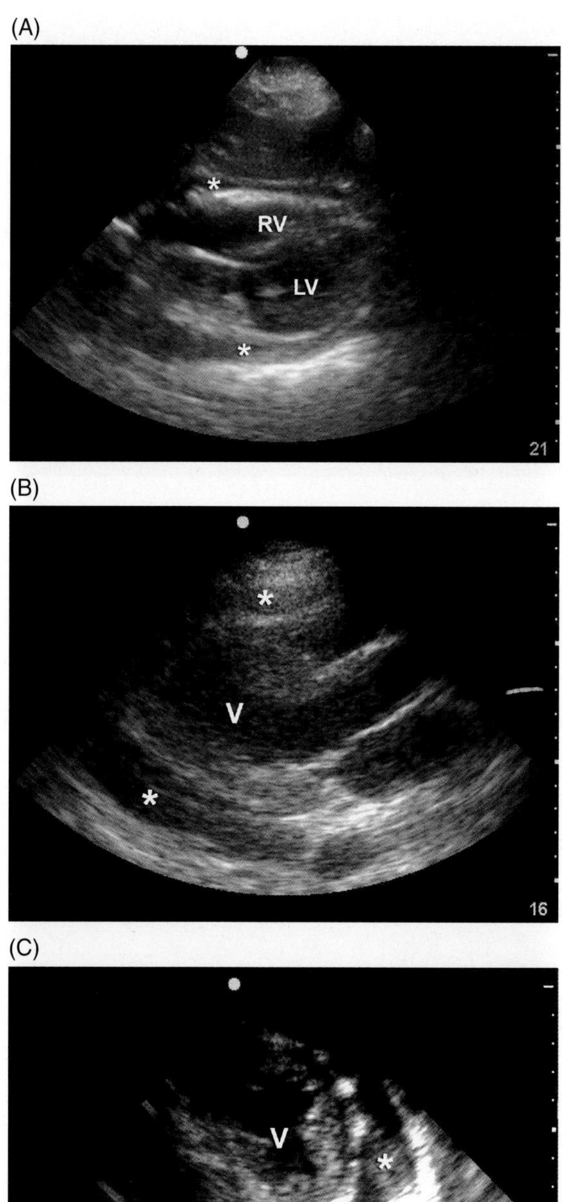

Figure 3.22

Pericardial fluid (*) in three different views. (*A*) Subxiphoid view, with right ventricle (RV) and left ventricle (LV) visible. (*B*) Parasternal long-axis view, with fluid surrounding the left ventricle (V). (*C*) Parasternal short-axis view, with fluid surrounding the left ventricle (V).

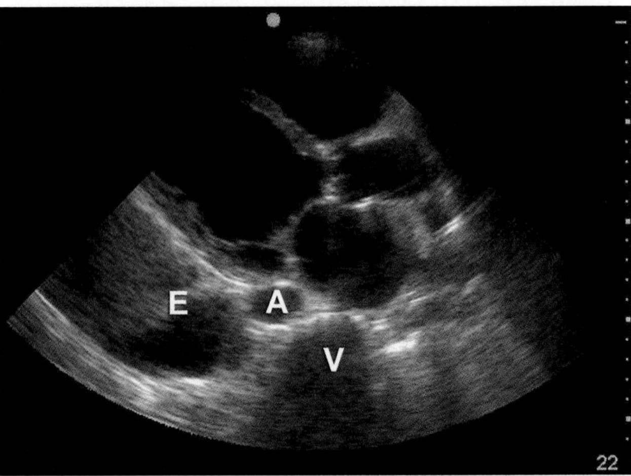

Figure 3.23
Parasternal long-axis view demonstrating a pleural effusion (E). Note that the effusion does not cross past the aorta (A), located superficial to the vertebral body (V). If the effusion were pericardial, it would be evident between the heart and the aorta. Dilated ventricles and left atrium are evident in this view as well.

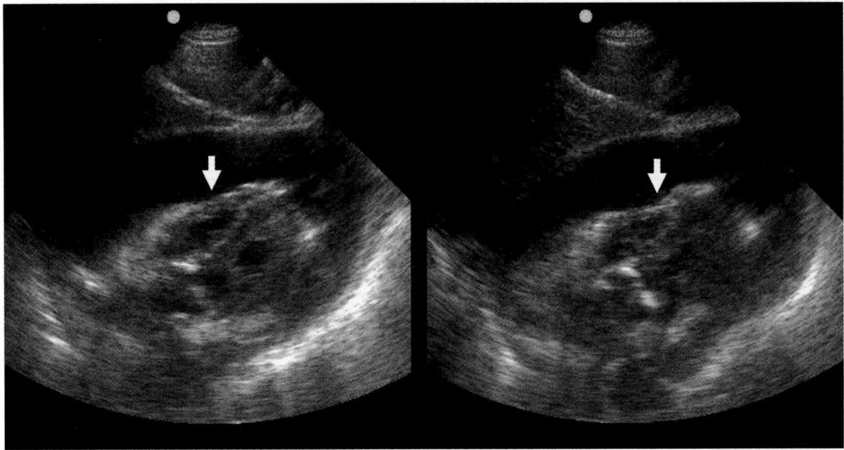

Figure 3.24
Subxiphoid view of the heart showing pericardial fluid with right ventricular scalloping. Note the bowing in of the anterior wall of the right ventricle (arrows), more prominent during diastole (*right*).

demonstrates diastolic collapse of the right ventricle or right atrium – also referred to as "scalloping" of the right ventricle (Figures 3.24 and 3.25). Left atrial or left ventricular collapse can occur in localized left-sided compressions. Finally, a dilated inferior vena cava (IVC) without inspiratory collapse (plethora) is highly suggestive of tamponade [4]. Remember that these findings should be taken in light of the patient's overall clinical picture. Cardiac tamponade should be suspected in the setting of a circumferential pericardial effusion in any hemodynamically unstable patient.

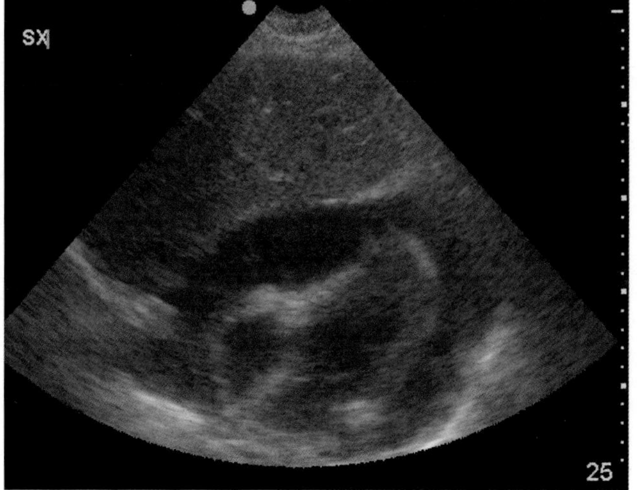

Figure 3.25 Circumferential effusion seen on subxiphoid four-chamber view with right ventricle almost fully collapsed. Courtesy of Dr. Andrew Liteplo, Massachusetts General Hospital, Boston, MA.

Hemopericardium

Identification of any pericardial fluid in the setting of penetrating injury to the thorax or upper abdomen requires aggressive resuscitation. Hemopericardium is the most common feature of penetrating cardiac injuries. In acute massive hemopericardium, there is insufficient time for defibrination to occur. The hemopericardium organizes and may partially clot, resulting in a pericardial hematoma. The hematoma may appear echogenic (gray) instead of echo-free (black) and thus be more challenging to identify, but deformation of the right ventricle when hemopericardium is suspected is a pertinent clue to the diagnosis. The use of bedside cardiac ultrasound in the trauma setting has been shown to be lifesaving because the time to mobilization of the operating room for thoracotomy or the time to initiation of emergency department thoracotomy are both dramatically decreased with the ability of the emergency physician or trauma surgeon to make the diagnosis at the bedside [5,6].

Other potential sources of cardiac perforation include central line placement, pacemaker insertion, cardiac catheterization, sternal bone-marrow biopsies, and pericardiocentesis. The right atrium is the most common site of perforation from catheter placement. Perforation, as well as direct catheter infusion of fluids, can also cause tamponade.

Global cardiac function

There have been multiple studies evaluating the ability of non-echocardiologists to use bedside transthoracic cardiac ultrasound to estimate left ventricular ejection fraction (EF) or global cardiac function [7–14]. Formal EF calculations can be performed using several different methods and range from simple observation to a variety of two-plane calculation formulas to measurements

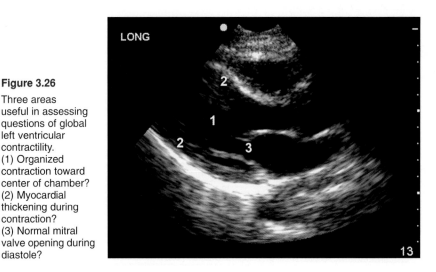

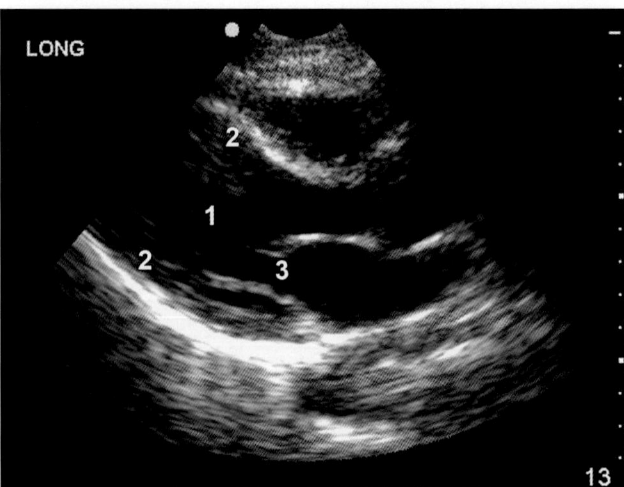

Figure 3.26
Three areas useful in assessing questions of global left ventricular contractility.
(1) Organized contraction toward center of chamber?
(2) Myocardial thickening during contraction?
(3) Normal mitral valve opening during diastole?

using M-mode. In addition, there are software packages that machines have to estimate EF by tracing the borders of ventricular cavities in diastole and systole. There are also studies, however, that have shown that visual estimation of EF is as good as or better than calculated EF [15–17]. When faced with caring for a critically ill patient who is hypotensive, decisions must be made regarding the use of volume or inotropic support. In these patients, global cardiac function assessments can be particularly beneficial [18–21]. Kaul *et al.* even demonstrated that transthoracic cardiac ultrasound can provide information that is comparable to a pulmonary artery catheter in 86% of patients [21].

For the non-cardiologist looking to estimate ejection fraction, global assessments of contractility should evaluate three major aspects of cardiac function (Figure 3.26):

1. Is the ventricle contracting symmetrically toward its center?
   This necessitates a gestalt assessment of overall contractility. Imagine the chamber from the perspective of a mechanical pump. Would the degree of "squeeze" visualized be expected to pump out most of the blood in the chamber? This cannot occur efficiently if the walls do not move simultaneously toward the center, if parts of the wall do not contribute to the contractions, or if little movement is noted. It should be noted that this is an oversimplification of wall motion assessment by experienced echocardiographers and is altered by bundle-branch blocks, improper windows, and a host of other factors. Yet it should assist the novice in a broad overall assessment.
2. Is the myocardium thickening as it shortens?
   Healthy myocardium should thicken as it contracts, just as the biceps would. Myocardium which moves but does not change in thickness may represent scar; this does not contribute effectively to EF. If minimal

contractility or shortening is visible with enlarged chamber sizes, a "low" EF state can be assumed.

3. Is the mitral valve opening normally during diastole?
   Since the circulatory system is closed, blood pumped out of the heart will be replaced by blood coming into the heart. Assuming normal valve function, a mitral valve which opens widely (nearly hitting the septum during diastole) implies that lots of blood is rushing into the ventricle, and therefore lots of blood was just pumped out. With a low EF, little systolic flow means there will be little diastolic flow.

Again it should be noted that these three criteria are simplified and are inaccurate in the setting of non-standard probe positions, many dysrhythmias, or valve abnormalities.

The suspicion for low EF may additionally be supported by the finding of dilated atria (Figure 3.27). Lack of forward flow in the ventricles (from congestive heart failure or obstruction) causes the normally low-pressure atria to dilate.

Cardiac arrest

In the emergency setting, the palpation and/or auscultation of peripheral pulses can be difficult to assess in cardiac arrest or hypotensive patients [22]. Although asystole, ventricular fibrillation, and ventricular tachycardia are usually evident on the cardiac monitor, the diagnosis of pulseless electrical activity (PEA) depends on the determination of a pulse. Cardiac ultrasound is helpful not only because it can detect cardiac motion, but also because it can detect a pericardial effusion or evidence of a dilated right ventricle consistent with pulmonary embolism – two possible causes of PEA [23].

Sonographic asystole will show an absence of ventricular contraction. Absence of cardiac contractions despite resuscitative efforts can help the clinician formulate a prognosis and determine when resuscitative efforts should be stopped. However, rare contractions of the atria and/or mitral valve may continue despite a terminal event, so it is important to base prognosis on ventricular contractions. One other important point is to ensure that artificial respirations and compressions are held during the ultrasound, because respiratory effort can occasionally appear as ventricular movement. Blaivas and Fox, in their study of ultrasound in cardiac arrest, suggest that patients who arrive in emergency departments with cardiac standstill confirmed on ultrasound have little to no chance of survival [24]. Given that the prognosis for asystole compared to PEA during cardiac arrest is so disparate, differentiating between the two with bedside ultrasonography can be quite useful.

M-mode can assist in documenting the absence of cardiac activity. The M-mode line should be placed across the ventricular wall of the left ventricle in the parasternal long-axis or subxiphoid position. When the graph of motion over time shows a flat line, this can be a still-image representation of asystole (Figure 3.28).

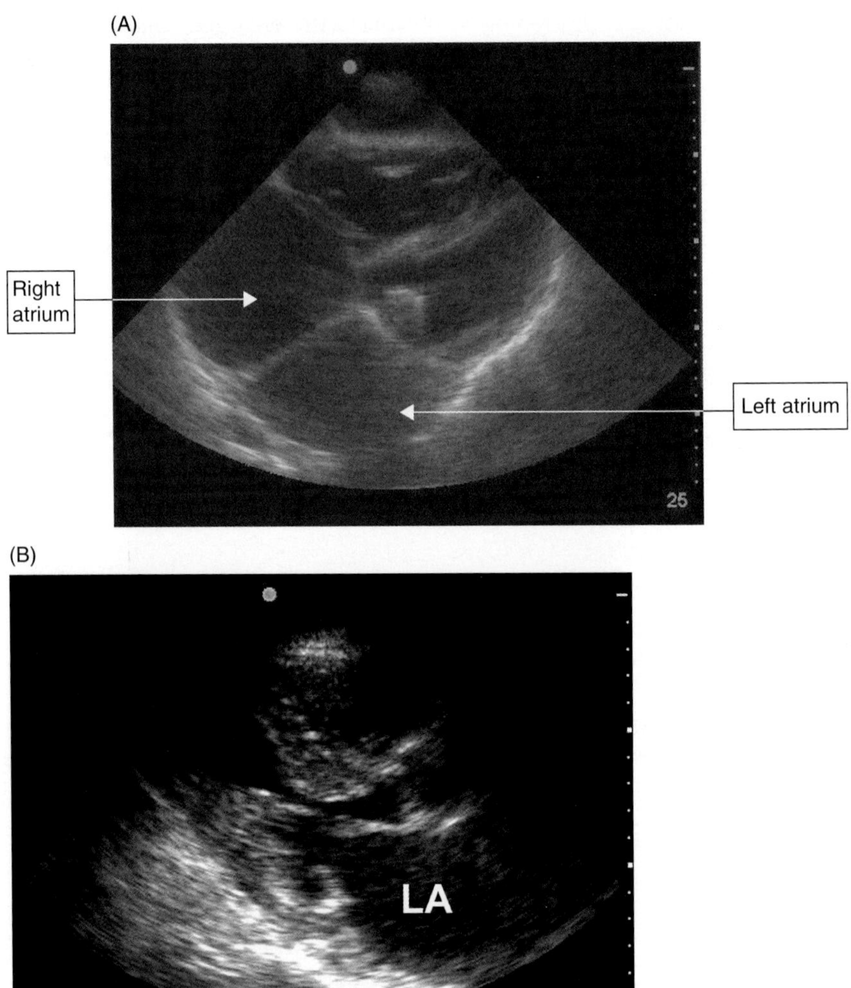

Figure 3.27
(*A*) This subxiphoid four-chamber view shows enlarged right and left atria suggestive of high intravascular volume states. (*B*) This parasternal long-axis view in a patient with hypertrophic obstructive cardiomyopathy (HOCM) demonstrates a dilated left atrium (LA).

Pulmonary embolism

Bedside cardiac ultrasound is not sufficiently accurate for the diagnosis of pulmonary embolism (PE) by itself, but there are sonographic findings that may help expedite intervention. Remember that in the normal heart pressures in the right ventricle are lower than in the left. This is why the right ventricular

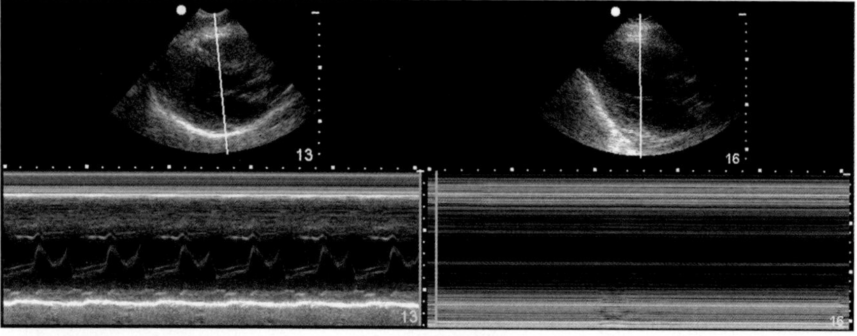

Figure 3.28
The heart on the left has M-mode waveforms, indicating contractility. The heart on the right has flat M-mode lines, indicating asystole and no contractions.

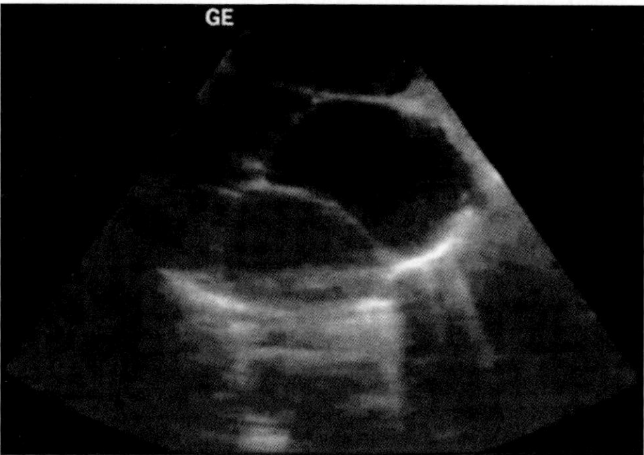

Figure 3.29
This subxiphoid view shows a very enlarged right ventricle – in fact, it is difficult to tell the right from the left ventricle because they are both the same size. This image was obtained from a patient with a saddle pulmonary embolus who required lysis. Courtesy of Emergency Ultrasound Division, St. Luke's–Roosevelt Hospital Center, New York, NY.

wall is thinner and more responsive to sudden increases in pressure. The normal right ventricle, therefore, looks triangular (Figure 3.17) and is smaller than the left ventricle because of this lower pressure. When the pressure in the right ventricle rises, the right ventricular wall will bow outward, and the right ventricle will appear to be the same size as or larger than the left ventricle (Figure 3.29) [2,25]. In the parasternal long-axis view, the normal circular appearance of the left ventricle can become D-shaped as abnormally high right ventricular pressures deform the septum out from the right ventricle (Figure 3.30). If a patient has a massive PE and is hemodynamically unstable, there may not be time to obtain tests such as computed tomography scanning or transesophageal echocardiography. Therefore, in the right clinical setting, the detection of a dilated, stiff right ventricle may provide evidence for consideration of lysis [3,26–29].

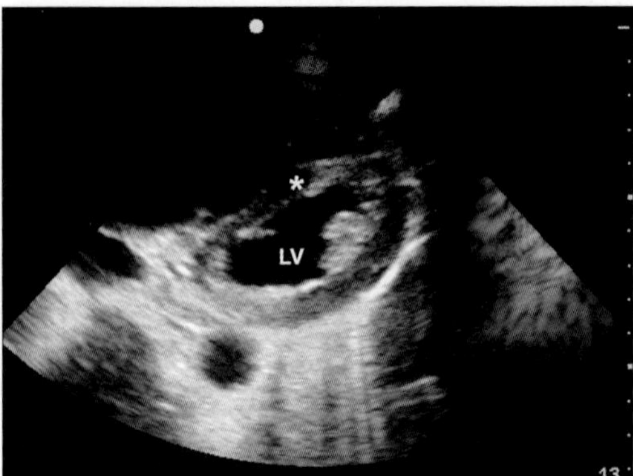

Figure 3.30
The parasternal short-axis view in a patient with elevated right ventricular pressure. Note the flattened septum (*), which deforms the normal circular appearance of the left ventricle (LV) into a D-shape.

Sample clinical protocols

Figures 3.31 and 3.32 show protocols for ultrasound use in cardiac arrest and penetrating thoracic injury.

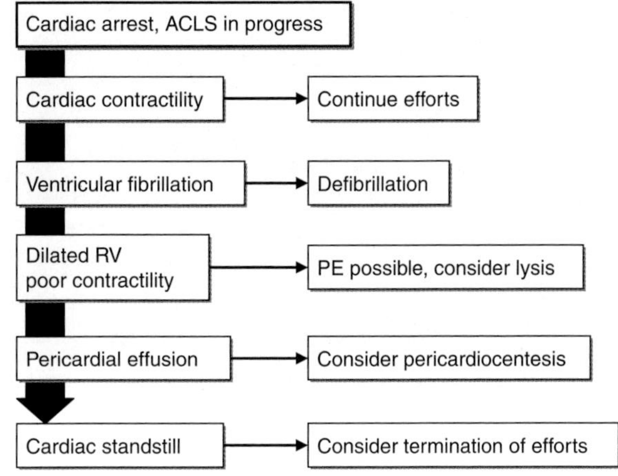

Figure 3.31
Protocol for ultrasound use in cardiac arrest.

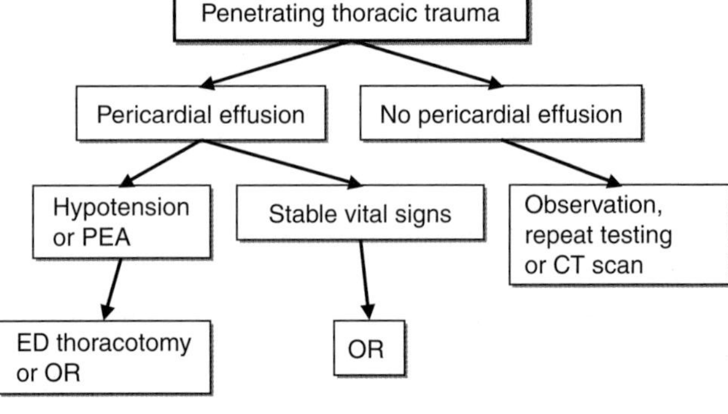

Figure 3.32
Protocol for ultrasound use in penetrating thoracic injury.

Literature review

Reference	Methods	Results	Notes
Blaivas & Fox 2001 [24]	169 emergency department (ED) patients undergoing ACLS resuscitation, bedside cardiac US during code by emergency physicians (EPs).	Cardiac standstill on initial echocardiogram in patients with ongoing CPR had 100% positive predictive value (PPV) for death.	Provided data for bedside cardiac US findings indicative of poor outcomes and of when to stop ACLS resuscitation.
Plummer *et al.* 1992 [5]	Penetrating trauma patients randomized to ED US vs. "standard of care" evaluation (cardiac US called in).	Diagnosis and disposition expedited in ED US group, also noted survival benefit if patients had ED US.	Mortality benefit of ED US in penetrating cardiac injury.
Kaul *et al.* 1994 [21]	Blinded interpreters evaluated cause of hypotension (cardiac vs. non-cardiac) in critical ICU patients receiving both 2-D cardiac US and PA catheters.	Cardiac US and PA catheter evaluations agreed on cause of hypotension in 86% (36/42) patients evaluated. Fewer complications with US, and it was performed faster.	Proves the utility of bedside cardiac US in more rapidly evaluating etiology of hypotension, with fewer complications.
Amico *et al.* 1989 [16]	Comparison of multiple methods for calculating the ejection fraction with subjective visual estimation.	Best correlation of methods studied between expert observers was with visual estimate.	Support for determination of left ventricular ejection fraction by expert visual estimation.
Moore *et al.* 2002 [8]	Comparison of visual estimations of ejection fraction grouped as normal, depressed, and severely depressed by echocardiographers and trained EPs.	Cardiology and EP ventricular function estimation had similar interobserver correlation ($r = 0.86$) to two cardiology estimations ($r = 0.84$).	Showed non-echocardiologists and cardiologists make similar estimates of global cardiac function.
Randazzo *et al.* 2003 [7]	Comparison of EP-estimated ejection fraction (poor, moderate, normal) and central venous pressure (low, moderate, high) with formal US. EPs were ACEP level III trained (3 h formal course).	86% overall agreement in ejection fraction estimation. 70.2% agreement in central venous pressure.	With minimal training, overall agreement in broad categorical EF and CVP assessment is still good.

Reference	Methods	Results	Notes
Alexander *et al.* 2004 [11]	Comparison of medical house staff cardiac US interpretations after 3 h training course with that of formal US.	Agreement was 75% for LV dysfunction and 98% for pericardial effusions.	Medical house staff with very limited training can diagnose LV dysfunction and pericardial effusions on bedside US.
Kobal *et al.* 2005 [13]	Comparison of medical students' ultrasound cardiac evaluation after 18 h of training with physical exam of the heart performed by board-certified cardiologists.	Students correctly identified 75% of the pathologies vs. 49% found by cardiologists. Diagnostic accuracy of students vs. cardiologists was superior in detecting valvular disease, left ventricular dysfunction, enlargement and hypertrophy.	If medical students can do it . . .

New directions

There are many new directions that bedside cardiac ultrasound could take in the next few years. As three-dimensional cardiac ultrasound technology becomes more widespread, and as the cost of three-dimensional cardiac ultrasound machines decreases, it is easy to imagine that ejection fraction calculations could be made much more accurately. Machine automated protocols for estimating global cardiac function could even become standard. Estimations of volume status and central venous pressure could likewise be accurately generated by three-dimensional cardiac ultrasound and could finally replace invasive monitoring [30,31].

As this technology spreads throughout critical care medicine, it is likely that ultrasound-guided protocols for evaluating critically ill hypotensive patients could be helpful in many critical care settings, and it is expected that with the diffusion of this technology, research in this area will continue. An expanding role for transesophageal cardiac ultrasound may even be realized as more intensivists and emergency physicians become familiar with the technology [32].

References

1. Cheitlin MD, Alpert JS, Armstrong WF, *et al.* ACC/AHA guidelines for the clinical application of echocardiography. *Circulation* 1997; **95**: 1686–744.
2. Otto CM. Echocardiographic evaluation of left and right ventricular systolic function. In Otto CM (ed.), *Textbook of Clinical Cardiac Ultrasound*, 2nd edn. Philadelphia, PA: Saunders; 2000: 120–1.

3. Goldhaber S. Pulmonary embolism thrombolysis: broadening the paradigm for its administration. *Circulation* 1997; **96**: 716–18.
4. Munt BI, Kinnaird T, Thompson CR. Pericardial disease. In Otto CM (ed.), *Textbook of Clinical Cardiac Ultrasound*, 2nd edn. Philadelphia, PA: Saunders; 2000: 649.
5. Plummer D, Brunette D, Asinger R, Ruiz E. Emergency department echocardiography improves outcome in penetrating cardiac injury. *Ann Emerg Med* 1992; **21**: 709–12.
6. Rozycki GS, Feliciano DV, Ochsner MG, *et al.* The role of ultrasound in patients with possible penetrating cardiac wounds: a prospective multicenter study. *J Trauma* 1999; **46**: 543–51.
7. Randazzo MR, Snoey ER, Levitt MA, Binder K. Accuracy of emergency physician assessment of left ventricular ejection fraction and central venous pressure using cardiac ultrasound. *Acad Emerg Med* 2003; **10**: 973–7.
8. Moore CL, Rose G, Tayal V, *et al.* Determination of left ventricular function by emergency physician cardiac ultrasound of hypotensive patients. *Acad Emerg Med* 2002; **9**: 186–93.
9. DeCara JM, Lang RM, Koch R, *et al.* The use of small personal ultrasound devices by internists without formal training in cardiac ultrasound. *Eur J Echocardiogr* 2003; **4**: 141–7.
10. Lemola K, Yamada E, Jagasia D, Kerber RE. A hand-carried personal ultrasound device for rapid evaluation of left ventricular function: use after limited echo training. *Cardiac ultrasound* 2003; **20**: 309–12.
11. Alexander JH, Peterson ED, Chen AY, *et al.* Feasibility of point-of-care cardiac ultrasound by internal medicine house staff. *Am Heart J* 2004; **147**: 476–81.
12. Mangione S, Nieman LZ. Cardiac auscultatory skills of internal medicine and family practice trainees: a comparison of diagnostic proficiency. *JAMA* 1997; **278**: 717–22.
13. Kobal SL, Trento L, Baharami S, *et al.* Comparison of effectiveness of hand-carried ultrasound to bedside cardiovascular physical examination. *Am J Cardiol* 2005; **96**: 1002–6.
14. Kimura BJ, Pezeshki B, Frack SA, DeMaria AN. Feasibility of "limited" echo imaging: characterization of incidental findings. *J Am Soc Echocardiogr* 1998; **11**: 746–50.
15. Mueller X, Stauffer JC, Jaussi A, Goy JJ, Kappenberger L. Subjective visual echocardiographic estimate of left ventricular ejection fraction as an alternative to conventional echocardiographic methods: comparison with contrast angiography. *Clin Cardiol* 1991; **14**: 898–907.
16. Amico A, Lichtenberg GS, Reisner SA, *et al.* Superiority of visual versus computerized echocardiographic estimation of radionuclide left ventricular ejection fraction. *Am Heart J* 1989; **118**: 1259–65.
17. Stamm RB, Carabello BA, Mayers DL, Martin RP. Two-dimensional echocardiographic measurement of left ventricular ejection fraction: prospective analysis of what constitutes an adequate determination. *Am Heart J* 1982; **104**: 136–44.

18. Sanfilippo AJ, Weyman AE. The role of cardiac ultrasound in managing critically ill patients. *J Crit Illn* 1988; **3**: 27–44.
19. Rose JS, Bair AE, Mandavia D, Kinser DJ. The UHP ultrasound protocol: a novel ultrasound approach to the empiric evaluation of the undifferentiated hypotensive patient. *Am J Emerg Med* 2001; **19**: 299–302.
20. Jones AE, Tayal VS, Sullivan DM, Kline JA. Randomized, controlled trial of immediate versus delayed goal-directed ultrasound to identify the cause of nontraumatic hypotension in emergency department patients. *Crit Care Med* 2004; **32**: 1703–8.
21. Kaul S, Stratienko AA, Pollack SJ, *et al.* Value of two-dimensional cardiac ultrasound for determining the basis of hemodynamic compromise in critically ill patients: a prospective study. *J Am Soc Echocardiogr* 1994; **7**: 598–606.
22. Calinas-Correia J, Phair I. Is there a pulse? *Resuscitation* 1999; **41**: 201–2.
23. Tayal VS, Kline JA. Emergency cardiac ultrasound to detect pericardial effusion in patients in PEA and near-PEA states. *Resuscitation* 2003; **59**: 315–18.
24. Blaivas M, Fox JC. Outcome in cardiac arrest patients found to have cardiac standstill on the bedside emergency department echocardiogram. *Acad Emerg Med* 2001; **8**: 616–21.
25. Kasper W, Meinertz T, Henkel B, *et al.* Echocardiographic findings in patients with proved pulmonary embolism. *Am Heart J* 1986; **112**: 1284–90.
26. Kasper W, Konstantinides S, Geibel A, *et al.* Prognostic significance of right ventricular afterload stress detected via cardiac ultrasound in patients with clinically suspected proven pulmonary embolism. *Heart* 1997; **77**: 346–9.
27. Ribeiro A, Lindmarker P, Juhlin-Dannfelt A, Johnsson H, Jorfeldt L. Echocardiography Doppler in pulmonary embolism: right ventricular dysfunction as a predictor of mortality rate. *Am Heart J* 1997; **134**: 479–87.
28. Jardin F, Dubourg O, Gueret P, Delorme G, Bourdarias JP. Quantitative two-dimensional cardiac ultrasound in massive pulmonary embolism: emphasis on ventricular interdependence and leftward septal displacement. *J Am Coll Cardiol* 1987; **10**: 1201–6.
29. Grifoni S, Olivotto I, Cecchini P, *et al.* Utility of an integrated clinical, echocardiographic and venous ultrasonographic approach for triage of patients with suspected pulmonary embolism. *Am J Cardiol* 1998; **82**: 1230–5.
30. Clark TJ, Sheehan FH, Bolson EL. Characterizing the normal heart using quantitative three-dimensional cardiac ultrasound. *Physiol Meas* 2006; **27**: 467–508.
31. Jacobs LD, Salgo IS, Goonewardena S, *et al.* Rapid online quantification of left ventricular volume from real-time three-dimensional echocardiographic data. *Eur Heart J* 2006; **27**: 460–8.
32. Beaulieu Y. Bedside echocardiography in the assessment of the critically ill. *Crit Care Med* 2007; **35**: S235–49.

4 First trimester ultrasound

Introduction

Ectopic pregnancy (EP) is the leading cause of maternal mortality in the United States and is estimated to have a prevalence of 8% in pregnant patients presenting to the emergency department for any complaint [1,2]. Indeed, the incidence of ectopic pregnancy has been rising since the mid 1980s [3]. Therefore, any female of child-bearing age who comes to the emergency room with abdominal pain, vaginal bleeding, near-syncope, or syncope has ectopic pregnancy on the differential. This is a "can't miss" diagnosis. Given the volume of female patients presenting with these complaints, an algorithm incorporating first trimester ultrasound can be time-saving for the physician and patient, but it must increase efficiency without compromising safety.

The evaluation for ectopic pregnancy differs from other indications for bedside ultrasound. Evaluation of the uterus seeks to confirm an intrauterine pregnancy (IUP), ruling out ectopic gestation by exclusion. Visualization of the actual ectopic pregnancy is not the goal. In contrast, evaluation of the aorta, heart, and other organs typically confirms pathology (aneurysm, asystole, hydronephrosis) via direct visualization.

There are instances where an extrauterine gestation will be seen on bedside ultrasound or free fluid will be seen in a hypotensive pregnant female and ectopic pregnancy will be diagnosed or inferred. This will be the exception, however, to how bedside ultrasound is used for this application. Bedside ultrasonography instead will be used to increase the number of IUP cases that can be definitively diagnosed and discharged in the emergency department without further imaging.

One other important subgroup of patients that should be mentioned is those women who are undergoing in-vitro fertilization (IVF) or assisted reproduction and who present to the emergency department with pain or vaginal bleeding. Because the risk of heterotopic pregnancy in these women is higher than in women without assisted reproduction, it is the view of the authors that these patients should *always* have formal ultrasonography done by gynecology or radiology and should always have a formal gynecology consultation [4–7]. Others have suggested that there are other subgroups of patients (history of ectopic pregnancy, known fallopian tube scarring) with unacceptably high rates of heterotopic pregnancy who should also always undergo formal sonography and consultation, but this recommendation is not universally followed.

Focused questions for first trimester ultrasound

The questions for first trimester ultrasound are as follows:

1. Is there an intrauterine pregnancy?
   a. Is there an intrauterine yolk sac, fetal pole, or fetal heartbeat?
   b. Anything else (including an intrauterine gestational sac) is *not* an intrauterine pregnancy, and a formal study or a formal consultation should be performed.

In addition, female patients of child-bearing age who present with atraumatic abdominal pain and shock should always undergo a FAST exam to evaluate for abdominal hemorrhage. In this patient population a positive FAST should prompt treatment and resuscitation for ruptured ectopic pregnancy.

Terminology

Terminology used when describing first trimester pregnancy can be confusing, and it is important that emergency physicians are precise when describing their findings. Miscommunication can lead to emotional distress and unsafe assumptions. The following list defines terms commonly used in first trimester pregnancy:

- **Spontaneous abortion** and **miscarriage** – synonymous terms in early pregnancy that refer to spontaneous passage of the products of conception (POC) through the cervical os.
- **Threatened abortion** – a pregnancy prior to 20 weeks of gestation accompanied by cramping and vaginal bleeding.
- **Incomplete abortion** – a condition in which some POC remain within the uterus after miscarriage.
- **Complete abortion** – a condition in which all POC have passed through the os and none remain in the uterus.
- **Inevitable abortion** – a condition in which the patient's cervix is dilated and POC are often seen exiting the cervical os.
- **Missed abortion** – refers to the clinical situation in which an intrauterine pregnancy is present but no longer developing normally. The gestation is termed a missed abortion only if the diagnosis of incomplete abortion or inevitable abortion is excluded. Patients with this condition may present with an anembryonic gestation (empty sac or blighted ovum) or with fetal demise prior to 20 weeks' gestation.
- **Blighted ovum** – an ambiguous term that formerly indicated that no embryo ever developed. This term was synonymous with

the term *anembryonic gestation*. Recent advances in ultrasound scanning have shown that a very early embryo usually develops. Therefore, *embryonic resorption* has become the more modern and appropriate term.

- **Embryonic demise** – refers to a pregnancy in which no fetal heartbeat or motion is seen despite a clearly visible embryo of a gestational size where a fetal heartbeat would be expected.

Again, these terms are important to the emergency physician only in terms of clear communication. The purpose of performing bedside emergency first trimester ultrasound is to diagnose an intrauterine pregnancy in patients with an acceptably low risk of heterotopic pregnancy (non-IVF, no history of ectopic pregnancy) so they can be discharged and followed up as outpatients safely. If an intrauterine pregnancy is not diagnosed, most emergency department patients should be referred for formal sonography and gynecology consultation.

hCG levels

Another area of much confusion and debate is the correlation of serum human chorionic gonadotropin (hCG) levels with ultrasound findings. The first important rule for the emergency physician is that there is no hCG level at which a patient can be ruled out for ectopic pregnancy. Ectopic pregnancies have been described with levels < 30 IU/mL, and very frequently < 1000 IU/mL [8,9]. Therefore, pelvic sonography should be done for any patient who is pregnant regardless of beta-hCG [8–10]. The concept of a discriminatory zone becomes more significant after pelvic sonography is complete. The discriminatory zone is the level of beta-hCG at which an intrauterine pregnancy should be seen 100% of the time. Transvaginal ultrasound is able to visualize intrauterine pregnancies earlier, and the discriminatory zone is usually accepted as 1500 IU/mL. The discriminatory zone for transabdominal ultrasound is usually believed to be between 4000 and 6500 IU/mL because it uses a lower-frequency probe and thus images with less resolution [11]. Therefore, if an ultrasound is indeterminate and the serum hCG is above the discriminatory zone, the suspicion for ectopic pregnancy should be increased [12]. However, serum quantitative hCG levels are mostly helpful in following a patient over time, and there is no level at which a patient will not require an ultrasound (except zero).

Anatomy

There are several anatomic relationships that can help guide the sonographic evaluation of the female pelvis (Figure 4.1). The bladder is anterior to the

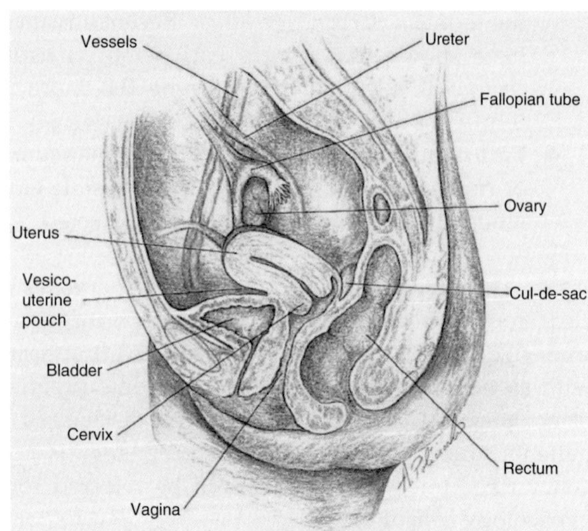

Figure 4.1
Normal female anatomy. Image reproduced from *Gray's Anatomy* (image out of copyright).

uterus unless it is empty, when the anteverted uterus can fold over an underfilled bladder. The ovaries are usually found at the end of the fallopian tubes and are anterior and medial to the iliac vessels (Figure 4.2). If the bladder is full, it is a good acoustic window for visualizing the uterus transabdominally. However, it is easier to visualize the uterus transvaginally with an empty bladder because then the uterus will be anteflexed in most cases over the vaginal introitus.

Technique

There are two approaches to performing the sonographic exam of an early pregnancy: transabdominal and transvaginal. Usually, a transabdominal scan is done first while the patient still has a full bladder. The patient then can empty her bladder prior to the transvaginal scan if the transabdominal scan was non-diagnostic for intrauterine pregnancy. In patients with unclear gestational age, it is even more important to perform an abdominal scan first. Occasionally, a second trimester fetus will be visualized transabdominally, and a non-sterile pelvic exam (which would increase the risk of infection) can be avoided.

Transabdominal scanning technique

Probe selection

Use a 3.5 MHz curvilinear transducer for the transabdominal scan.

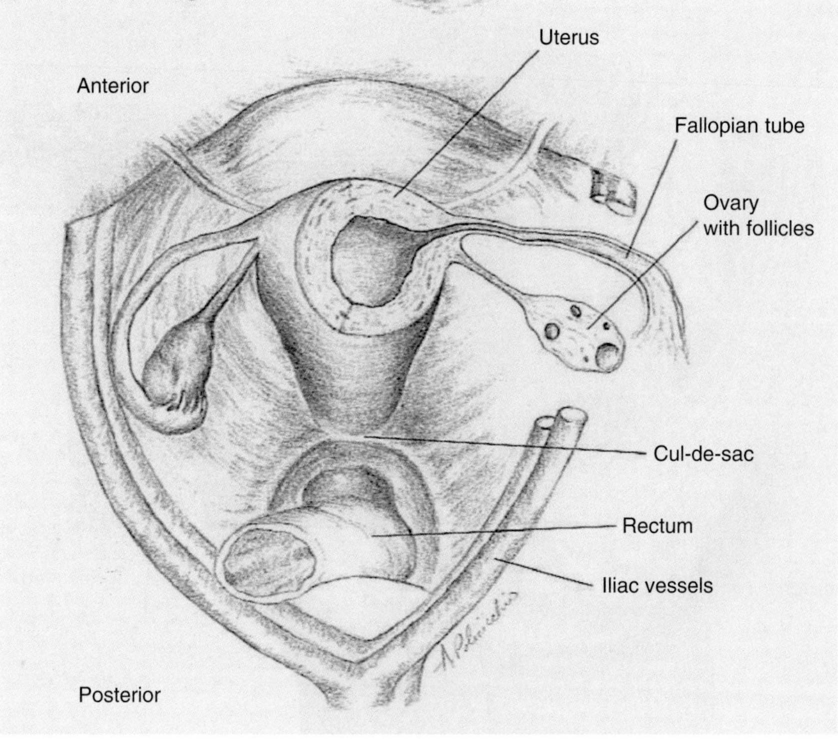

Figure 4.2

Normal female anatomy. Note the relation between the ovaries and the iliac vessels; ovaries are found superior and medial to vessels on ultrasound imaging. Image reproduced from *Gray's Anatomy* (image out of copyright).

Views

At least two views are necessary for complete evaluation of the uterus: a transverse view and a longitudinal view, both demonstrating the endometrial stripe (and uterine contents, if any).

Like the suprapubic window used in the FAST and renal exams, the transabdominal ultrasound of the patient with an early pregnancy is easier with a full urinary bladder. An inadequately filled bladder is one of the most common causes of a technically inadequate transabdominal exam.

Begin by placing the probe above the pubic symphysis (Figure 4.3A). Start in the midline, and use both the transverse and the sagittal/longitudinal orientations. Again, careful angulation and movement off the midline may be necessary to obtain optimal views of the structure being evaluated (and to see the endometrial stripe). Remember that when scanning transversely the probe marker is to the patient's right (Figure 4.3B), and

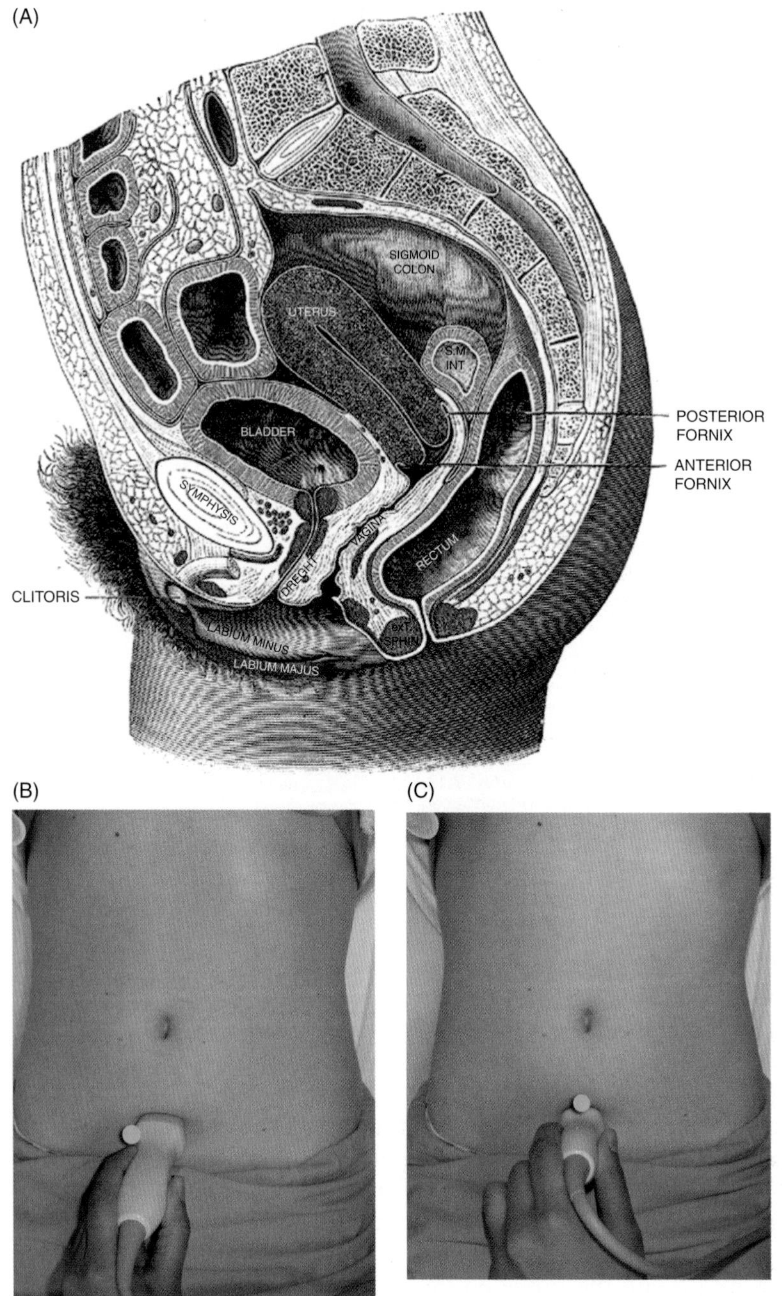

Figure 4.3

Probe positioning and anatomy in transabdominal scanning. (*A*) The anatomy underneath the probe; image reproduced from *Gray's Anatomy* (image out of copyright). (*B*) Transverse probe position (probe marker to patient's right). (*C*) Longitudinal probe position (probe marker to patient's head).

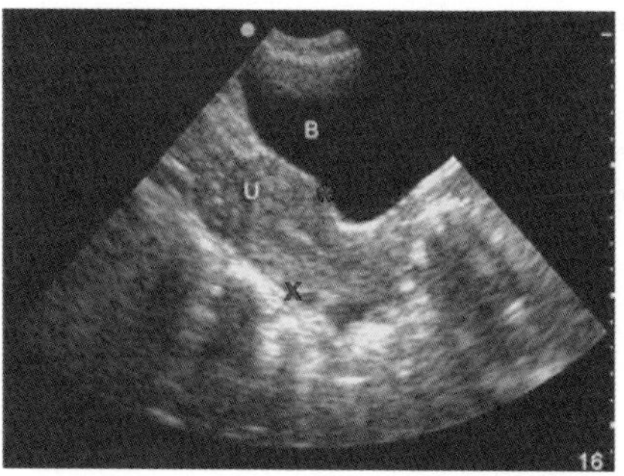

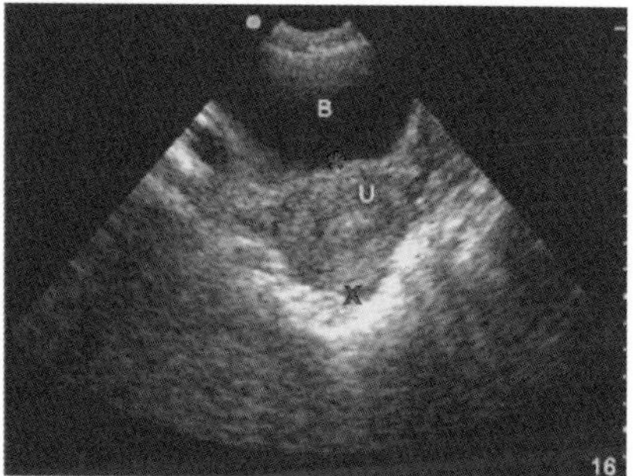

Figure 4.4

Transabdominal images of non-pregnant female pelvis: longitudinal (*left*) and transverse (*right*) images of a normal uterus. B, bladder; U, uterus; *, uterovesicular space; X, pouch of Douglas.

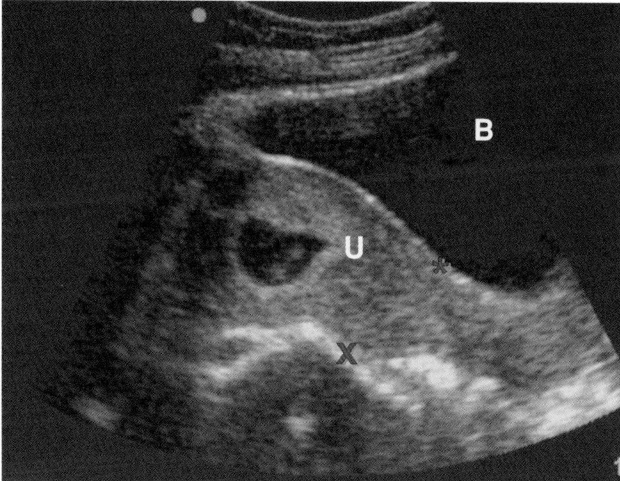

Figure 4.5

Transabdominal imaging of pregnant female pelvis – longitudinal image of a normal uterus. B, bladder; U, uterus; *, uterovesicular space; X, pouch of Douglas.

when scanning longitudinally the probe marker is to the patient's head (Figure 4.3C). When an image of the transverse uterus is identified, fanning superiorly and inferiorly in order to visualize the entire uterus in a two-dimensional sweep is essential. When a sagittal or longitudinal view of the uterus is obained it is essential to fan side to side to visualize the complete structure.

Figure 4.4 shows transabdominal images of a non-pregnant female pelvis, and Figure 4.5 is a transabdominal longitudinal image of a uterus with IUP, with the bladder noted anteriorly and the uterus and rectum posteriorly. The uterovesicular pouch is anterior to the uterus, and the pouch of Douglas is posterior to the uterus.

Transvaginal scanning technique

Probe selection

Most manufacturers have a high-frequency intracavitary or transvaginal probe that is specifically made for transvaginal scanning. The frequency ranges are usually from 5 to 9 MHz.

Views

Again, at least two views are necessary for complete evaluation of the uterus: one transverse view and one longitudinal view, both demonstrating the endometrial stripe (and uterine contents, if any).

After performing a transabdominal scan, the patient should empty her bladder to facilitate the transvaginal scan. As with all invasive procedures, before proceeding to the transvaginal exam, the physician should counsel the patient about the exam and obtain consent. The probe must be cleaned and sterilized, and the probe tip covered with a small amount of conductive gel; a sterile condom or cover is then placed over the probe and sterile gel is placed on the outer condom tip. Holding the probe with the indicator or marker to the ceiling, the probe is inserted into the vaginal canal (Figures 4.6 and 4.7A).

The first view, with the marker pointing to the ceiling, should give the image in Figure 4.8A. It is important to fan through the entire body of the uterus; in the longitudinal plane, make sure to fan the probe side to side and see the entire uterus (the endometrial stripe should disappear and reappear as you fan). To bring the cervix into the viewing window, bring the transducer handle toward the ceiling. This will angle the tip toward the posterior fornix of the vaginal canal, which is where the cervix is located in most women (Figure 4.8A).

After scanning in the longitudinal plane, turn the probe marker to the patient's right (Figure 4.7B). You will then see the uterus in a transverse plane

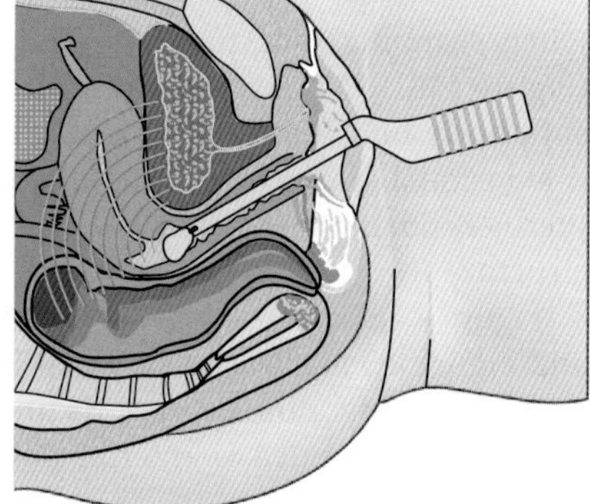

Figure 4.6
Probe positioning in transvaginal scanning. Sagittal or longitudinal transvaginal probe positioning, with the probe marker pointed to the ceiling.

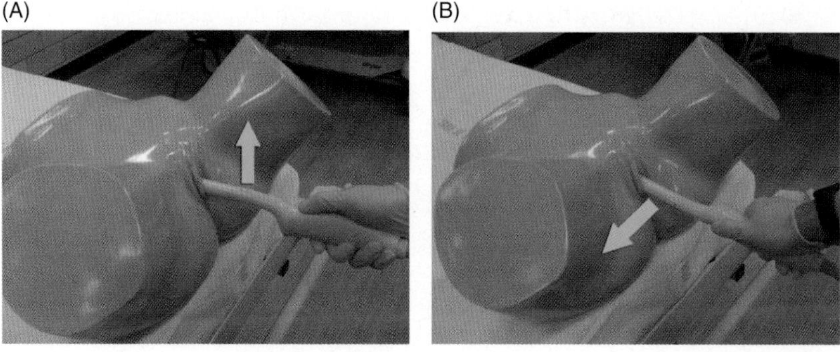

Figure 4.7

Probe positioning in transvaginal scanning. (*A*) Sagittal or longitudinal transvaginal probe positioning, with the probe marker pointed to the ceiling. (*B*) Transverse transvaginal probe positioning, with the probe marker to the patient's right.

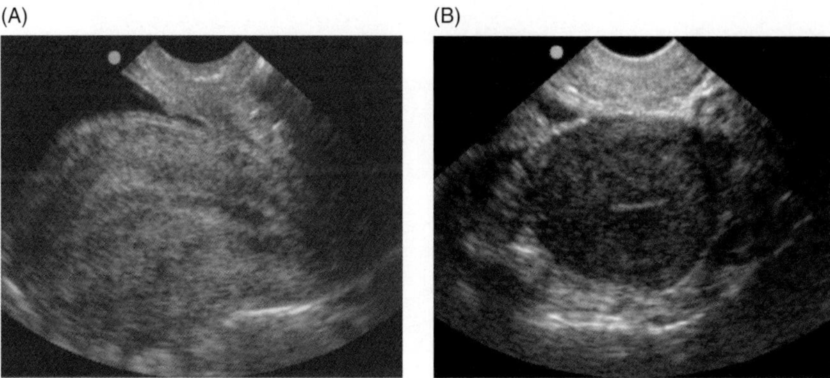

Figure 4.8

Transvaginal views of the uterus: (*A*) longitudinal and (*B*) transverse. Anechoic fluid in the left-hand corner of the longitudinal view is the bladder. To image the cervix on the longitudinal image, the handle of the probe would be brought up and the probe tip angled toward the posterior fornix.

(Figure 4.8B). Again, it is important to fan through the entire uterus, so fan the probe anteriorly and posteriorly to see the entire fundus. The endometrial stripe should again disappear and reappear as you fan. At this point, the fallopian tubes can be traced out to visualize the ovaries. If you see the iliac vessels, then the ovaries should be anterior and medial. The ovaries will often have multiple follicles, which look like multiple cysts (Figure 4.9). This can help identify them. However, the emergency physician should remember that he or she is doing this scan to identify an intrauterine pregnancy. Performing a complete ovarian ultrasound is beyond the scope of this text.

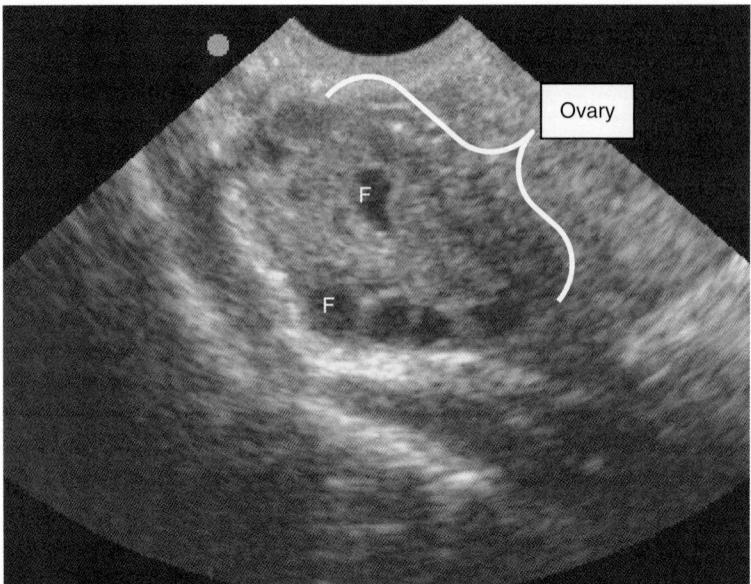

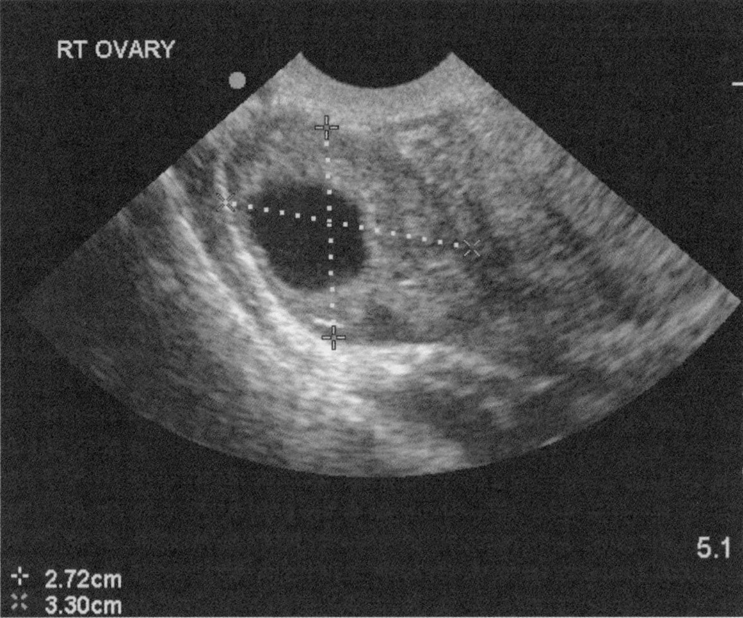

Figure 4.9

Two normal transvaginal views of the ovary. Most women will have multiple visualized follicles (F) – some may be quite prominent, depending on luteal stage.

Scanning tips

Trouble with the transabdominal view

Unable to see the uterus?

- Try sliding the probe to the left or right. Sometimes the uterus is not midline.
- Adjust (increase) the depth. If the depth is too shallow the uterus and the pouch of Douglas will be out of view.

Disoriented as to position of the uterus and bladder?

- Most women have an anteverted uterus. Thus if the bladder is full the bladder will push the fundus more sagittal and in the transverse plane the bladder will be above the uterus. However, if the bladder is less full, the fundus can occasionally be on top of the bladder and thus in the transverse plane the uterus will be anterior to the bladder. By scanning longitudinally as well, it is easy to distinguish these two and to ensure there is no free fluid.
- If a woman has a retroverted uterus it can be hard to find in the transverse plane. To get oriented always try a longitudinal view – and increase the depth to make sure you see the entire fundus.

Trouble with the transvaginal view

Unable to get oriented?

- Think of placing the ultrasound probe in the same position as the speculum. By angling gently posterior and increasing the depth usually you can get a familiar picture to come into view.
- If there is nothing familiar coming into view, slowly fan side to side with your probe marker to the ceiling. Again, often the uterus is located slightly off midline.
- Dont forget to measure the myometrial mantle. The pregnancy should be located in the endometrial cavity with at least 8 mm of myometrium surrounding it to support a viable pregnancy. If the myometrial rim seems narrow obtain consultation or formal imaging, as this can be a sign of an irregularly placed or cornual ectopic.

Normal images in early pregnancy

As mentioned previously, to be conservative and to practice with the greatest safety, only an intrauterine yolk sac, fetal pole, or intrauterine fetal heartbeat

(A)

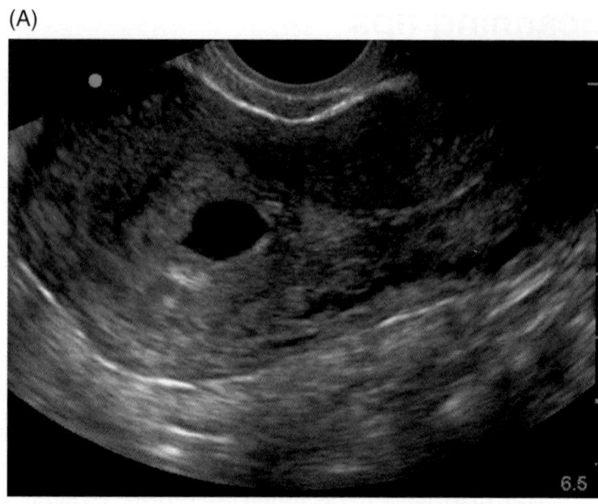

(B)

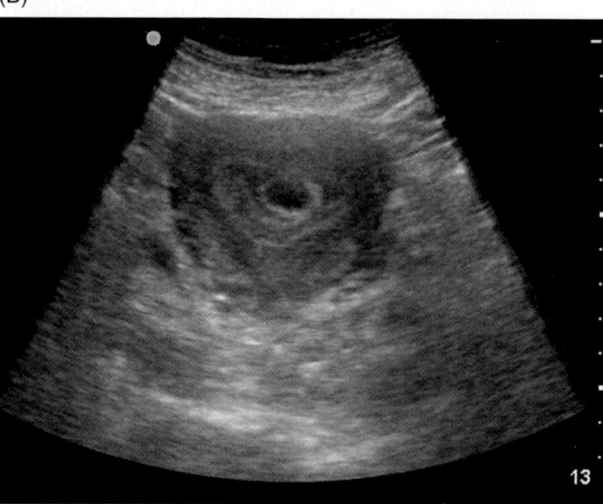

Figure 4.10
Double decidual sign. The hyperechoic layer surrounding the gestational sac can be seen in both (*A*) longitudinal and (*B*) transverse views. However, because there is no yolk sac visualized within the gestational sac, this cannot be definitively called an intrauterine pregnancy.

should be identified as an intrauterine pregnancy on bedside ultrasound scans. The reason for this is that although a gestational sac can be an early marker of a normal gestation, it can also be the result of hormonal stimulation caused by an ectopic pregnancy, known as "pseudogestational sac of ectopic pregnancy" [3,13]. This finding is seen in up to 10–20% of all ectopic pregnancies [13]. Therefore, it is not recommended to use this finding as a sign of normal gestation. The "double decidual sign" has also been described as a reliable marker for early intrauterine pregnancy (Figure 4.10). This is a sac with echogenic and hypoechoic rings surrounding it. However, even in the radiology and obstetric literature, there is debate as to the accuracy of this finding, and it is not present in all cases. Thus, before the appearance of a yolk sac, an IUP should not be definitively diagnosed by bedside emergency ultrasound.

(A)

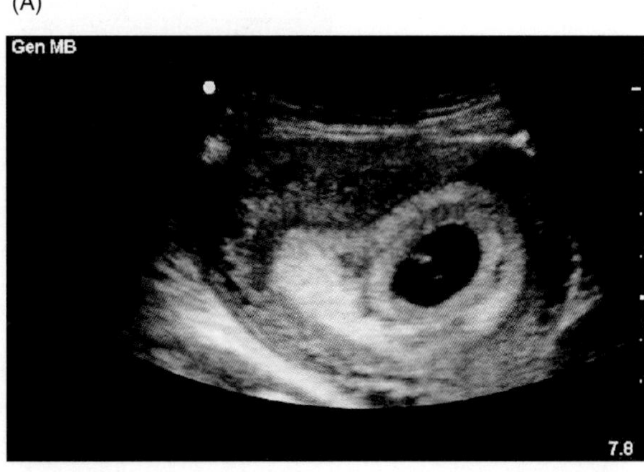

(B)

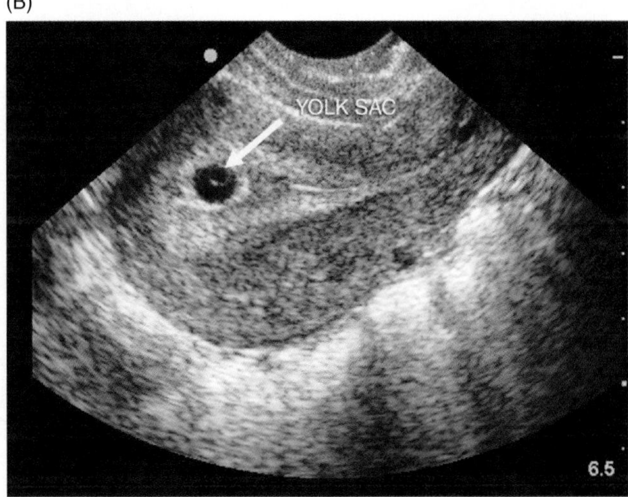

Figure 4.11
In (*A*), the double decidual sign is clearly seen. More importantly, a yolk sac is seen in both (*A*) and (*B*). This "sac within the sac" (yolk sac) is the first definitive sign of an intrauterine pregnancy.

When first visible, the gestational sac contains no identifiable structures. By the time its diameter reaches 5–8 mm, the yolk sac ("sac within the sac") should be detectable (Figure 4.11).

By the end of the sixth menstrual week, the mean diameter of the gestational sac grows by 1 mm/day, the yolk sac appears, and embryonic cardiac activity may be seen between the yolk sac and the wall of the chorionic sac even before the embryo is measurable. At this point, the tiny embryo is surrounded by a small amniotic membrane. This complex, located between the yolk sac and the chorionic wall, is termed the fetal pole (Figure 4.12).

The embryo grows by about 1 mm/day in crown–rump length, and by the end of the seventh menstrual week the embryo measures 5–10 mm

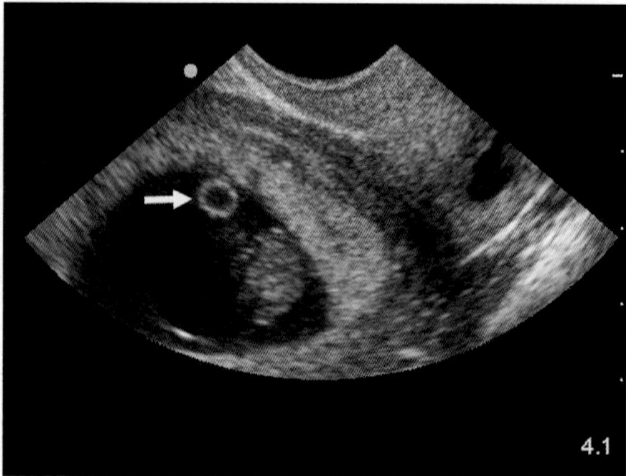

Figure 4.12
Transvaginal image of the yolk sac and fetal pole.

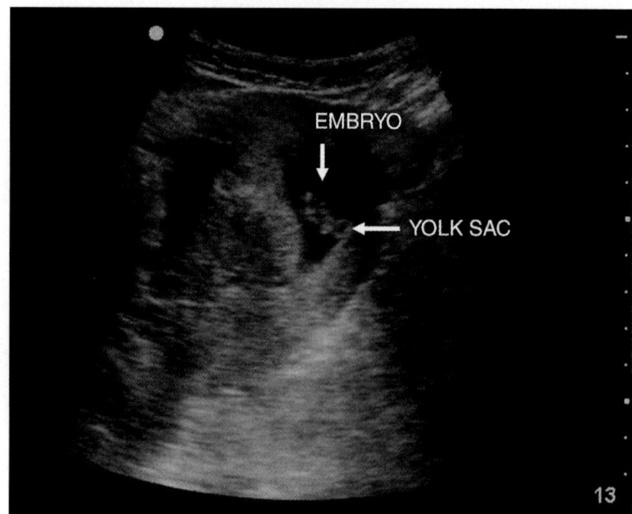

Figure 4.13
Embryo and yolk sac on a transabdominal sagittal window.

(Figures 4.13 and 4.14) and should exhibit cardiac motion on both transvaginal and transabdominal scanning.

The gold standard for the diagnosis of a living intrauterine pregnancy is the visualization of embryonic cardiac activity. This may be seen as early as 41–43 menstrual days (6 weeks) or when the mean sac diameter is 12–16 mm. Physicians must use M-mode to highlight cardiac motion (Figure 4.15) because it uses less acoustic power than Doppler and thus theoretically transmits less acoustic energy to the fetus (see Chapter 1). The alternating black and gray bands represent chamber movement. Heart rate is calculated

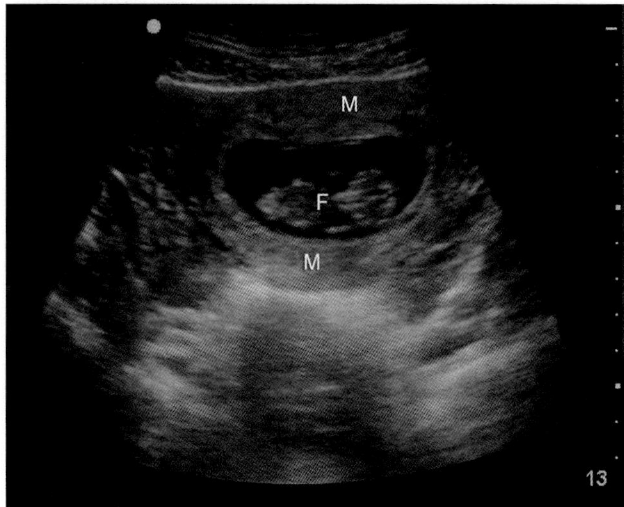

Figure 4.14
Intrauterine pregnancy. Fetus (F) surrounded by myometrial mantle (M).

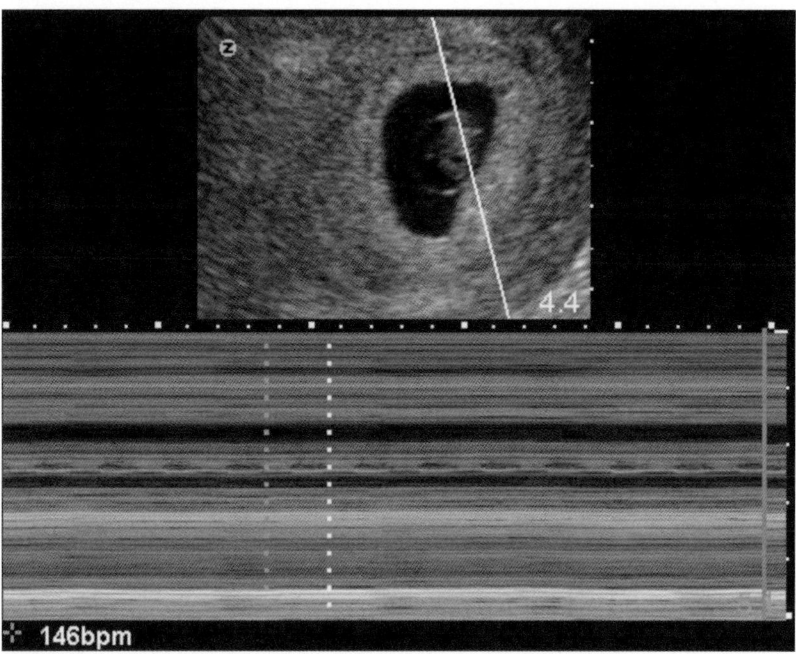

Figure 4.15
Fetal heart rate (FHR) by M-mode (FHR 146 seen on bottom of screen).

by measuring one cycle length and determining the cycles per second based on that measurement. In addition, many bedside ultrasound machines will have an automatic fetal heart-rate calculation function in their M-mode menu.

Ectopic pregnancy

Ectopic pregnancy occurs in about 2% of all pregnancies in the United States. However, some studies have reported an incidence of 7.5–13% among symptomatic patients who present to the emergency department [1–3].

Transvaginal ultrasound can detect the embryo in ectopic pregnancies. The presence of an adnexal mass and/or cul-de-sac fluid in a patient with no intrauterine gestation and measurable circulating hCG is highly specific for the diagnosis of ectopic pregnancy. Absence of ectopic sonographic findings does not exclude the diagnosis, because up to 30% of women with extrauterine gestations have no sonographic evidence of an adnexal mass or pelvic intraperitoneal fluid [1–3,12–19]. The majority (95%) of ectopic pregnancies occur in the fallopian tubes. Ovarian, abdominal, cervical, and interligamentary ectopics are rare. However, these non-fallopian ectopics carry a higher mortality because they rupture at a later gestational age, and thus hemorrhage is more rapid. To prevent mistaking a cervical or corneal ectopic for an intrauterine pregnancy, one must determine that a thick enough "myometrial mantle" exists to sustain the gestation within the uterus. Thus, the thinnest stripe of myometrium seen surrounding the gestation should be measured (Figure 4.16). Anything < 8 mm is concerning for a cervical or corneal/interstitial ectopic pregnancy, and proper consultation should be arranged [1–3].

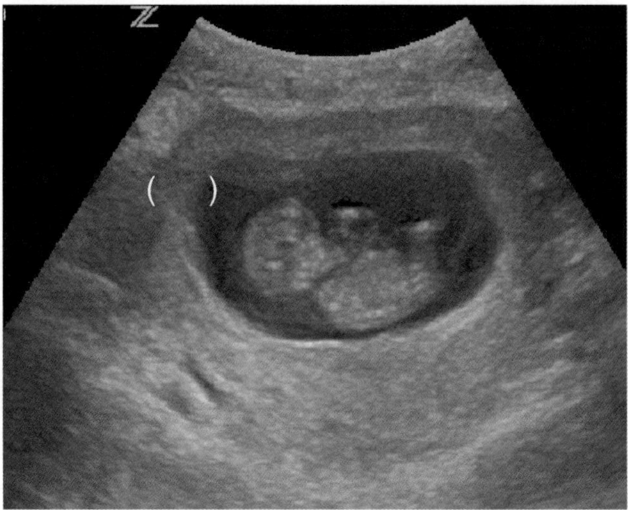

Figure 4.16 Where to measure the myometrial mantle. Image courtesy of Dr. Greg Press, University of Texas – Houston, Hermann Memorial Hospital, Houston, TX.

Abnormal images

Figures 4.17–4.23 show images of abnormal pelvic ultrasound scans.

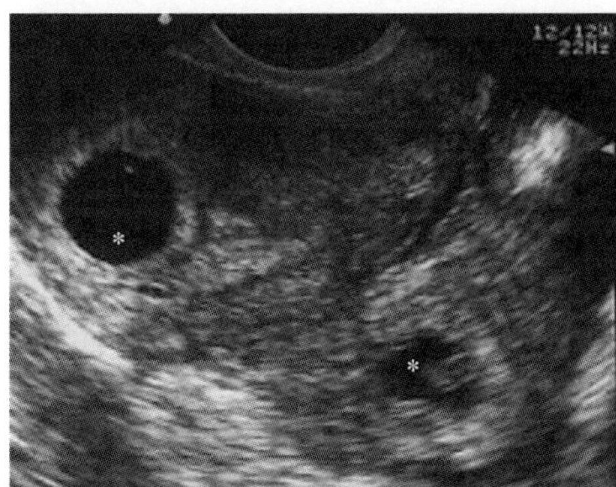

Figure 4.17

Heterotopic pregnancy. Two gestational sacs are seen (*). The sac in the lower right-hand corner of the screen is outside the uterine cavity. Courtesy of Dr. Greg Press, University of Texas – Houston, Hermann Memorial Hospital, Houston, TX.

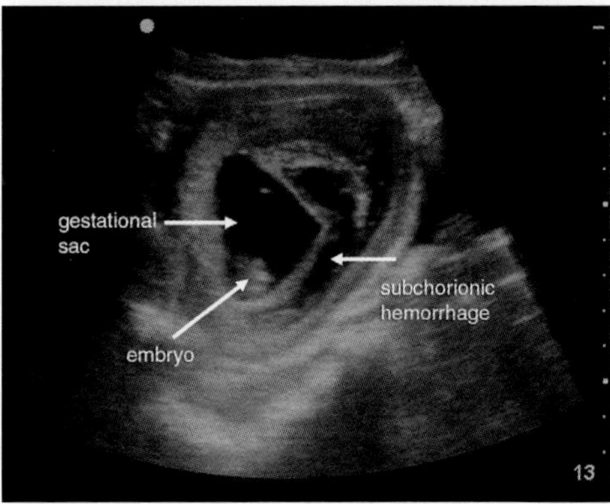

Figure 4.18

Subchorionic hemorrhage. The anechoic fluid separating the gestational sac from the myometrium is clearly seen. These patients should pursue formal consultation because they are at a higher risk of hemorrhage and miscarriage.

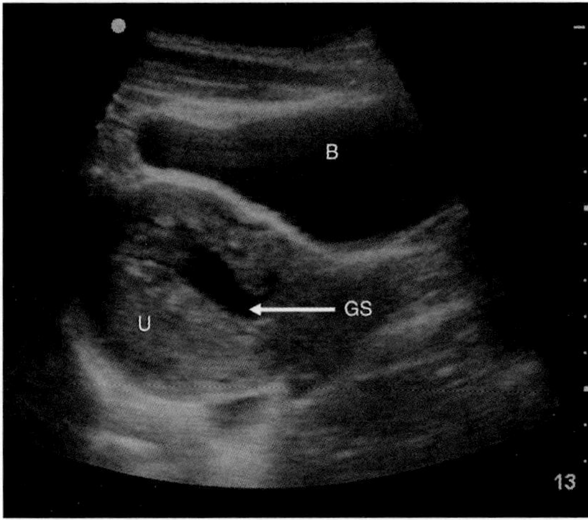

Figure 4.19

Large, irregularly shaped gestational sac. Because no yolk sac or fetal pole is seen, this is likely embryonic resorption and a missed abortion. However, pseudogestational sac of ectopic pregnancy cannot be ruled out on this image alone, and proper consultation should be obtained. B, bladder; GS, gestational sac; U, uterus.

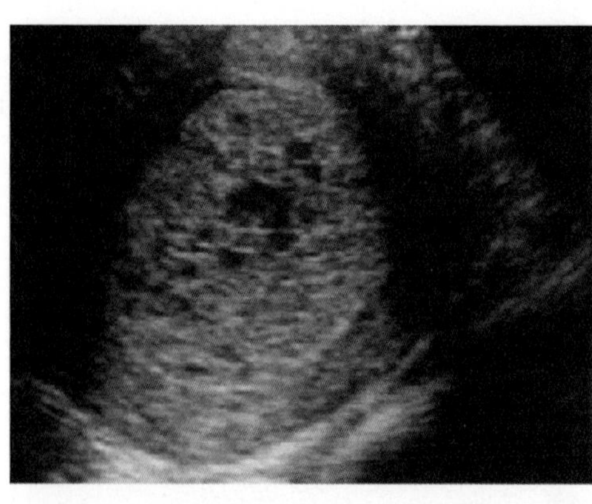

Figure 4.20

Molar pregnancy. The large uterus appears filled with heterogeneous material in the form of hundreds of tiny follicles. Because a significant number of such patients have high hCG levels and undergo malignant transformation of this tissue, they should pursue formal consultation.

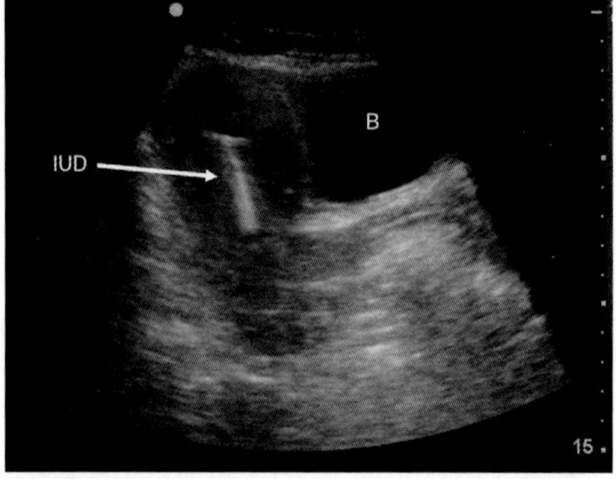

Figure 4.21

Intrauterine device (IUD) for contraception. Reverberation artifact is seen. Placement is normal (mid-uterus at endometrial stripe).
B, bladder.

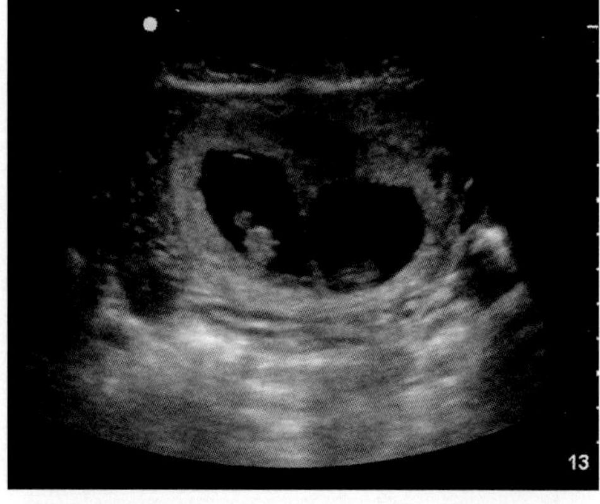

Figure 4.22

Twin gestation.

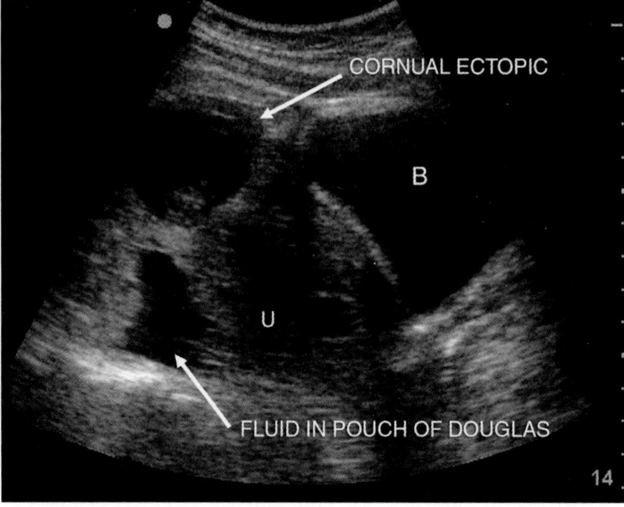

Figure 4.23
Cornual or interstitial ectopic. Pregnancy is implanted at the edge of the myometrium. A pseudogestational sac is seen just anterior to the uterus (U). Free fluid is also noted. B, bladder. Courtesy of Dr. Robert Miller, North Shore Medical Center, Salem, MA.

Sample clinical protocol

Algorithms using transvaginal sonography and a beta-hCG discriminatory zone (Table 4.1) have been developed to improve diagnostic accuracy and clinical consistency. There are several variations of this algorithm, although the recommendations are generally similar (1–3,12).

The protocol illustrated in Figure 4.24 is a typical algorithm incorporating several key decision points (pelvic ultrasound, Rh type, hCG level, etc.) into a care plan for patients with possible ectopic pregnancy.

Table 4.1 Discriminatory zone findings on transabdominal (TA) and transvaginal (TV) scanning

	TA	TV	hCG level
Gestational sac	5.5–6 weeks	4.5–5 weeks	1700–6000
Yolk sac	6–6.5 weeks	5–5.5 weeks	8000–15 000
Fetal pole	7 weeks	5.5–6 weeks	13 000–15 000
Cardiac activity	7 weeks	6 weeks	16 000–25 000
Fetal parts	> 8 weeks	8 weeks	29 000–39 000

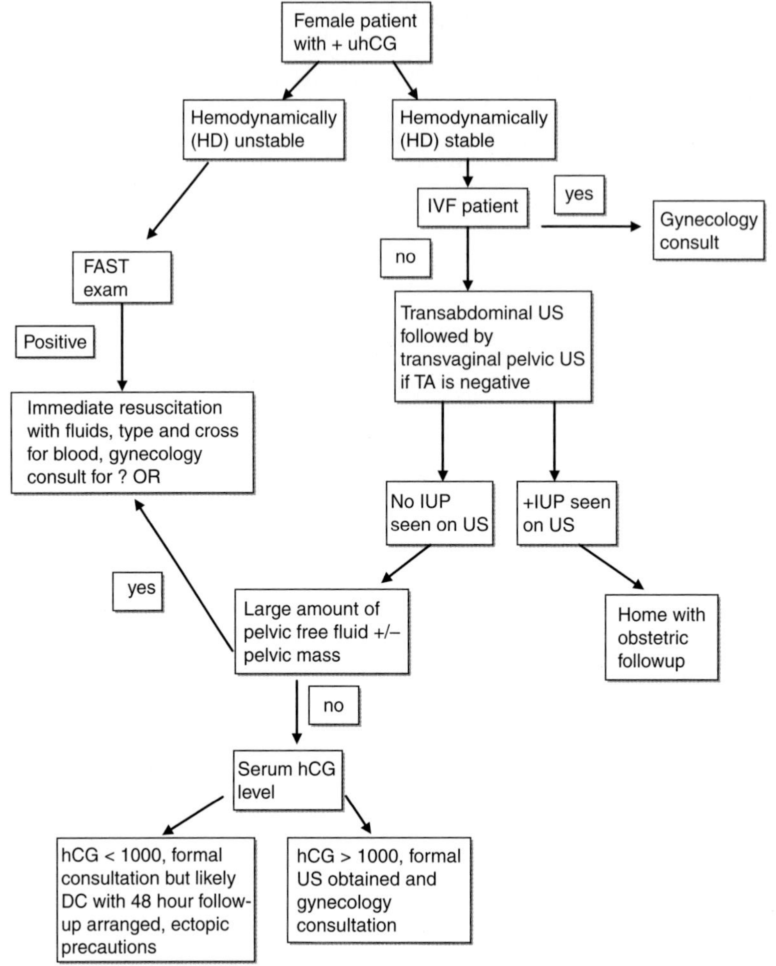

Figure 4.24
Sample clinical protocol for evaluation of possible ectopic pregnancy.

Literature review

Reference	Methods	Results	Notes
Blaivas *et al.* 2000 [14]	Retrospective chart review of 1419 emergency department (ED) patients undergoing US to rule out ectopic pregnancy.	For patients with intrauterine pregnancy (IUP), length of stay 21% (daytime) to 28% (evening) shorter when emergency physicians (EPs) perform US vs. radiology.	Time saving with EP-performed bedside US.

Reference	Methods	Results	Notes
Burgher *et al.* 1998 [20]	Retrospective review of 84 patients undergoing evaluation for ectopic pregnancy by EPs and ob/gyn.	Shorter length of stay, no missed ectopics in group evaluated by EPs.	Time saving with EP-performed bedside US, low risk of missed ectopic.
Durston *et al.* 2000 [16]	Retrospective study evaluating test ordering practices after introduction of EP-performed pelvic sonography.	Specificity of EP-performed sonography ruling in IUP was 95%. Increased availability of US improves quality of ectopic pregnancy detection at expense of number of US done.	Proposed that EP physicians screen all patients with first trimester cramping or bleeding and immediately refer for formal study all indeterminate scans for best results.
Moore *et al.* 2007 [21]	Prospective evaluation of 242 female patients suspected of ectopic pregnancy.	EP-performed US included RUQ view of Morison's pouch. 10/28 patients with ectopic pregnancy had fluid in Morison's pouch, yielding increased likelihood ratio (LR = 112) for OR.	By performing bedside US in patients suspected of ectopic pregnancy, fluid in RUQ predicts need for OR and can expedite workup and perhaps decrease need for other testing.
Condous *et al.* 2004 [22]	Evaluation of the prevalence and natural history of ovarian pathology in pregnancy.	161/3000 pregnant women undergoing first trimester US had ovarian pathology. 4/3000 women (0.13%) required acute intervention for ovarian pathology during their pregnancy.	Further evidence that focused assessment for intrauterine pregnancy is safe.

New directions

As emergency physicians have become more proficient with first trimester scanning, new protocols have been proposed to address the large number of patients with indeterminate scans who are clinically and hemodynamically stable. Patients with indeterminate first trimester scans have three possible outcomes: (1) the pregnancy is too early and is below the discriminatory zone level for ultrasound detection, (2) the pregnancy is an ectopic pregnancy, or (3) the pregnancy is a missed or incomplete abortion [18]. Often, patients with indeterminate scans and hemodynamic stability are sent home to be followed up in 48 hours for a repeat serum quantitative hCG level to assess the viability of the pregnancy.

Tayal *et al.* [23] proposed an algorithm that would decrease the number of patients requiring formal gynecology consultation before discharge in the indeterminate ultrasound group. They suggested that patients with indeterminate bedside ultrasound scans who (1) have no adnexal tenderness,

(2) have no pelvic free fluid seen on ultrasound, (3) are hemodynamically stable, and (4) have an hCG level < 1500 are safe for discharge without gynecology consultation but with a plan for follow-up in 48 hours for repeat evaluation.

Although this is not recommended for departments that are new to bedside scanning, this protocol further highlights the progress of ultrasound. As technology becomes more routine and techniques are mastered, the diagnostic envelope continues to be pushed forward.

References

1. Reardon RF, Martel ML. First trimester pregnancy. In Ma OJ, Mateer JR (eds.), *Emergency Ultrasound*. New York, NY: McGraw-Hill; 2003: 239–76.
2. Moore C, Promes SB. Ultrasound in pregnancy. *Emerg Med Clin North Am* 2004; **22**: 697–722.
3. Lyons E, Levi C, Dashefsky S. The first trimester. In Rumack C, Wilson S, Carboneau J (eds.), *Diagnostic Ultrasound*, Vol 2. St. Louis, MO: Mosby-Year Book; 1998: 978–1011.
4. Richards SR, Stempel LE, Carlton BD. Heterotopic pregnancy: reappraisal of incidence. *Am J Obstet Gynecol* 1982; **142**: 928–30.
5. Reece EA, Petrie RH, Sirmans MF, Finster M, Todd WD. Combined intrauterine and extrauterine gestations: a review. *Am J Obstet Gynecol* 1983; **146**: 323–30.
6. Bright DA, Gaupp FB. Heterotopic pregnancy: a reevaluation. *J Am Board Fam Pract* 1990; **3**: 125–8.
7. Gamberdella FR, Marrs RP. Heterotopic pregnancy associated with assisted reproductive technology. *Am J Obstet Gynecol* 1999; **160**: 1520–2.
8. Dart RG, Kaplan B, Cox C. Transvaginal ultrasound in patients with low beta-human chorionic gonadotropin values: how often is the study diagnostic? *Ann Emerg Med* 197; **30**: 135–40.
9. Chambers SE, Muir BB, Haddad NG. Ultrasound evaluation of ectopic pregnancy including correlation with human chorionic gonadotropin levels. *Br J Radiol* 1990; **63**: 246–50.
10. DiMarchi JM, Kosasa TS, Hale RW. What is the significance of the human chorionic gonadotropin value in ectopic pregnancy? *Obstet Gynecol* 1989; **74**: 851–5.
11. Kadar N, Bohrer M, Kemmann E, Shelden R. The discriminatory human chorionic gonadotropin zone for endovaginal sonography: a prospective randomized study. *Fertil Steril* 1994; **61**: 1016–20.
12. Gracia CR, Barnhart KT. Diagnosing ectopic pregnancy: decision analysis comparing six strategies. *Obstet Gynecol* 2001; **97**: 464–70.
13. Yeh HC, Goodman JD, Carr L, Rabinowitz JG. Intradecidual sign: a US criterion of early intrauterine pregnancy. *Radiology* 1986; **161**: 463–7.
14. Blaivas M, Sierzenski P, Plecque D, Lambert M. Do emergency physicians save time when locating a live intrauterine pregnancy with bedside ultrasonography? *Acad Emerg Med* 2000; **7**: 988–93.

15. Brennan DF. Diagnosis of ectopic pregnancy. *J Fla Med Assoc* 1997; **84**: 549–56.
16. Durston WE, Carl ML, Guerra W, Eaton A, Ackerson LM. Ultrasound availability in the evaluation of ectopic pregnancy in the ED: comparison of quality and cost-effectiveness with different approaches. *Am J Emerg Med* 2000; **18**: 408–17.
17. Kaplan BC, Dart RG, Moskos M, *et al.* Ectopic pregnancy: prospective study with improved diagnostic accuracy. *Ann Emerg Med* 1996; **28**: 10–17.
18. Tayal VS, Cohen H, Norton HJ. Outcome of patients with an indeterminate emergency department first-trimester pelvic ultrasound to rule out ectopic pregnancy. *Acad Emerg Med* 2004; **11**: 912–17.
19. Stovall TG, Kellerman AL, Ling FW, Buster JE. Emergency department diagnosis of ectopic pregnancy. *Ann Emerg Med* 1990; **19**: 1098–103.
20. Burgher SW, Tandy TK, Dawdy MR. Transvaginal ultrasonography by emergency physicians decreases patient time in the emergency department. *Acad Emerg Med* 1998; **5**: 802–7.
21. Moore C, Todd WM, O'Brien E, Lin H. Free fluid in Morison's pouch on bedside ultrasound predicts the need for operative intervention in suspected ectopic pregnancy. *Acad Emerg Med* 2007; **14**: 755–8.
22. Condous G, Khalid A, Okaro E, Bourne T. Should we be examining the ovaries in pregnancy? Prevalence and natural history of adnexal pathology detected at first trimester sonography. *Ultrasound Obstet Gynecol* 2004; **24**: 62–6.
23. Tayal VS, Forgash AJ, Norton HJ. Outcomes for ectopic pregnancy patients with indeterminate pelvic ultrasounds using a modified CMC pregnancy ultrasound protocol with selective non-IUP gynecologic consultation. *Ann Emerg Med* 2006; **48**: S105–6.

5 Abdominal aorta ultrasound

Introduction

With the possible exception of pericardial tamponade, there is no other condition in which the rapid diagnostic capabilities of bedside sonography are of such striking benefit as abdominal aortic aneurysm (AAA) [1,2]. Emergency bedside ultrasonography enables the physician to confirm a high-risk diagnosis, decreasing the time needed to mobilize resources or even transfer the patient to a referral center if necessary. This one exam will save lives if incorporated into the regular practice of emergency and critical care physicians involved in the evaluation of acutely ill patients [1].

There is a wide array of symptoms related to unstable AAA. Patients can have back pain, flank pain that sounds like ureteral colic, syncope, abdominal pain, gastrointestinal bleeding, or any variety of these. Because of this, and because of the ease of a screening abdominal aortic ultrasound, it is recommended that all patients with the aforementioned presenting symptoms and risk factors for AAA undergo an ultrasound screening exam. This is particularly true if a patient with flank pain is found to have unilateral hydronephrosis. An expanding abdominal aneurysm can compress the ureter so that hydronephrosis results. It is far better to perform a screening evaluation in at-risk patients with flank pain than to miss this life-threatening diagnosis.

Focused questions for aorta ultrasound

The questions for aorta ultrasound are as follows:

1. Is the abdominal aorta >3 cm in diameter?
2. Are the iliac arteries >1.5 cm in diameter?

If the answers to these questions are no, then the aorta ultrasound evaluation is normal. However, one must be careful to examine the entire length of the abdominal aorta and to evaluate in two planes, as described in this chapter.

If the answer to either of these questions is yes, then an aneurysm has been diagnosed, and the physician's next step depends on the clinical picture of the patient. A vascular surgeon should be called immediately for unstable patients and operative repair expedited. For stable but symptomatic patients, further evaluation with a CT scan can be arranged to better define anatomy and facilitate operative repair. Outpatient referral for vascular surgery evaluation can be arranged if the aneurysm is asymptomatic and the diameter is <5 cm [3–5].

Anatomy

The normal abdominal aorta (Figure 5.1) has a proximal-to-distal taper, and a loss of that taper with a diameter > 3 cm indicates the presence of an AAA. An iliac diameter > 1.5 cm is indicative of an iliac aneurysm. All measurements are from outer wall to outer wall (it is better to overestimate in this case than underestimate!). Significant abdominal aneurysms (i.e., high risk of rupture) are ordinarily ≥ 5 cm in diameter, with a fusiform shape [5]. Much research has been done to correlate diameter with risk of rupture: AAAs < 4 cm have a 2% per year risk of rupture, AAAs 4–5 cm have a 3–12% per year risk of rupture, and AAAs > 5 cm have a 25–41% risk of rupture [2].

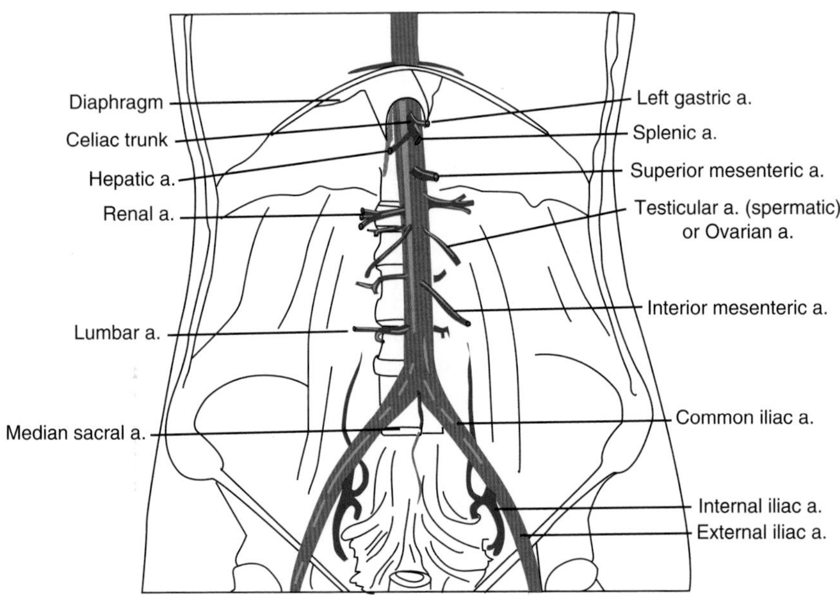

Figure 5.1
Normal anatomy of the abdominal aorta.

Technique

Probe selection

Using a standard 3.5 MHz transducer, the abdominal aorta can usually be visualized in its entirety – down to the iliacs. A curvilinear-array probe will often give the best penetration, especially in patients with a larger body habitus.

Views

We recommend that the entire length of the aorta should be imaged in real time for a complete exam. In order to document these findings, it is helpful to specifically image the following five areas:

1. Transverse view of the proximal aorta
2. Transverse view of the mid aorta
3. Transverse view of the distal aorta
4. Transverse view of the distal aorta showing the bifurcation into both iliac arteries
5. Longitudinal/sagittal view of the aorta

The most helpful landmark for aorta scanning is the vertebral body shadow – remember that both the aorta and the vena cava will be just anterior to the vertebrae. The aorta will be a bright white circle filled with black located right on top of the vertebral body. One common mistake is to set the depth on the ultrasound machine too shallow to find the vertebrae. It is recommended to set the depth as deep as the machine will allow until the vertebral shadow is found. The depth can then be decreased to visualize the aorta near the center of the screen. On-screen, the vena cava is usually noted to be just to the left of the aorta. This corresponds to the patient's right side when the probe marker faces the patient's right. Because it is a low-pressure system, the vena cava often appears triangular or teardrop-shaped. The vena cava may pulsate because it is adjacent to the pulsatile aorta (or because of brisk venous return), so do not use visually observed pulsations to distinguish the two. The best way to distinguish between the vena cava and the aorta is to show the compressibility of the vena cava. The walls of the vena cava are also much thinner and less echogenic. If your machine has spectral Doppler, the waveforms of each vessel can also help to distinguish artery from vein.

Proximal aorta

Starting proximally, position the probe in the transverse orientation with the probe marker to the patient's right (Figure 5.2). The probe should be in the

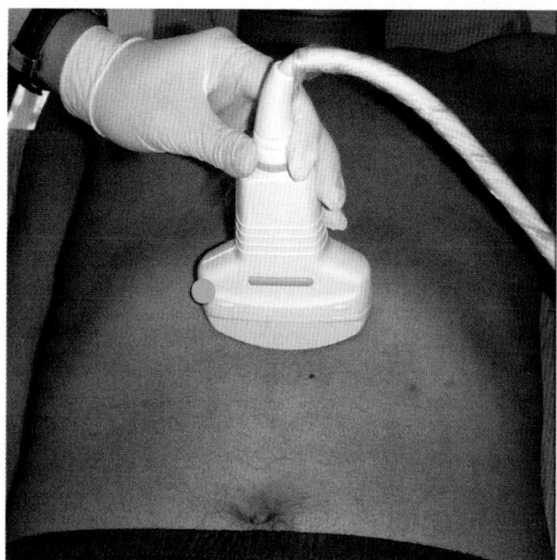

Figure 5.2
Probe positioning for transverse imaging. The probe marker (green dot) faces the patient's right side.

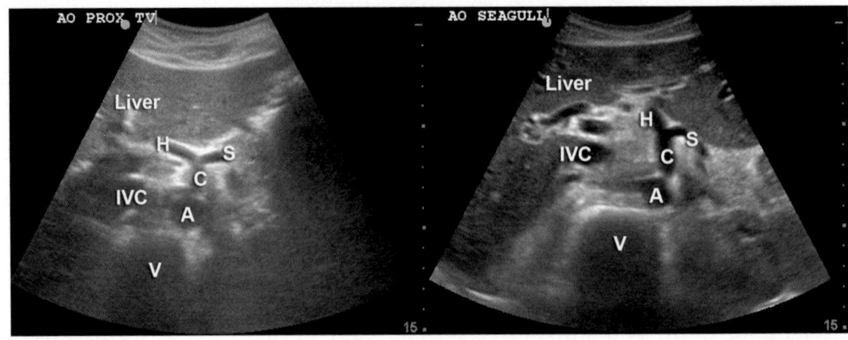

Figure 5.3
Most proximal abdominal aorta view including the celiac trunk. Two variations on the anatomy are seen. Deep to the liver (and using it as a window) the celiac trunk (C), hepatic artery (H), and splenic artery (S) branches are seen. In addition the aorta (A), inferior vena cava (IVC), and vertebral body shadow (V) are visualized.

epigastric area just distal to the subxiphoid process and perpendicular to the patient's abdominal wall.

When scanning the proximal aorta, the left lobe of the liver is often included in the field. The most proximal level of the abdominal aorta includes the celiac trunk (Figure 5.3). However, it can often be difficult to get a view this proximal and to visualize the celiac artery. Clinically, it is exceedingly rare to have an isolated AAA that only involves the abdominal aorta from the celiac trunk to the superior mesenteric artery, so it is not essential that this branch is visualized for screening purposes. The appearance of the hepatic and splenic arteries arising from the celiac trunk looks like a seagull, and thus this view is often called "the seagull sign." The gastric arterial branch is rarely seen in AAA screening images.

Figure 5.4 shows the more commonly seen proximal view with the bright echogenic superior mesenteric artery (SMA) just anterior to the aorta. The splenic vein is seen traveling anterior to the SMA. It is even possible to see a glimpse of the renal vein as it travels under the SMA to fuse with the inferior vena cava (IVC).

Figure 5.5 shows another view of the proximal aorta, measured with calipers. The SMA is visible immediately above the aorta as a small bright echogenic-surrounded vessel. A collapsed IVC can be seen on the left (which is the patient's right), along with a good view of the vertebral shadow.

Figure 5.6 shows the view just distal to Figure 5.5. Here, the left renal artery can be seen as it merges with the aorta. Most of the time it is difficult to visualize the renal arteries with bedside ultrasound, which is why surgeons often appreciate the anatomic detail provided by a CT scan for operative planning.

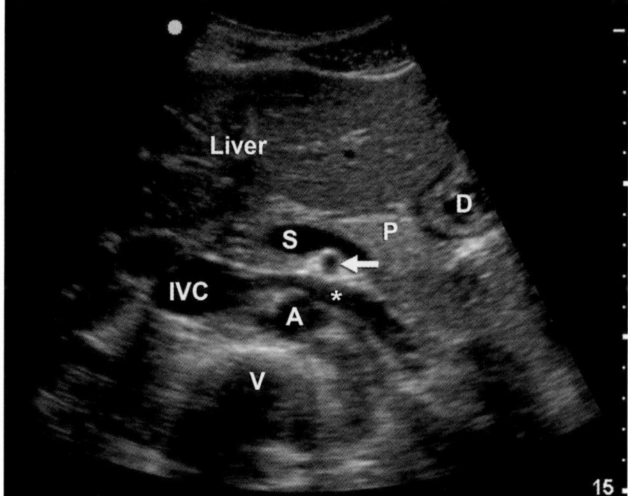

Figure 5.4
Standard proximal view of the abdominal aorta visualizing the aorta (A), IVC, and vertebral body shadow (V). The left renal vein (*) traverses between the aorta and the superior mesenteric artery (arrow). In this view the splenic vein (S) and a portion of the pancreas (P) and duodenum (D) are also seen.

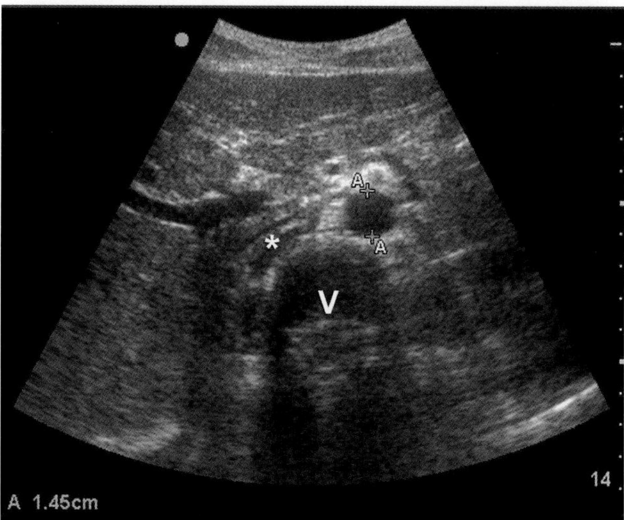

Figure 5.5
Standard proximal view of the normal aorta (with calipers measuring the diameter). The vertebral body shadow (V) is seen, and in this image the IVC (*) is flat.

Mid aorta

A transverse view of the mid aorta (Figure 5.7) is obtained by moving the probe caudally along the midline while maintaining a transverse orientation (probe marker to patient's right). This view lacks unique landmarks. Remember that most AAAs are infrarenal, and this portion of the aorta should be thoroughly imaged.

Distal aorta

As the probe approaches the umbilicus, the distal aorta is imaged as it bifurcates (Figure 5.8). In most cases, the bifurcation of the aorta is located at

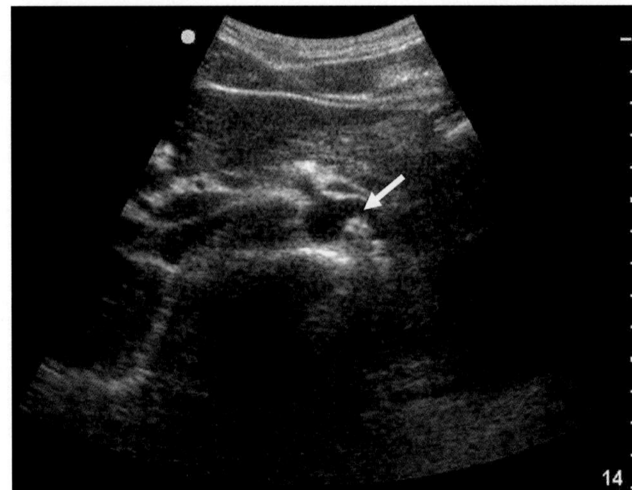

Figure 5.6
Abdominal aorta with left renal artery (arrow) visualized.

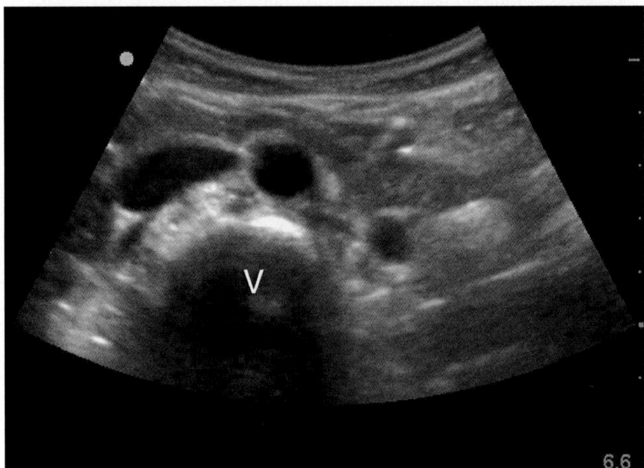

Figure 5.7
Mid aorta (round) and IVC (elliptical) above the vertebral body shadow.

the level of the umbilicus (near L4). Careful adjustment of the angle of the probe with regard to the abdominal wall will often reveal where the aorta splits into the iliac arteries. Often, a small rocking motion angling toward the feet will be all that is required to image the split.

Longitudinal view

Obtaining a long axis/sagittal plane view of the aorta is most easily obtained from the proximal to mid-aortic view positions. However, it should be viewed as distal as possible, given the higher rate of AAA distal to the renal arteries. Begin by locating the aorta in the short-axis/transverse plane, then slowly rotate the probe 90 degrees with the marker toward

(A)

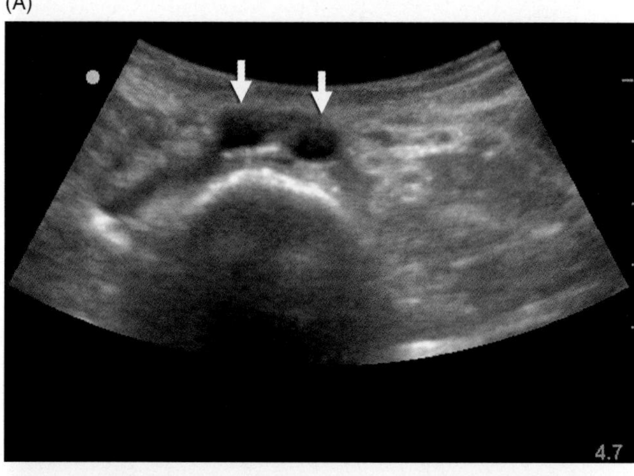

(B)

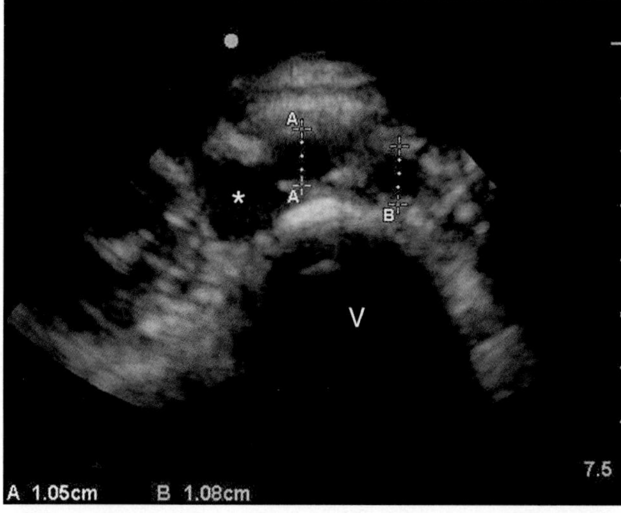

Figure 5.8
Distal bifurcation of the aorta into the iliac arteries (arrows in *A*, calipers in *B*) above the vertebral body shadow (V). *, inferior vena cava).

the patient's head to obtain the longitudinal view (Figure 5.9). Again, careful side-to-side adjustment of the angle of the probe with regard to the abdominal wall will ensure that the aorta's greatest diameter is visualized (Figures 5.10 and 5.11).

It is also important to remember that a tubular structure (the aorta) is being imaged by a plane (the ultrasound beam). Thus, the transverse view is more accurate in terms of ensuring that the true cross-section of the aorta is visualized. When imaging longitudinally, it is easy to see how a falsely small cross-section of the aorta could be measured if the plane of the beam is just off midline (Figure 5.11). The reason to image in two planes is to ensure that saccular outpouchings of the aortic wall are not missed.

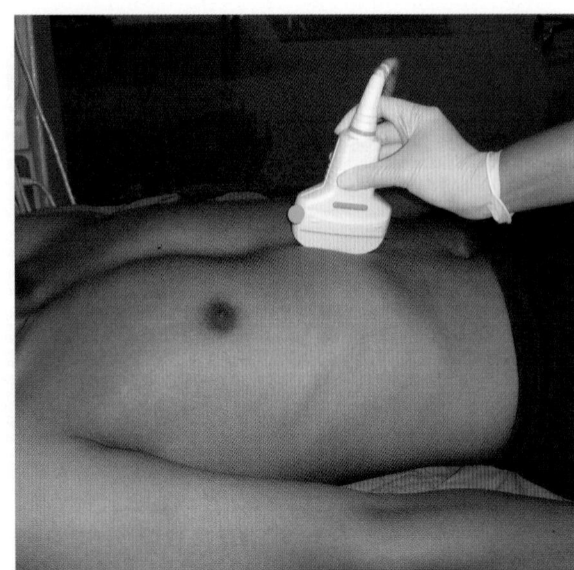

Figure 5.9
Probe positioning for longitudinal imaging. The probe marker (green dot) faces cephalad.

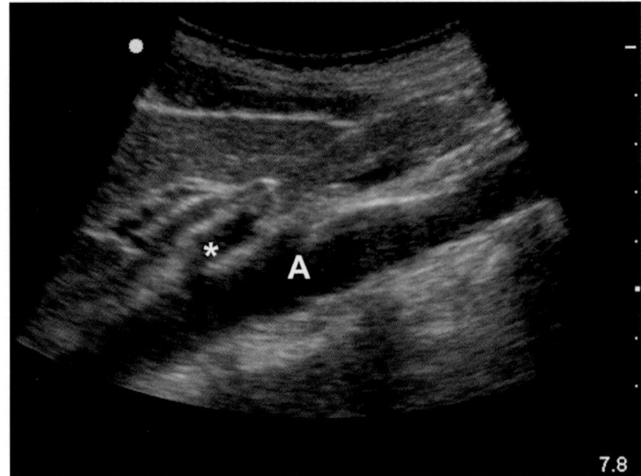

Figure 5.10
Longitudinal aorta (A) with SMA branch point (*) visible.

Aorta versus vena cava

Differentiating between the IVC and the aorta (Figure 5.12) may seem straightforward, but a few points are worth remembering. Of course, holding the probe marker to the patient's right will generally reveal the aorta on the right of the screen (the side without the screen marker, thus indicating the patient's left). In addition, the aorta is a thicker-walled structure than the vena cava and often develops calcifications as sequelae of atherosclerotic plaque. Thus, it may appear to have brightly

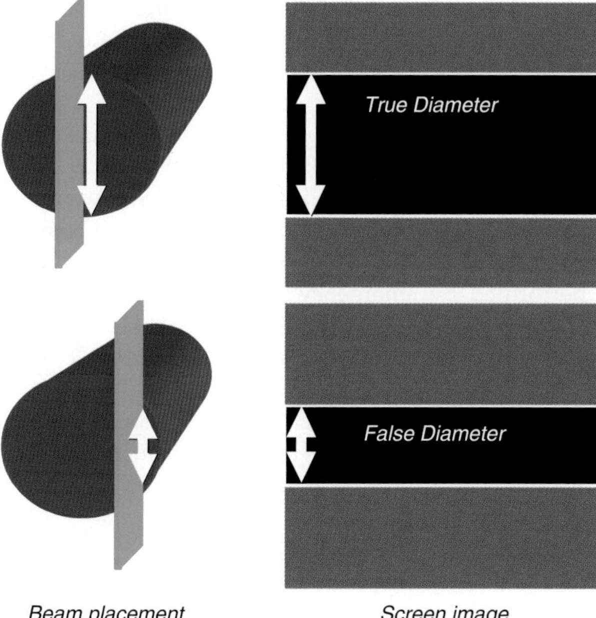

Figure 5.11
Beam placement determines apparent diameter through a cylinder.

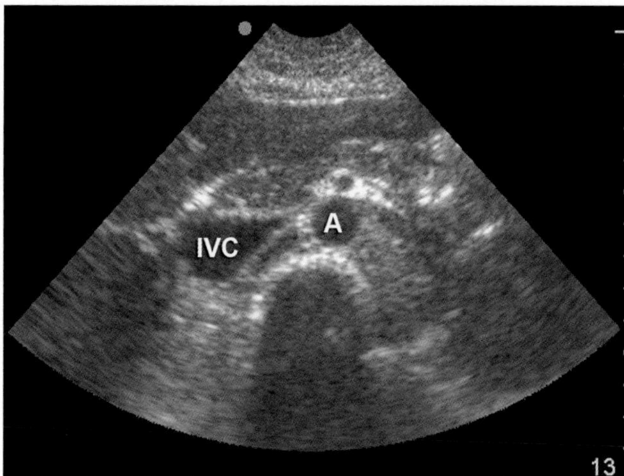

Figure 5.12
Inferior vena cava (IVC) versus aorta (A).

echogenic walls. The aorta is generally round, while the IVC is often elliptical or teardrop-shaped. The SMA will generally be visible proximally immediately above the aorta, not the IVC. The aorta is actively pulsatile; however, as mentioned, transmission of pulsations to the IVC from the aorta and the right ventricle can make this distinction difficult. The aorta is not compressible with probe pressure, whereas the vena cava is. The normal aorta tapers as it progresses distally, whereas the vena cava gets somewhat larger as it approaches the renal vessels. Finally, with deep inspirations (sniff test) the IVC will change caliber, whereas the aorta will not.

Adequate visualization of the entire length of the aorta is required to exclude AAA. If the diameter of the aorta (from outer wall to outer wall) appears normal over this length, then this excludes a ruptured AAA with an essentially 100% negative predictive value [6–9], although false-positive screening exams have been reported [10]. Several studies of bedside AAA screening evaluations performed by emergency physicians have reported high rates of technically limited studies ranging from 8% to 33% [11–13], with that number likely influenced by operator experience and difficult body habitus [13].

Again, remember that an aortic diameter >3 cm and an iliac artery diameter >1.5 cm are considered abnormal. Do not forget to evaluate the iliac arteries – aneurysmal dilatation and rupture of the iliacs can carry significant morbidity and mortality.

Scanning tips

Trouble with aorta scanning

Bowel gas in the way?

- Apply pressure to minimize artifact caused by bowel gas interposed between the probe and the aorta. Occasionally, it will be necessary to hold constant pressure to force peristalsis of the overlying bowel out of the field of view. If obesity and/or bowel gas still degrade the quality of the images, rolling the patient into a left lateral decubitus position may help mechanically shift the bowel out of the way of the ultrasound beam.
- Jiggle the probe with gentle pressure over the offending bowel to encourage peristalsis and afford a clearer view of the aorta.
- Try imaging the transverse aorta from an angle. If bowel gas obscures the right side of your screen, move the probe to your left and angle the beam toward the aorta to visualize it from an angle. As long as the beam remains transverse, this should not alter the size of the aorta as it appears on the screen (Figure 5.13).

Can't see the aorta at all?

- Have the patient roll onto his or her left side, and use the liver as an acoustic window to try and view the aorta this way.
- Increase the depth to the maximum to see if you can find the vertebral shadow.

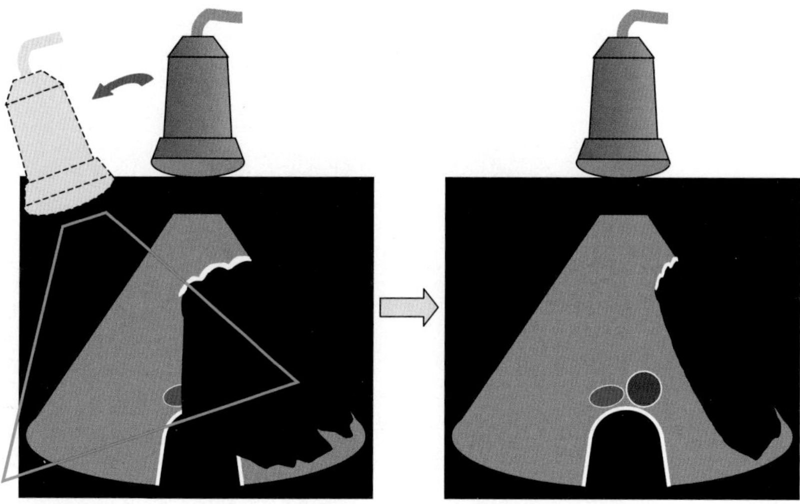

Figure 5.13
Probe angles to avoid bowel gas when imaging the abdominal aorta.

Abnormal images

AAA

Figure 5.14 is a transverse view of the mid-abdominal aorta in an elderly patient presenting with back pain. The depth markers on the screen reveal that this is larger than 3.0 cm in diameter, and therefore aneurysmal. Note that the blackened center (lumen) is the only area through which blood flows. The thickened outer dimension of the aorta is the result of a clot and atherosclerotic plaque that are adherent to the wall.

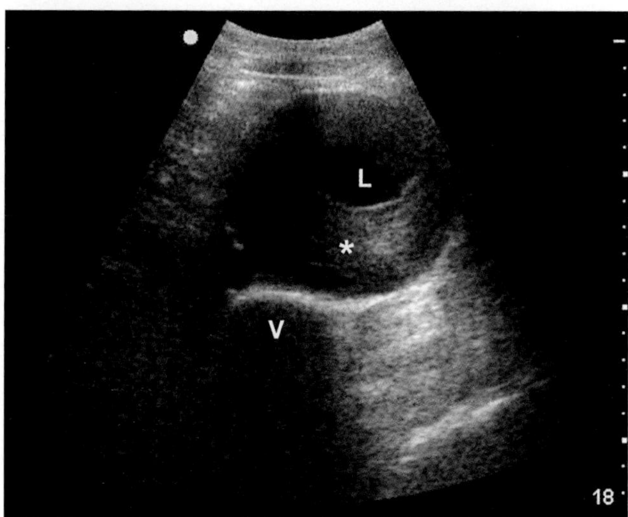

Figure 5.14
AAA with thrombus (*) and lumen (L) visible as well as vertebral body shadow (V).

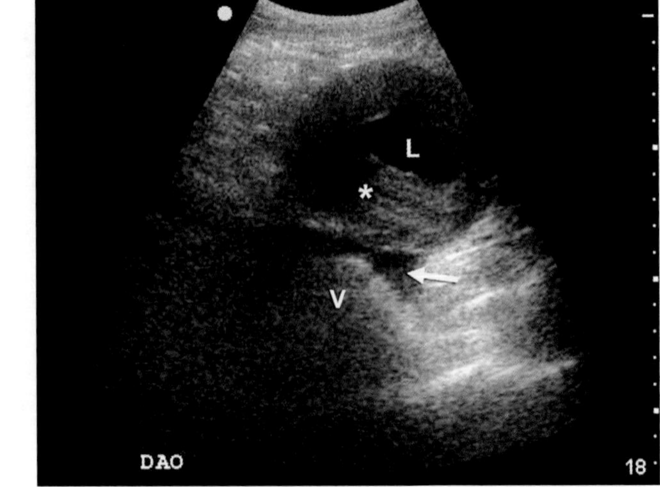

Figure 5.15

Thrombus (*) and lumen (L) within aorta are visible above vertebral body shadow (V). In this image hemorrhage from leaking AAA is evident as well (arrow).

(A)

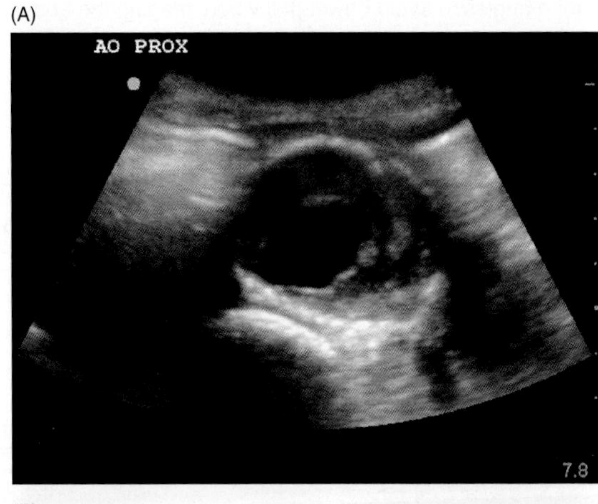

(B)

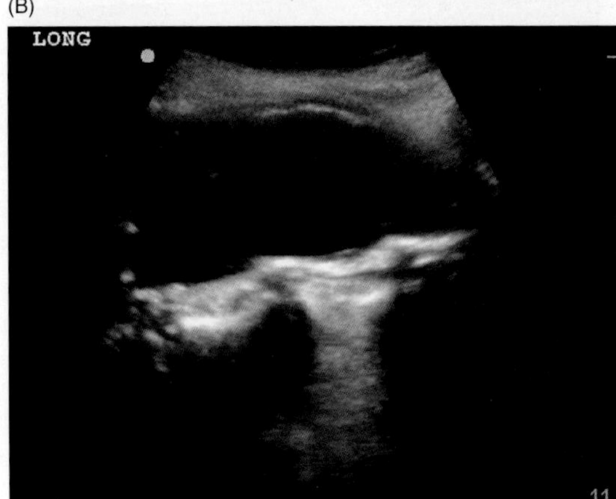

Figure 5.16

The same AAA seen in (*A*) transverse and (*B*) longitudinal views.

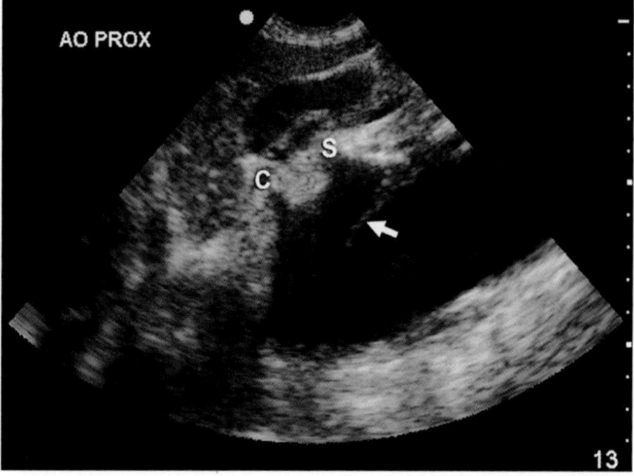

Figure 5.17
Longitudinal view of proximal AAA with the celiac (C) and superior mesenteric (S) arteries branching off. In this view an aortic dissection flap (arrow) is evident as well.

In the next examples of AAA (Figures 5.15 and 5.16), lumen clot is visualized as a somewhat more heterogeneous gray lining of the aorta. Caution must be used when measuring the diameter so as not to be fooled into measuring only the patent lumen but to include the luminal clot in the diameter measurement. It should be appreciated that the aorta is actually significantly larger than the vertebral shadow, which is a visual clue that the diameter is likely dilated.

Figure 5.17 shows a longitudinal view of an abdominal aortic aneurysm. It is easy to appreciate the fusiform shape in these views.

Aortic dissection

CT is a much more accurate test for dissection, and only rarely will bedside ultrasound be able to image the flap of an aortic dissection. However, if images similar to those in Figures 5.18 to 5.20 are seen (in particular, the

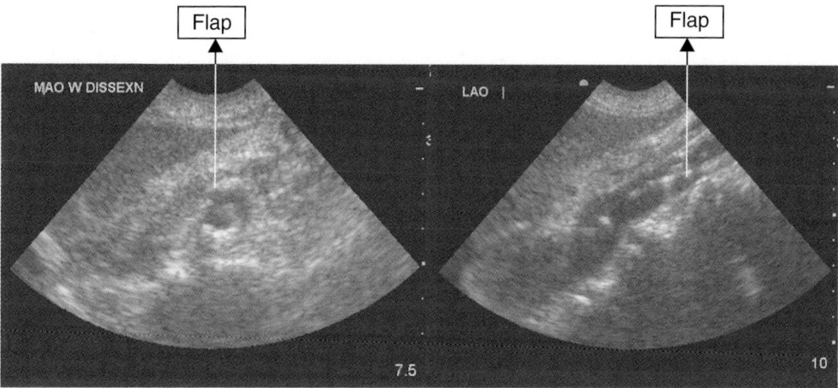

Figure 5.18
Transverse and longitudinal view of aorta with flap visible within the lumen.

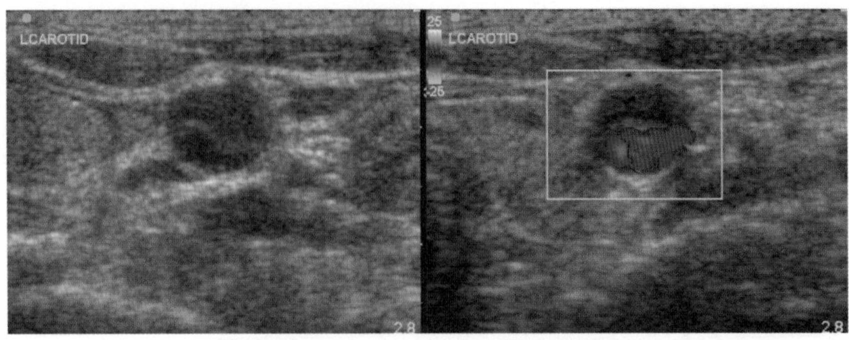

Figure 5.19

This dissection also extended into the carotid, as a flap is seen (*left*) and confirmed with Doppler flow (*right*).

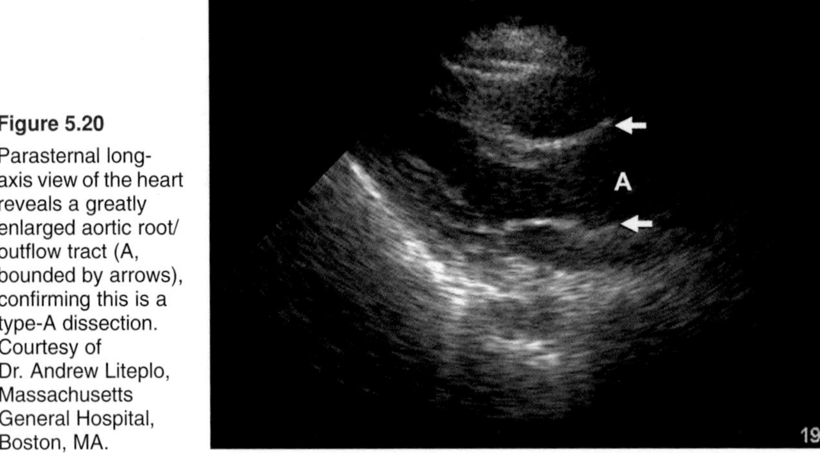

Figure 5.20

Parasternal long-axis view of the heart reveals a greatly enlarged aortic root/outflow tract (A, bounded by arrows), confirming this is a type-A dissection. Courtesy of Dr. Andrew Liteplo, Massachusetts General Hospital, Boston, MA.

dilated aortic root as seen in Figure 5.20), the physician should have a very high suspicion for aortic dissection. Immediate consultation and definitive imaging should be arranged.

Sample clinical protocol

A sample protocol for incorporating ultrasound into the evaluation for AAA is detailed in Figure 5.21. Note that the test is most useful in a stable patient when AAA is excluded via a technically adequate (i.e., complete) study, or in an unstable patient in whom a large AAA is found. Further imaging is warranted for any technically limited bedside study, or in a stable patient without a clear diagnosis.

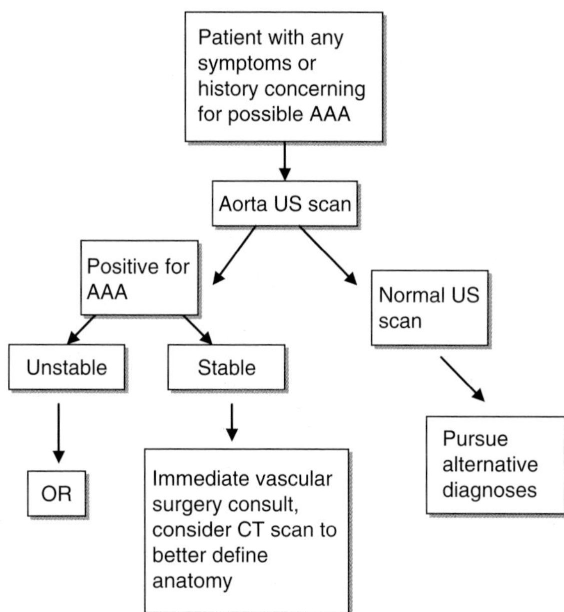

Figure 5.21
Sample clinical protocol for the evaluation of suspected AAA.

Literature review

Reference	Methods	Results	Notes
Plummer *et al.* 1998 [1]	Randomized patients to US vs. standard of care diagnostics and compared time to diagnosis and operating room (OR).	US improved time to diagnosis (5.4 min vs. 83 min) and improved time to disposition for patients requiring operative intervention (12 min vs. 90 min).	Provided support for improved diagnosis and disposition for patients with symptomatic AAA who received bedside US.
Limet *et al.* 1991 [4]	Analysis of expansion rate and incidence of rupture in AAA.	AAA < 4 cm have 2% per year risk of rupture, 4–5 cm have 3–12% per year risk of rupture, and > 5 cm have 25–41% per year risk of rupture.	Further defines diameter at which AAA needs urgent vs. emergent treatment.
Tayal *et al.* 2003 [6]	Prospective study of accuracy and outcome of bedside US in diagnosis of AAA.	29/125 patients diagnosed with AAA over 2 years. PPV 93% (27/29) and NPV 100%. Immediate OR for 10/27 without confirmatory study – all with intraoperative confirmation of AAA.	PPV and NPV numbers provide strong support for emergency department (ED) US as AAA screening test. Additional data for more rapid disposition (10/27 for immediate OR).

Reference	Methods	Results	Notes
Costantino *et al.* 2005 [9]	Accuracy comparison of emergency physician (EP)-performed US vs. CT, MRI, or operative findings.	EP-performed US had a sensitivity of 94% and a specificity of 100%. Regression of EP-performed US AAA diameter was strongly correlated ($r^2 = 0.92$).	More evidence supporting the accuracy of US performed by emergency physicians.
Salen *et al.* 2003 [10]	Prospective observational study of test characteristics of EP-performed bedside US in diagnosis of AAA. If AAA found by EP, radiology US was performed.	125 suspected AAA cases. PPV 75% compared to radiology US, MRI, or laparotomy (6 true positives, 2 false positives by EPs).	Gold standard only applied to patients who screened positive for AAA by emergency physicians.

References

1. Plummer D, Clinton J, Matthew B. Emergency department ultrasound improves time to diagnosis and survival in ruptured abdominal aortic aneurysm [abstract]. *Acad Emerg Med* 1998; **5**: 417.
2. Ernst CB. Abdominal aortic aneurysm. *N Engl J Med* 1993; **328**: 1167–72.
3. Cronenwett JL, Murphy TF, Zelenock GB, *et al.* Actuarial analysis of variables associated with rupture of small abdominal aortic aneurysms. *Surgery* 1985; **98**: 472–83.
4. Limet R, Sakalihassan N, Albert A. Determination of the expansion rate and incidence of rupture of abdominal aortic aneurysms. *J Vasc Surg* 1991; **14**: 540–8.
5. Ouriel K, Green RM, Donayre C, *et al.* An evaluation of new methods of expressing aortic aneurysm size: relationship to rupture. *J Vasc Surg* 1992; **15**: 12–18.
6. Tayal VS, Graf CD, Gibbs MA. Prospective study of accuracy and outcome of emergency ultrasound for abdominal aortic aneurysm over two years. *Acad Emerg Med* 2003; **10**: 867–71.
7. LaRoy LL, Cormier PJ, Matalon TA, *et al.* Imaging of abdominal aortic aneurysms. *AJR Am J Roentgenol* 1989; **152**: 785–90.
8. Pleumeekers HJ, Hoes AW, Mulder PG, *et al.* Differences in observer variability of ultrasound measurements of the proximal and distal abdominal aorta. *J Med Screen* 1998; **5**: 104–8.
9. Costantino TG, Bruno EC, Handly N, Dean AJ. Accuracy of emergency medicine ultrasound in the evaluation of abdominal aortic aneurysm. *J Emerg Med* 2005; **29**: 455–60.

10. Salen P, Melanson S, Buro D. ED screening to identify abdominal aortic aneurysms in asymptomatic geriatric patients. *Am J Emerg Med* 2003; **21**: 133–5.
11. Blaivas M, Theodoro D. Frequency of incomplete abdominal aorta visualization by emergency department bedside ultrasound. *Acad Emerg Med* 2004; **11**: 103e5.
12. Moore CL, Holliday RS, Hwang JQ, Osborne MR. Screening for abdominal aortic aneurysm in asymptomatic at-risk patients using emergency ultrasound. *Am J Emerg Med* 2008; **26**: 883–7.
13. Hoffmann B, Bessman ES, Um P, Ding R, McCarthy ML. Successful sonographic visualisation of the abdominal aorta differs significantly among a diverse group of credentialed emergency department providers. *Emerg Med J* 2010 Aug 2 [Epub ahead of print].

6 Renal and bladder ultrasound

Introduction

The kidney and bladder are two of the most sonographically accessible organs. The evidence for using ultrasound to make lifesaving diagnoses in this application is not as apparent as it is for cardiac or aortic ultrasound (except, of course, if flank pain and hydronephrosis are the result of a rapidly expanding AAA – see Chapter 5). Indeed, it is accurate to say that computed tomography (CT) is dramatically more sensitive and specific in detecting ureteral stones and that ultrasound has a very low specificity for identifying ureteral stones [1–4]. However, despite the advantages of CT for nephrolithiasis, there is still a role for ultrasound in evaluating the urinary tract in the emergency setting. In the most straightforward case, ultrasound identification of mild or moderate unilateral hydronephrosis in a patient with known renal colic and normal renal function testing (and a normal aortic screening evaluation) can obviate further radiologic testing. As patients and clinicians become sensitized to the amount of radiation patients are exposed to from repeated CT diagnostic imaging tests, the benefits of a non-ionizing point-of-care test become more obvious. Especially in patients with known renal colic, obviating further radiation exposure by first utilizing bedside ultrasound is currently being evaluated as a new paradigm or standard of care. In addition, patients who have relative contraindications to radiation exposure (pregnancy, pediatric patients) can also have ureteral obstruction evaluated by ultrasound. Renal ultrasonography easily and rapidly obtains evidence for or against high-grade obstruction, thereby expediting decisions regarding management and disposition [5,6].

In addition, determination of bladder volume is another important indication for urinary tract ultrasound. Before catheterizing a patient to evaluate for postrenal obstruction or urinary retention secondary to neurologic events, an ultrasound can give an estimation of bladder volume and indicate whether catheterization is even necessary. Pediatric patients can also have bladder volume evaluated with ultrasound. If they have a contracted bladder, catheterization or suprapubic taps should be postponed until after hydration to ensure invasive procedures are done with maximal chance of success [7]. Finally, ultrasound-guided suprapubic taps have shown fewer complications and superior outcomes [8]. Pediatric applications are discussed in more detail in Chapter 13.

Focused questions for renal and bladder ultrasound

The questions for renal and bladder ultrasound are relatively straightforward:

1. Is there hydronephrosis?
2. Is the bladder distended?

Anatomy

The renal cortex has a homogeneous appearance on ultrasound, and it is slightly less echogenic (less bright) than the neighboring liver in normal physiologic states. The renal medulla, which forms the pyramids that point toward the pelvis of the kidney, is significantly less echogenic than the surrounding cortex. In some patients, the renal pyramids are surprisingly prominent and hypoechoic. Do not mistake such pyramids for renal cysts or hydronephrosis. The pyramids are discrete anechoic spaces that do not connect with each other or the renal pelvis (Figure 6.1). The renal pelvis appears as an echogenic or brighter central complex within the kidney. The hyperechoic stripe surrounding the kidney represents Gerota's fascia. Both kidneys are ordinarily 9–12 cm in length, 4–5 cm in width, and within 2 cm of each other in terms of size (Figure 6.2). Because the spleen is smaller than the liver, the left kidney will be positioned more superior and posterior than the right kidney.

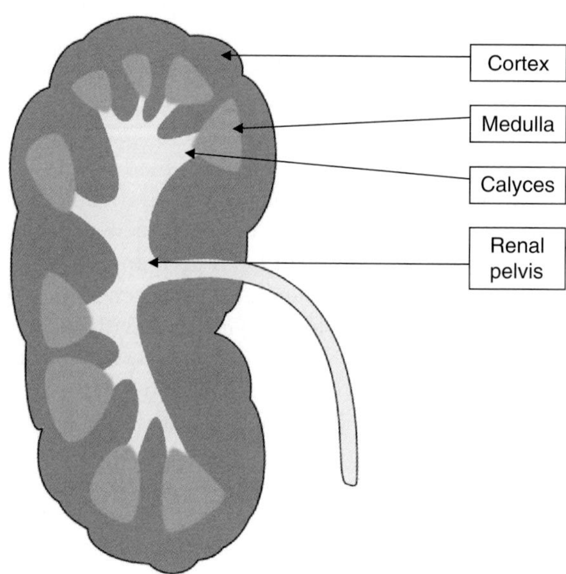

Figure 6.1
Renal anatomy. Image courtesy of Dr. Manuel Colon, Hospital of the University of Puerto Rico, Carolina, PR.

(A)

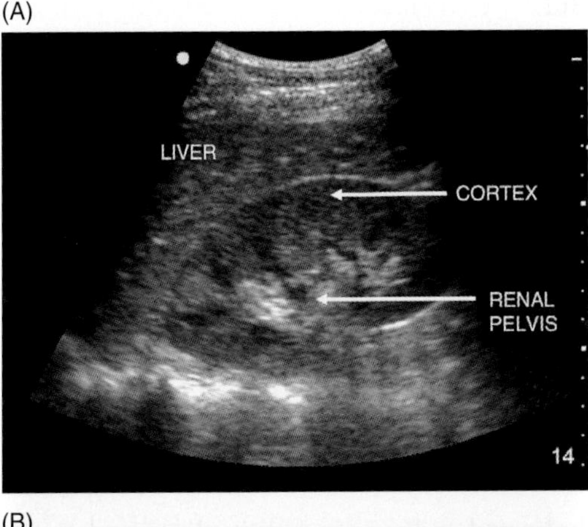

(B)

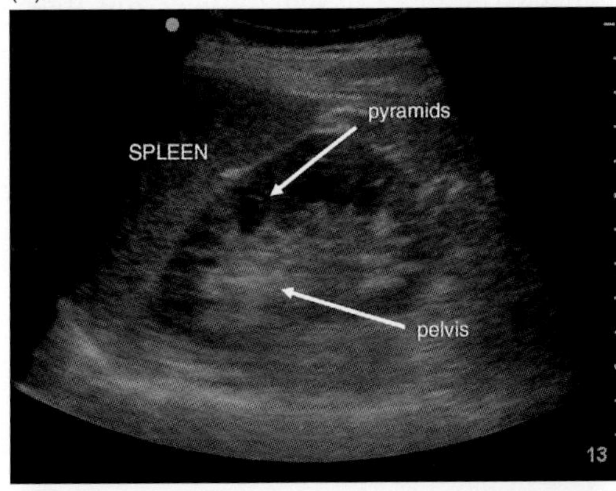

(C)

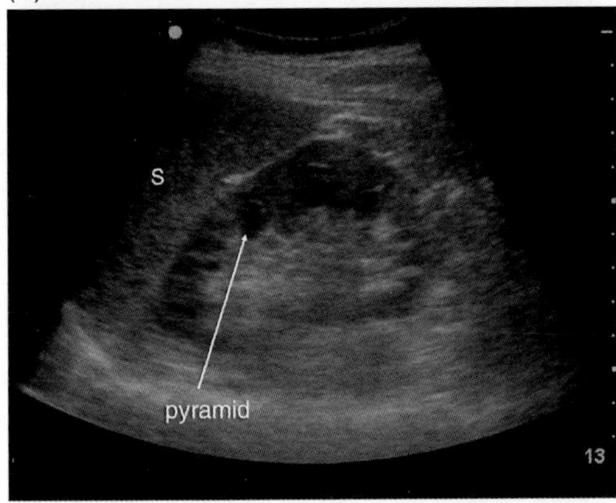

Figure 6.2

Three normal longitudinal views of the kidney. Prominent pyramids are seen in both *B* and *C*, but as the collecting system is still echogenic or brighter, and thus not dilated, these pictures show no hydronephrosis.

The normal ureter is not ordinarily visualized in the bedside scan, but when it is dilated it can sometimes be seen. It is often easier to identify the ureter in the transverse view.

Technique

Probe selection

The 2–5 MHz transducer is ordinarily used in adults, although good images can often be obtained in thin subjects using a higher-frequency probe.

Views

Images of both affected and unaffected kidneys in longitudinal and transverse planes should be obtained. As with other structures, it is absolutely necessary to carefully fan through the kidneys in both planes to examine the entire parenchyma. Finally, suprapubic transverse and longitudinal views of the bladder complete the urinary tract evaluation.

Although the technique for visualization of the kidneys was discussed in Chapter 2, we review the probe positioning here to reinforce the technique. To visualize the right kidney, begin with the patient in the supine position. Place the transducer along the right mid-axillary line, below the costal margin with the marker toward the patient's head (Figure 6.3A). Move the transducer incrementally from the costal margin to the iliac crest along the mid-axillary line to find the kidney. It will be necessary to rotate/twist the transducer on its vertical axis to obtain the kidney in its maximal length because of the kidney's oblique lie. Once an adequate longitudinal view is obtained, rotate the transducer on its vertical axis 90 degrees to obtain the transverse view. Again, scan the kidney from superior to inferior poles to

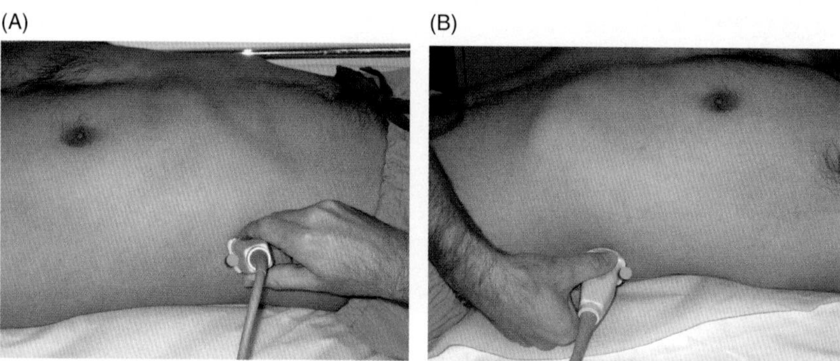

Figure 6.3
Probe positions useful in visualizing (*A*) the right and (*B*) the left kidney.

completely evaluate the parenchyma. When scanning longitudinally be sure to fan anterior to posterior. When scanning transversely fan from the superior to inferior pole.

To visualize the left kidney, the same technique is employed. However, because of interference from air in the stomach and intestine, it is often easier to obtain images using a more posterior window. Begin by placing the transducer along the left posterior axillary line (Figure 6.3B). Again, move the transducer between the costal margin superiorly and the iliac crest inferiorly to find the kidney. As with the right kidney, rotate/twist the transducer to find the kidney's longest axis before scanning through the entire kidney. Do not forget to obtain a transverse window and to fan throughout the transverse plane.

Scanning the left kidney is more difficult because of the left kidney's relatively cephalad positioning, which results in marked obscuration by rib shadows. Having the patient take a prolonged deep inspiration will bring the diaphragm, spleen, and left kidney down and may allow the sonographer to circumvent interfering rib shadows. You may also try positioning the patient in the right lateral decubitus position.

The bladder, which is ideally moderately filled at the time of examination, should be imaged with the transducer placed suprapubically. Again, the bladder should be scanned thoroughly in both longitudinal/sagittal and transverse planes. If your ultrasound machine is equipped with color Doppler technology, it is possible to record the presence or absence of ureteral jets. By using color Doppler techniques on the trigone of the bladder, you may observe a jet of urine entering the bladder (Figure 6.4). Observing

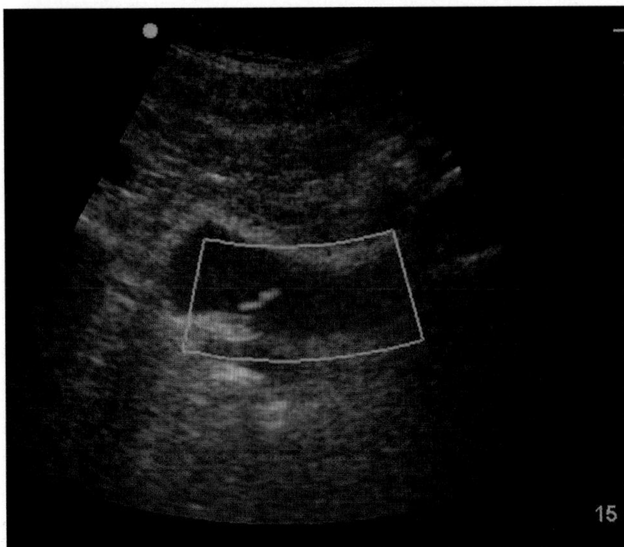

Figure 6.4
Transverse view of a filled bladder at the level of the trigone. Red color doppler flow in the center of the color Doppler field represents a ureteral jet.

bilateral ureteral jets *in a patient with normal hydration* provides evidence against the diagnosis of obstructive uropathy.

Bladder volume estimation

Bladder volume can be estimated by simple formulas that approximate the bladder to either an ellipsoid or a cylinder. For the clinical purposes of determining retention and/or postvoid residuals, these methods have good support in the literature and have good correlation with actual catheterization volumes [9–12]. The difficulty is that slightly different formulas have been used in different studies, and portable ultrasound machines use varying automated volume calculations. Initially, it is instructive to do the calculations by hand to ensure that the automated function is accurate on your machine. The quickest calculation to use (0.75 × width × length × height – see Figure 6.5) is based on research correlating these distance measurements with catheterized volume and seems to have the best correlation factor ($r = 0.983$) [12]. However, other studies have used the following formulas and also had good results: ellipsoid formula, $4/3\ \pi \times r_1 \times r_2 \times r_3$; cylinder formula, $3.14 \times r^2 \times$ height [10,11].

Scanning tips

Trouble with renal scanning

Pyramids versus hydronephrosis?

- Pyramids will be just below the cortex, and the kidney will still have a collapsed and hyperechoic pelvis and collecting system. They also do not connect one to another. Hydronephrosis should connect to a dilated renal pelvis.

Renal cyst versus hydronephrosis?

- Renal cysts are usually located in the cortex or periphery. They are smooth-walled and fluid-filled but do not connect to the pelvis or collecting system.

False positives

- Patients who are pregnant or have benign prostatic hyperplasia can have mild to moderate dilatation of their collecting system because of external compression of the ureters or overdistended bladders, respectively. The hydronephrosis in these cases should resolve after bladder emptying.

(A)

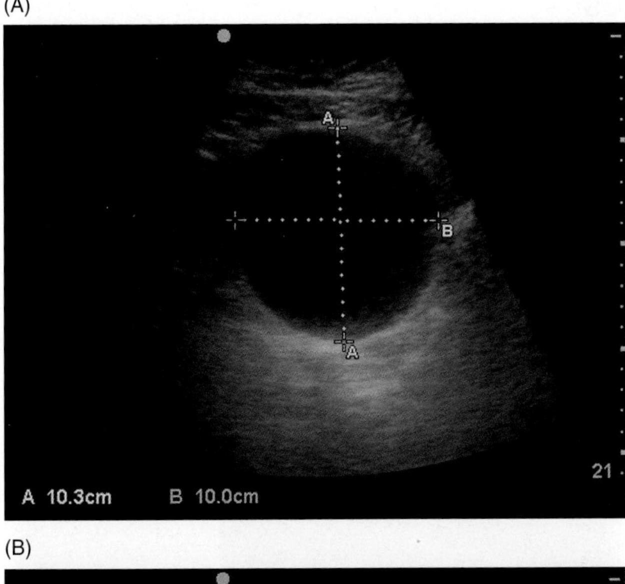

(B)

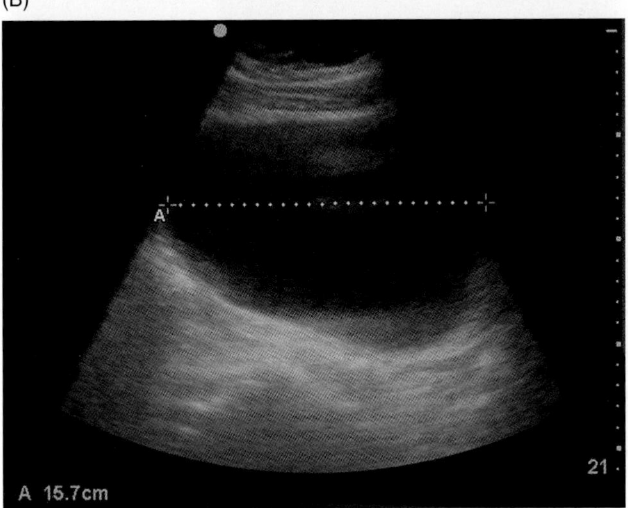

Figure 6.5

Bladder volume estimation: (*A*) measured width and height on transverse view; (*B*) measured depth on longitudinal view.

False negatives

- Patients who are severely dehydrated can have falsely negative renal scans for hydronephrosis. If there is clinical concern, a repeat renal scan should be done after some intravenous hydration.

Normal images

Figures 6.6–6.8 show examples of normal renal ultrasound scans.

(A)

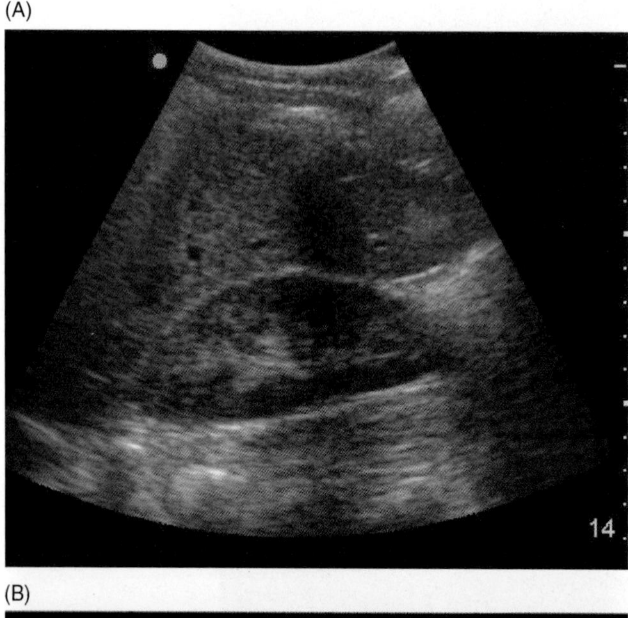

(B)

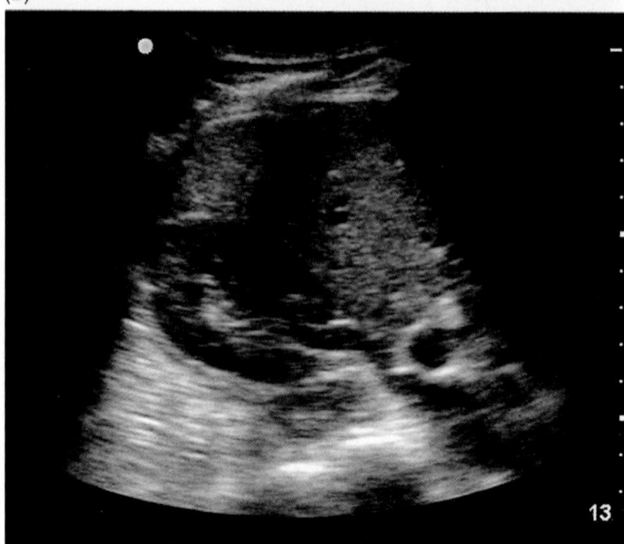

Figure 6.6

(A) Normal longitudinal view of the right kidney. Morison's pouch is well visualized here, too.
(B) Transverse view of the kidney.

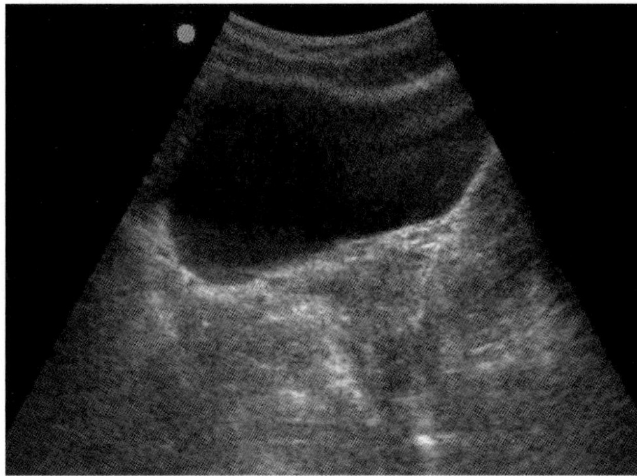

Figure 6.7
Transverse view of the bladder with no fluid seen outside the bladder wall.

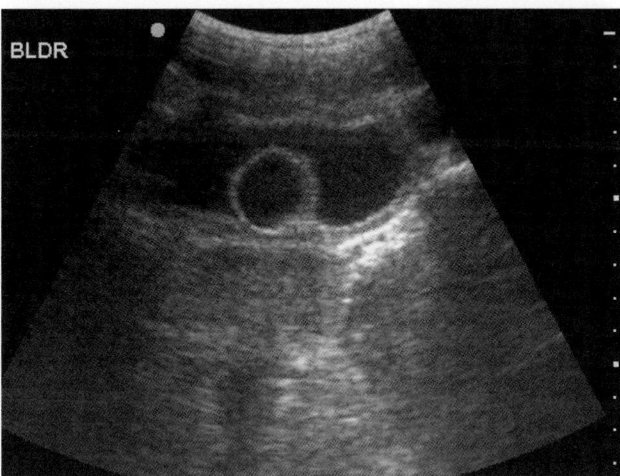

Figure 6.8
The bulb of the Foley catheter is visualized on ultrasound with a partially decompressed bladder.

Abnormal images

Hydronephrosis

According to Grainger and Allison's *Diagnostic Radiology* [13], the following grading system is used by radiologists/sonographers:

- Grade I – slight blunting of calyceal fornices
- Grade II – blunting and enlargement of calyceal fornices but easily seen shadows of papillae
- Grade III – rounding of calices with obliteration of papillae
- Grade IV – extreme calyceal ballooning

Figures 6.9–6.11 show images of different grades of hydronephrosis.

Chronic hydronephrosis can cause thinning of the renal medulla. Such distortion of the renal architecture is only seen in long-standing obstruction.

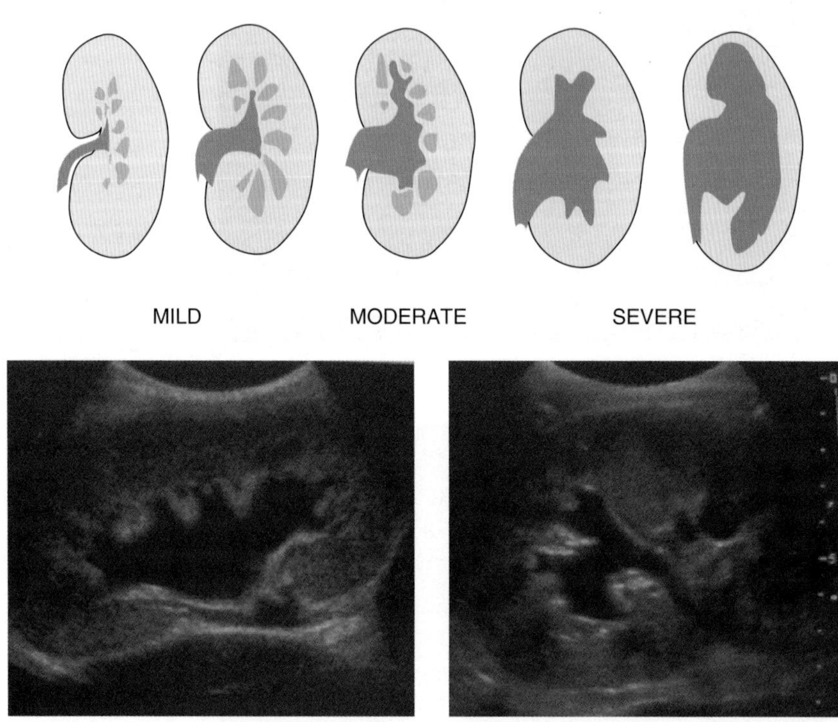

Figure 6.9

Grades of hydronephrosis (*top*). Longitudinal and transverse views of the kidney with moderate hydronephrosis (*bottom*).

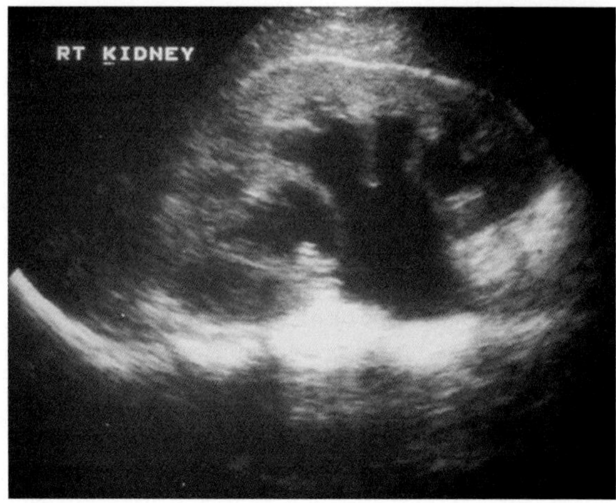

Figure 6.10

Dilated right renal pelvis with splaying of the renal calyces indicative of severe hydronephrosis.

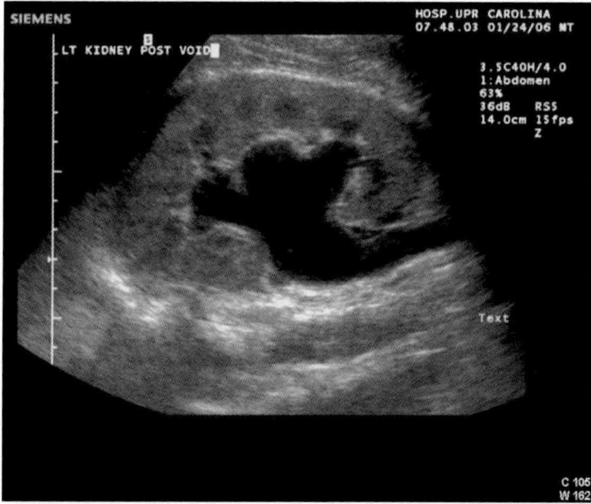

Figure 6.11

Another image of severe hydronephrosis. In this image, the pyramids can be seen as distinct from the dilated renal pelvis. Image courtesy of Dr. Manuel Colon, Hospital of the University of Puerto Rico, Carolina, PR.

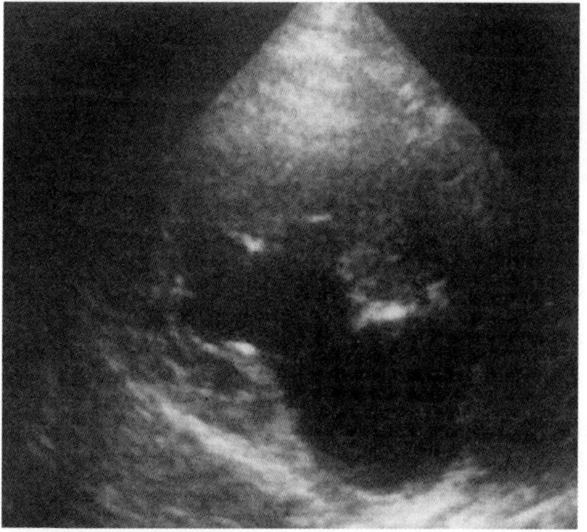

Figure 6.12

A very dilated proximal ureter and renal pelvis.

Bilateral evidence of hydronephrosis is less likely to be caused by two discrete ureteral events than by bladder outlet obstruction.

It is expected that pregnancy and an overdistended bladder cause hydronephrosis – sometimes to a large degree. Another common finding that can be confused with acute obstruction is that of an extrarenal pelvis. This is a developmental variant in which the collecting system lies predominantly outside the kidney.

Generally, in the normally hydrated patient, absence of any evidence of dilatation virtually rules out obstructive nephrolithiasis as the cause of severe pain (Figure 6.12).

Other pathologic images

To review, the focused questions of bedside renal and bladder ultrasound are to assess for the presence of hydronephrosis and to look for bladder volume. The following images of renal and bladder pathology may be seen during bedside screening, but these diagnoses should be made by formal scanning. If seen, these patients should be referred for further imaging either immediately or as an outpatient, depending on their clinical status.

Figure 6.13 shows renal and bladder stones.

Figure 6.14 shows a renal cyst. This is a smooth-walled, anechoic, fluid-filled structure far from the collecting system. The regularity of this structure is reassuring for non-malignant etiologies.

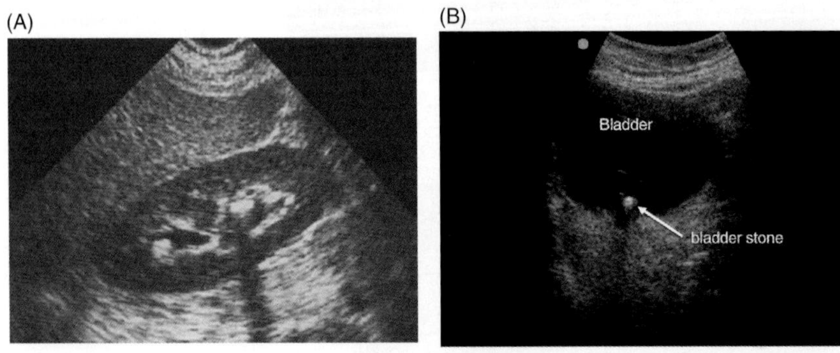

Figure 6.13

(*A*) The shadow of a renal calculus. However, because there is minimal dilatation of the collecting system, this stone is not likely responsible for renal colic. Courtesy of Emergency Ultrasound Division, St. Luke's–Roosevelt Hospital Center, New York, NY. (*B*) A stone in the bladder with shadowing behind.

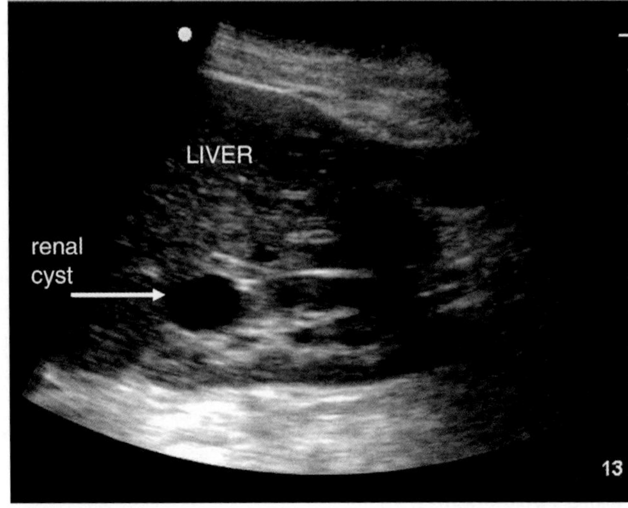

Figure 6.14
Renal cyst.

The kidney visualized in Figure 6.15 is full of irregular cysts. This is a patient with polycystic kidney disease.

As mentioned previously, most kidneys are darker or less echoic than adjacent live parenchyma. When the kidney is brighter or more echoic, it is most likely inflamed and/or infected; this is a marker for acute renal failure [14] (Figure 6.16).

As more bedside ultrasounds are performed, it is increasingly likely that asymptomatic pathology may be uncovered, including the diagnosis of renal cell carcinoma [15] (Figure 6.17A) or bladder cancer (Figure 6.17B). The

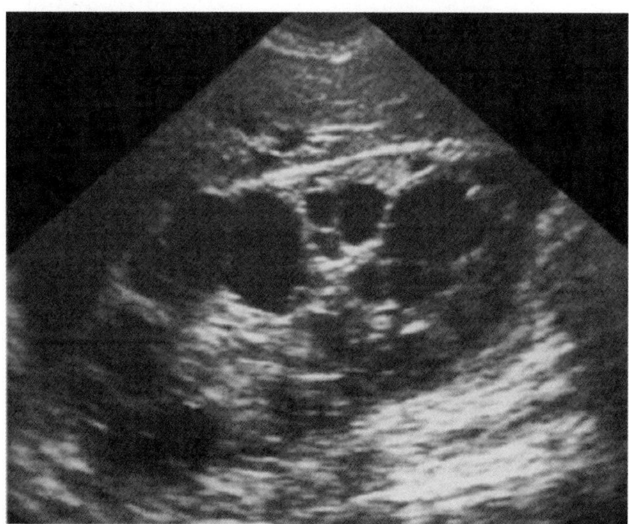

Figure 6.15 Polycystic kidney disease.

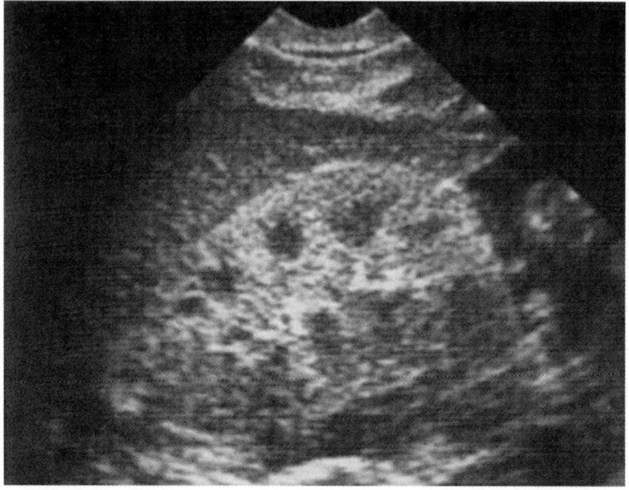

Figure 6.16 Acute renal failure.

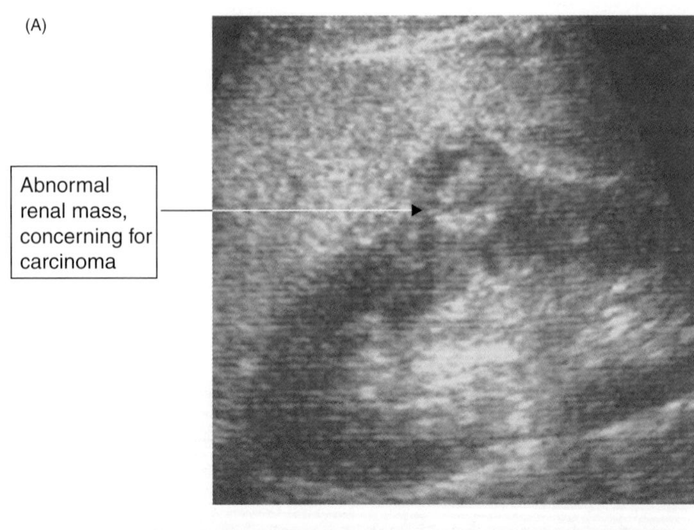

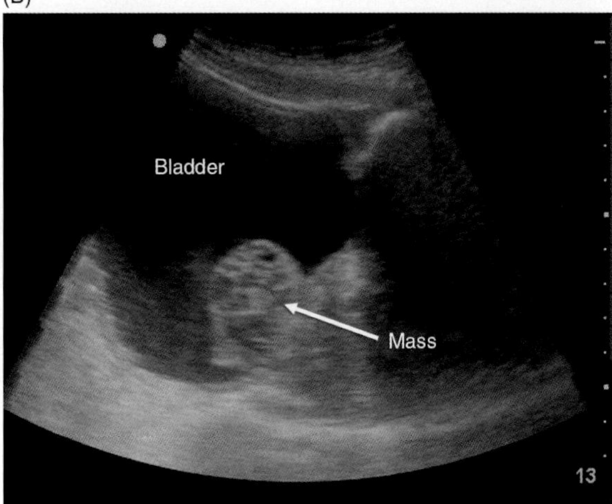

Figure 6.17
(*A*) Renal cell carcinoma.
(*B*) Bladder carcinoma.

important key to remember is that the renal cortex should always be smooth and regular. Whenever irregular masses or distortions are seen, patients should be informed and should have close follow-up with further radiologic imaging. While prostate hypertrophy can also be readily visualized on trans-abdominal ultrasound (Figure 6.18), it is important to remember that this bedside test is *not* sufficient to distinguish benign prostatic hypertrophy from prostate cancer, and patients should all be referred for appropriate follow-up testing.

As always, communication between bedside point-of-care sonographers and patients about the limited nature of the tests is essential. Bedside

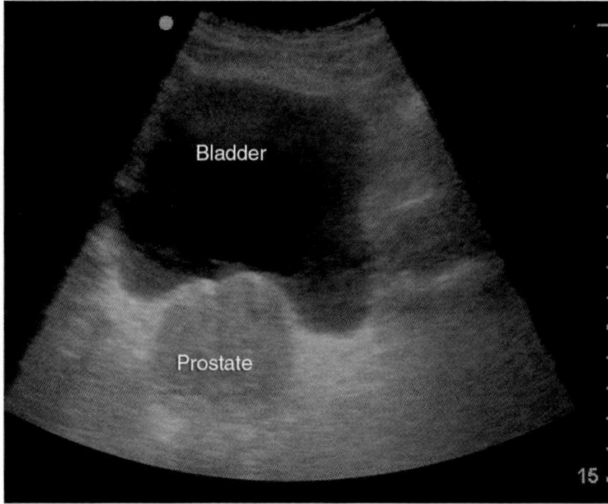

Figure 6.18
Prostate hypertrophy.

ultrasound is designed to answer focused questions. Any abnormality outside this scope of practice should be referred for formal testing.

Sample clinical protocol

Figure 6.19 shows a protocol for the use of renal and bladder ultrasound.

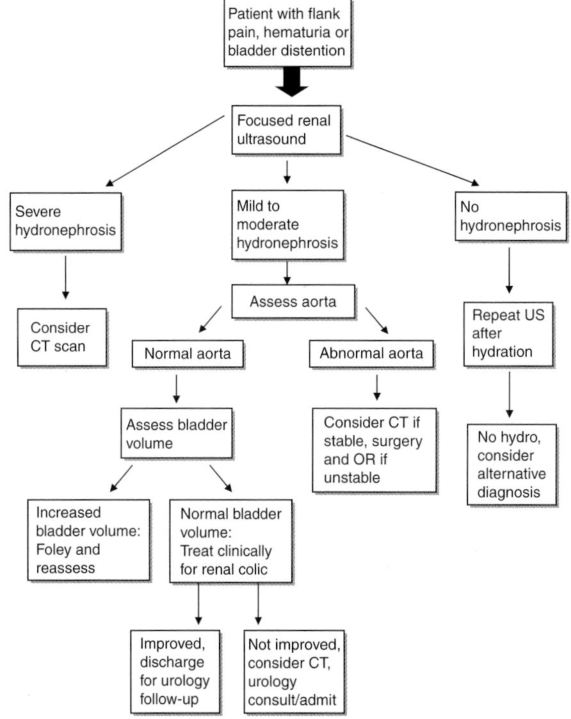

Figure 6.19
Sample clinical protocol.

Literature review

Reference	Methods	Results	Notes
Sheafor *et al.* 2000 [2]	Prospective comparison of helical CT and US in patients with renal colic.	CT much more sensitive in identifying stones (96% vs. 61%). Sensitivity for CT and US comparable in identifying hydronephrosis (100% vs. 92%).	Radiology literature showing advantages of CT but also that US is comparable when looking for hydronephrosis.
Chan 1993 [12]	Compare bladder volume estimations calculated using US with catheterized bladder volumes. Urinary retention suspected clinically.	Correlation of two measurements highly significant ($r = 0.983$).	Provided data supporting ultrasound use in calculating bladder volume.
Gaspari & Horst 2005 [6]	Evaluate sensitivity and specificity of renal US in diagnosing renal colic as compared to helical CT. Impact of hematuria on test characteristics was also evaluated.	In patients with hematuria, US was 87.8% sensitive and 84.8% specific for renal colic (86.8% and 82.4% without hematuria).	Ultrasound shows very good sensitivity and specificity for diagnosing renal colic.
Edmonds *et al.* 2010 [15]	Retrospective chart review of all patients, looking at ultrasound findings and need for urologic intervention.	2/352 patients (0.5%) with normal ultrasound required urologic intervention. 27/418 patients (6%) with ultrasound indicative of ureterolithiasis required intervention.	Patients with suspected renal colic who had a normal ultrasound very rarely required urological intervention.

New directions

One area of potential research for renal bedside ultrasound is assessing the outcomes and number of patients identified with renal cell cancer when performing renal scanning in the emergency department. As Mandavia *et al.* showed [16], incidental cancer identification is not unexpected given the volume of ultrasound scanning that is performed in most major trauma centers. In the future, perhaps patients will be screened for both AAAs and renal cell cancer when they come to the emergency department.

In addition, with increased attention of both the public and clinicians focused on limiting radiation exposure, the diagnostic evaluation of renal colic is primed for re-evaluation [17,18]. Outcome studies looking at ultrasound as an initial point-of-care screening test should assess the safety of this diagnostic strategy for patients and contrast that with cost and radiation exposure for traditional imaging strategies.

References

1. Colistro R, Torreggiani WC, Lyburn ID, *et al.* Unenhanced helical CT in investigation of acute flank pain. *Clin Radiol* 2002; **57**: 435–51.
2. Sheafor DH, Hertzberg BS, Freed KS, *et al.* Nonenhanced helical CT and US in the emergency evaluation of patients with renal colic: prospective comparison. *Radiology* 2000; **217**: 792–7.
3. Fowler KA, Locken JA, Duchesne JH, Williamson MR. US for detecting renal calculi with nonenhanced CT as a reference standard. *Radiology* 2002; **222**: 109–13.
4. Smith RC, Verga M, McCarthy S, Rosenfield AT. Diagnosis of acute flank pain: value of unenhanced helical CT. *AJR Am J Roentgenol* 1996; **166**: 97–101.
5. Mandavia DP, Aragona J, Chan L, Chan D, Henderson SO. Ultrasound training for emergency physicians: a prospective study. *Acad Emerg Med* 2000; **7**: 1008–14.
6. Gaspari RJ, Horst K. Emergency ultrasound and urinalysis in the evaluation of flank pain. *Acad Emerg Med* 2005; **12**: 1180–4.
7. Gochman RF, Karasic RB, Heller MB. Use of portable ultrasound to assist urine collection by suprapubic aspiration. *Ann Emerg Med* 1991; **20**: 631–5.
8. Kiernan SC, Pinckert TL, Keszler M. Ultrasound guidance of suprapubic bladder aspiration in neonates. *J Pediatr* 1993; **123**: 789–91.
9. Kiely EA, Hartnell GG, Gibson RN, Williams G. Measurement of bladder volume by real-time ultrasound. *Br J Urol* 1987; **60**: 33–5.
10. Roehrborn CG, Peters PC. Can transabdominal ultrasound estimation of postvoiding residual replace catheterization? *Urology* 1988; **31**: 445–9.
11. Ireton RC, Krieger JN, Cardenas DD, *et al.* Bladder volume determination using a dedicated, portable ultrasound scanner. *J Urology* 1990; **143**: 909–11.
12. Chan H. Noninvasive bladder volume measurement. *J Neurosci Nurs* 1993; **25**: 309–12.
13. Cronan JJ. Urinary obstruction. In Grainger RG, Allison DJ, Adam A, Dixon AK (ed.), *Diagnostic Radiology: a Textbook of Medical Imaging*, 4th edn. London: Churchill Livingstone; 1997: 1593–613.
14. Kawashima A, LeRoy AJ. Radiologic evaluation of patients with renal infections. *Infect Dis Clin North Am* 2003; **17**: 433–56.
15. Edmonds ML, Yan JW, Sedran RJ, McLeod SL, Theakston KD. The utility of renal ultrasonography in the diagnosis of renal colic in emergency department patients. *CJEM* 2010; **12**: 201–6.

16. Mandavia DP, Pregerson B, Henderson SO. Ultrasonography of flank pain in the emergency department: renal cell carcinoma as a diagnostic concern. *J Emerg Med* 2000; **18**: 83–6.
17. Smith-Bindman R, Lipson J, Marcus R, *et al.* Radiation dose associated with common computed tomography examinations and the associated lifetime attributable risk of cancer. *Arch Intern Med* 2009; **169**: 2078–86.
18. Griffey RT, Sodickson A. Cumulative radiation exposure and cancer risk estimates for emergency department patients undergoing repeat or multiple CT. *AJR Am J Roentgenol* 2009; **192**: 887–92.

7 Gallbladder ultrasound

Introduction

Gallbladder disease is well suited for emergency ultrasound investigations. Use of diagnostic ultrasound frequently leads to either confirmation of a presumptive diagnosis or rapid narrowing of the differential diagnoses. However, if biliary ultrasound findings are equivocal or conflict with initial clinical impressions, the emergency physician should be reminded that formal studies or other imaging modalities may be complementary. In this chapter, the application of bedside ultrasonography in the evaluation of the gallbladder is discussed.

Focused questions for gallbladder ultrasound

As with all emergency bedside ultrasound, it is important to focus on a few key questions while scanning. In gallbladder ultrasound, these questions are:

1. Are there gallstones?
2. Does the patient have a sonographic Murphy sign?

It is also useful to know the following:

3. Is the common bile duct dilated?
4. Is the anterior wall thickened?
5. Is there pericholecystic fluid?

However, the first two questions are far and away the most helpful and diagnostic [1,2].

Anatomy

It is important to remember that the gallbladder is not a fixed organ, so it can move to a variety of locations in the right upper quadrant (Figure 7.1). The gallbladder neck does have a fixed relationship to the main lobar fissure and the portal vein. The main lobar fissure connects the right portal vein to the gallbladder neck, and the fissure can be traced between the two (Figure 7.2). Another anatomic relationship that is reliable is that the bile duct is always anterior to the portal vein. Moreover, ducts appear to have brighter, more echogenic walls than veins or arteries on ultrasound, because they are fibrous and thicker than the thin walls of portal vessels or hepatic veins.

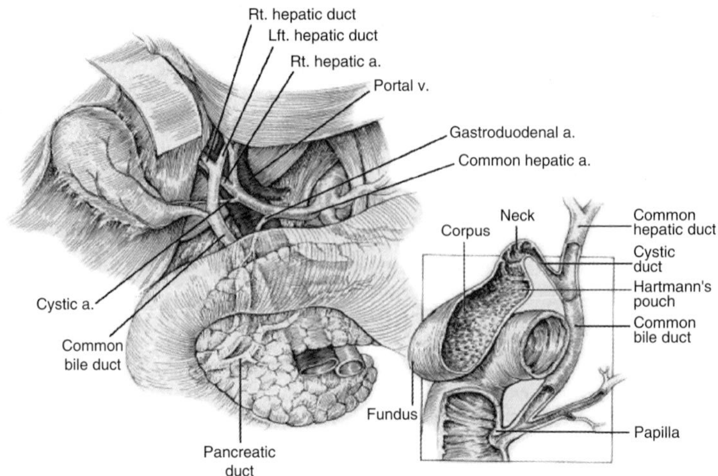

Figure 7.1

Gallbladder anatomy. Reproduced with permission from Townsend CM, Beauchamp DR, Evers MB, Mattox KL, Sabiston DC (eds.). In *Sabiston Textbook of Surgery*, 16th edn. Philadelphia, PA: Saunders; 2001: 1077, Figure 50–1.

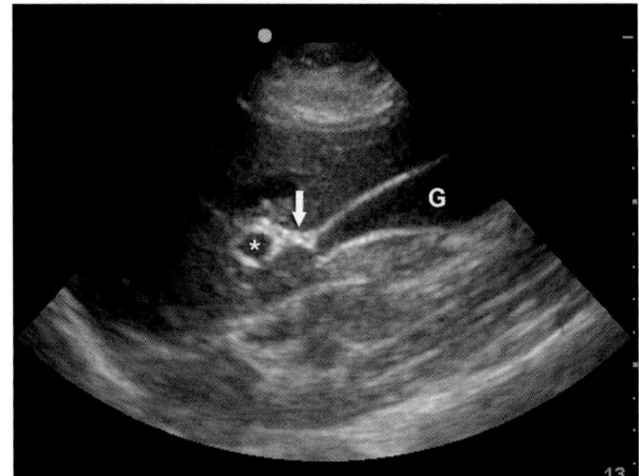

Figure 7.2

Relationship of gallbladder (G) and portal vein (*) with main lobar fissure (arrow).

Technique

Probe selection

When scanning the gallbladder, the curvilinear or abdominal probe with the curved footprint is most commonly used. Occasionally, a microconvex or phased-array probe with a smaller footprint is used to image a gallbladder located posterior to the ribs. The frequency range for both probe choices is usually 2.5–5.0 MHz.

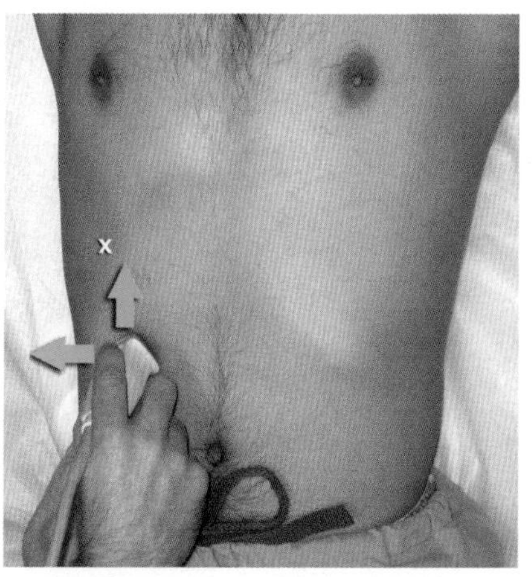

Figure 7.3
Probe positioning in gallbladder scanning. Transverse and longitudinal planes are illustrated (probe marker should be oriented toward green arrows) as well as one possible intercostal approach (X).

Views

Usually the patient is in the supine position, but the left lateral decubitus or upright sitting positions can be used in difficult cases.

Place the probe under the right costal margin, directed toward the right shoulder with the probe marker toward the patient's head (Figure 7.3). Sweep along the costal margin until an image of the gallbladder is obtained. If you are experiencing difficulty, you can have the patient take and hold a deep breath in order to bring the gallbladder down below the rib margin. If you continue to have difficulty, try placing the patient in the left lateral decubitus position.

An alternative approach is to hold the probe in a transverse view (marker toward the patient's right) at the costal margin in the mid-clavicular line. The probe is then tilted cephalad and caudad to locate the gallbladder. It is useful for the patient to hold a deep breath in this approach as well, or the probe can be placed in between the ribs above the costal margin in order to use the liver as a window and avoid bowel gas.

If the gallbladder still cannot be visualized (and it has been confirmed that it was never removed!), a third technique may be helpful. Begin by visualizing any portal vein tributary within the liver parenchyma. These are recognizable by their bright white walls (in contrast to hepatic vein tributaries, which have very little wall echogenicity). Trace the portal vein tributary back to the region where the left and right portal veins merge into the main portal vein. This region is very close to where the neck of the gallbladder should be visible. This anatomic relationship is simplified in Figure 7.4. In a transverse plane, fan cephalad and caudad with the probe; the right and left portal veins should be visualized merging and splitting as the probe moves, and nearby the gallbladder neck should be seen.

The next step is to obtain a true longitudinal view of the gallbladder. This is done by rotating the probe on its axis. Once this is done, try to demonstrate

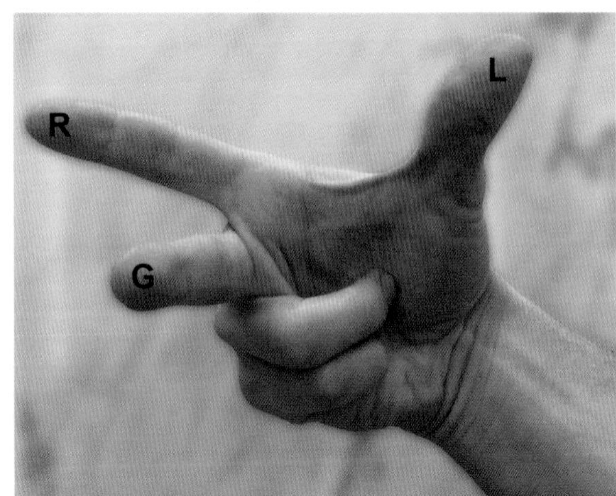

Figure 7.4

The position of your fingers can serve to illustrate the relative positions of the right portal vein (R), gallbladder (G), and left portal vein (L).

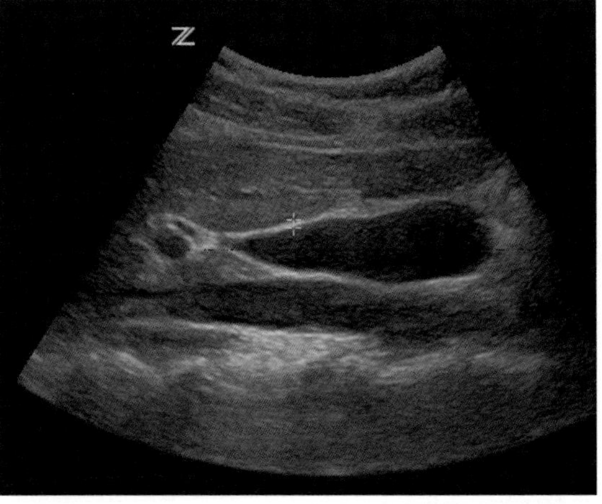

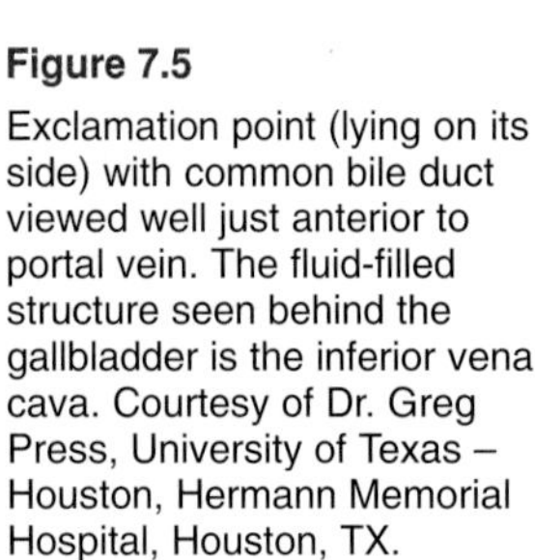

Figure 7.5

Exclamation point (lying on its side) with common bile duct viewed well just anterior to portal vein. The fluid-filled structure seen behind the gallbladder is the inferior vena cava. Courtesy of Dr. Greg Press, University of Texas – Houston, Hermann Memorial Hospital, Houston, TX.

the relationship with the portal triad. When you obtain a long-axis view of the gallbladder, main lobar fissure, and right portal vein, it will take on the appearance of an exclamation point (Figure 7.5). Obtaining this view helps confirm that the structure you are visualizing is indeed the gallbladder and not a loop of bowel, duodenum, or the inferior vena cava (IVC).

With a view of this characteristic exclamation point, gentle manipulation can reveal the common bile duct (CBD) – two bright/hyperechoic lines anterior to the portal vein. In some cases, the CBD and hepatic artery can be distinguished using color-flow Doppler. This can be helpful, because the hepatic artery and portal vein will light up, showing the blood flow within. The common bile duct will remain dark (i.e., no flow – Figures 7.6 and 7.7).

Next, scan the gallbladder in multiple longitudinal and transverse planes. It is important to fan through the entire gallbladder in a longitudinal and

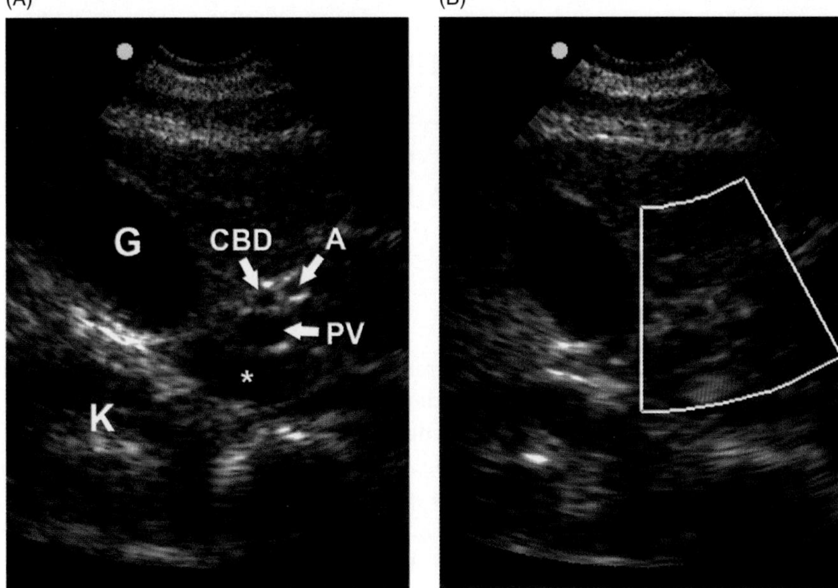

Figure 7.6

(*A*) The portal triad of common bile duct (CBD), hepatic artery (A), and portal vein (PV) is visible near the gallbladder (G) and superficial to the inferior vena cava (*). The kidney (K) is also visible. (*B*) The same image with Doppler flow demonstrated in all vessels and not within common bile duct.

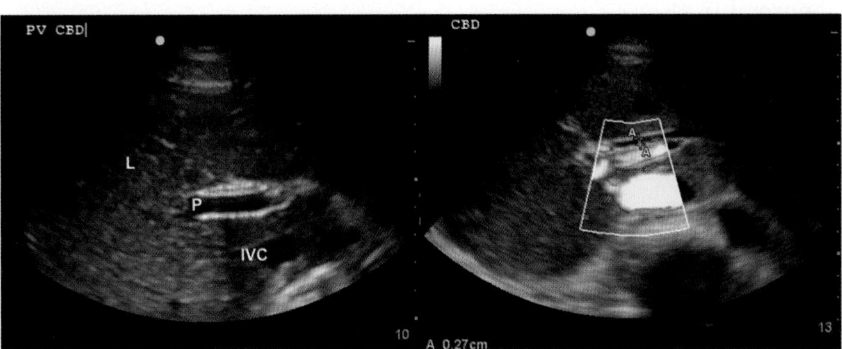

Figure 7.7

Longitudinal view of portal vein (P) within liver (L) and common bile duct (calipers, *right*). Note the lack of Doppler flow in the common bile duct, compared to the portal vein and inferior vena cava (IVC).

transverse plane to make sure you are not missing any stones. Often, the shadowing artifact is your only tip-off that a stone is present – even if you cannot see the white reflective wall of the stone itself. Follow the shadow, and you can usually find the stone.

Finally, if evaluating for acute cholecystitis, find the fundus of the gallbladder and use the probe tip to compress the fundus to assess the presence or absence of a "sonographic Murphy sign." This is probably the most specific sign of inflammation, and the technical challenge is to make sure that you are below the costal margin so that the probe pressure is directly compressing the fundus and not pushing on the ribs. A true sonographic Murphy sign shows deformation of the fundus with compression.

Measurements

As mentioned previously, two measurements are important when evaluating the gallbladder: the anterior gallbladder wall and the common bile duct.

A gallbladder wall that is thickened is a sign of inflammation. However, this is a non-specific finding, and many other pathologic processes, as well as a postprandial gallbladder, can give you falsely elevated measurements (Table 7.1). However, a complete exam does include this measurement. It is important that you measure the wall of the anterior gallbladder surface because of the acoustic enhancement artifact mentioned in Chapter 1 (shown again in Figure 7.8). Because sound waves travel through a fluid-filled structure, no attenuation occurs. Thus, when those sound waves hit the back of the gallbladder, they will be so strong that they will obscure an accurate picture of the wall thickness. For gallbladder wall thickness, greater than 3 mm is abnormal [3,4].

Table 7.1 Differential for thickened gallbladder wall [3,4]

Postprandial
Renal failure
Ascites
Hepatitis
Hypoalbuminemia
HIV/AIDS
Adenomyomatosis
Multiple myeloma
Cholecystitis
Congestive heart failure

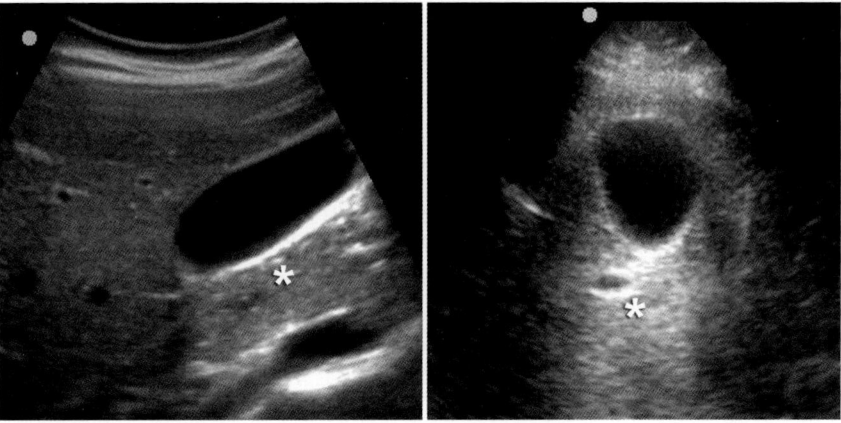

Figure 7.8

Posterior acoustic enhancement (area around asterisk) distal to the anechoic gallbladder, in two views. For more detailed explanation of this phenomenon, see Chapter 1.

Table 7.2 Common bile duct diameters [5]

CBD	Implication
2–5 mm	normal range
6–8 mm	clinical correlation required
6 mm	11% normal subjects
7 mm	4% normal subjects
>8 mm	abnormal

A common bile duct that is dilated is evidence of obstruction. This is the second measurement required for a complete evaluation. The common bile duct is typically less than 6 mm in transverse diameter [5]. The CBD diameter should be measured from inner wall to inner wall. The diameter can increase with age, and some authors have recommended that the diameter should be less than one-tenth of the patient's age. In patients who have had a cholecystectomy, the CBD may normally range up to 1 cm [5]. The range of CBD diameters and their implications is shown in Table 7.2.

Biliary obstruction, regardless of the etiology, will be demonstrated by a dilated biliary tree. Dilatation of the extrahepatic ducts implies CBD obstruction. This can eventually lead to intrahepatic duct dilatation. (Note that dilatation of the intrahepatic ducts *alone* suggests obstruction within the common hepatic duct or more proximal).

Scanning tips

Trouble with gallbladder scanning

Rib shadow in the way?

- Try angling the probe obliquely to sneak in between the ribs.
- Have the patient take a deep breath to lower the diaphragm and bring the gallbladder lower in the abdomen below the ribs.

Can't see the gallbladder at all?

- Try having the patient roll onto his or her left side to bring the gallbladder more anterior in the peritoneal cavity, or if the patient is sitting up have him or her lean forward.
- One unorthodox view is to have the patient get on his or her hands and knees and scan the abdomen this way so gravity works in your favor to pull the gallbladder toward the anterior abdominal wall.
- It is always easier to see the gallbladder if the patient has been NPO, because this causes the gallbladder to dilate. If feasible, you can wait for an hour to see if the dilating gallbladder will be easier to find.
- If any liver parenchyma is visible, try to trace the portal vein tributaries back to the main portal vein as described in the text. The gallbladder will reliably be located near the portal vein at this point. This technique is analogous to tracing retinal vessels back toward the optic disc in the eye exam.

Can't find the common bile duct?

- Have the patient take a deep breath or change position. Sometimes this makes things easier to find.
- If the patient has gallstones and has a sonographic Murphy sign, you have done your job with bedside ultrasound and do not need to spend more than a few minutes trying to confirm ductal dilatation.
- Use color Doppler to help distinguish the hepatic artery and portal vein from the common bile duct.

Unsure if the patient has a sonographic Murphy sign?

- Make sure that you are not pressing directly on the ribs and causing pain that way.
- Have the patient take a breath to see if you can get the fundus below the costal margin.

Object in the gallbladder isn't shadowing?

- Increase the probe frequency. Sometimes higher-frequency sound waves make shadowing more obvious.
- Move the patient. If the object does not respond to gravity, it is likely a polyp (or a tumor), and further imaging should be arranged.

Normal images

Figures 7.9–7.11 are examples of normal gallbladder anatomy and normal gallbladder ultrasound scans.

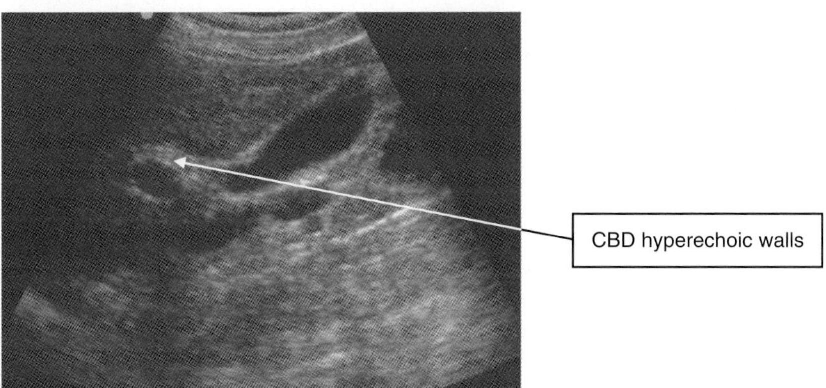

Figure 7.9
Normal gallbladder scan.

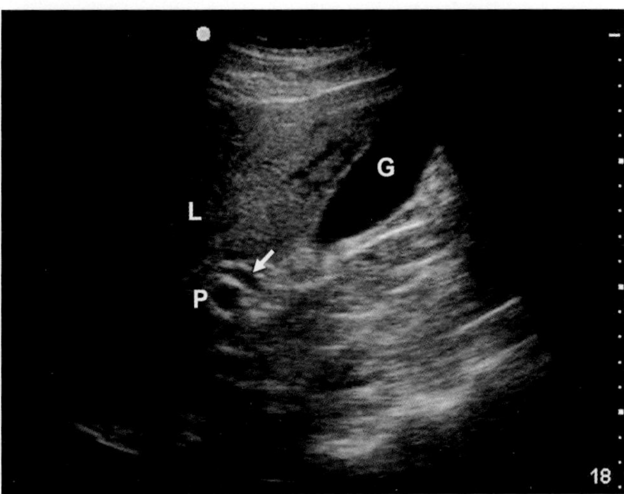

Figure 7.10
Normal gallbladder (G). Note the common bile duct (arrow) just anterior to portal vein (P), deep to liver (L).

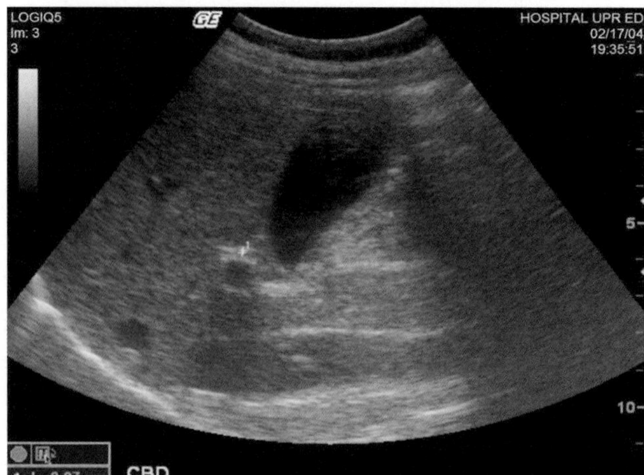

Figure 7.11
The common bile duct (calipers) is identified superficial to the portal vein

Abnormal images

Cholelithiasis

Cholelithiasis is the presence of gallstones within the gallbladder. This is distinct from the presence of inflammation of the gallbladder due to gallstones (cholecystitis – see below).

Gallstones appear as echogenic foci with acoustic shadowing (Figures 7.12–7.15). (Note that shadowing may be absent in gallstones that are <4 mm in diameter.) Most will layer in the most dependent portion of the gallbladder and will move when the patient is repositioned – unless they are impacted or are of high cholesterol content.

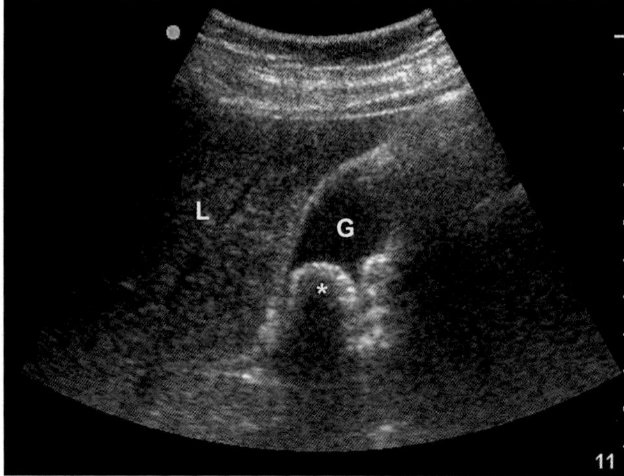

Figure 7.12
Large gallstone (*) within gallbladder (G). Liver (L) is visible on the left of the screen.

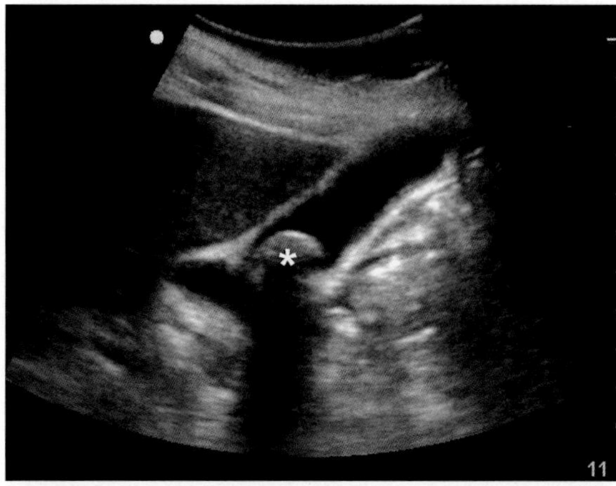

Figure 7.13
Large stone (*) in gallbladder neck.

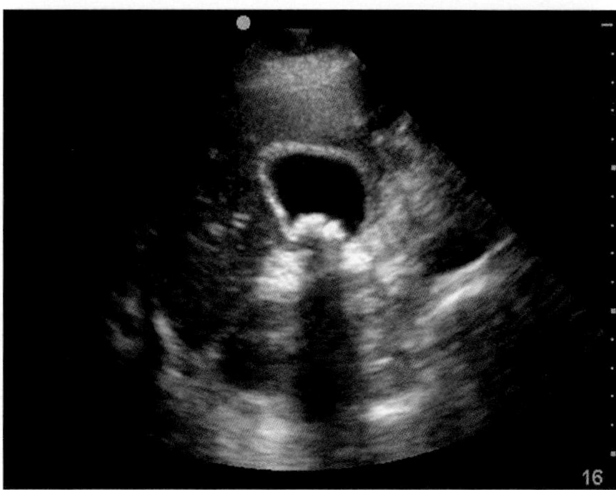

Figure 7.14
Transverse view of gallbladder with stones and shadowing.

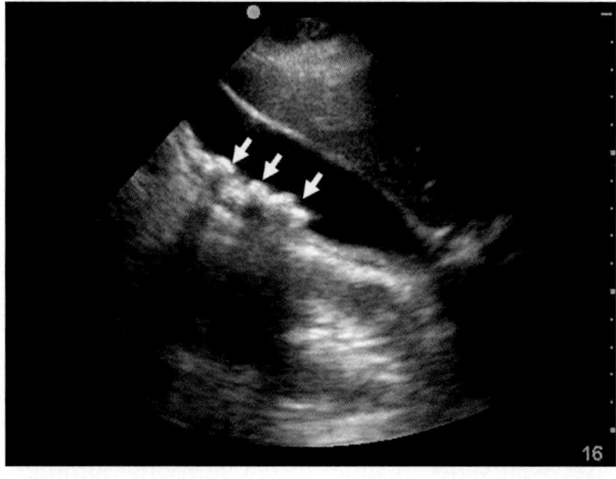

Figure 7.15
Longitudinal view of gallbladder with multiple small stones (arrows) and shadowing.

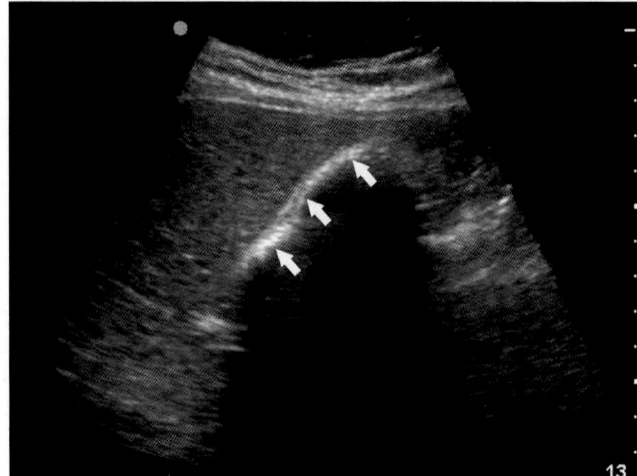

Figure 7.16
Wall-echo-shadow (WES) sign. The anterior wall of the gallbladder (and leading edge of gallstones) is noted with small arrows.

One distinct finding is the wall-echo-shadow (WES) sign, which can be seen in gallstone-filled gallbladders (Figure 7.16) [6]. It is characterized by the following:

- Anterior echogenic line within the near wall of the gallbladder
- An anechoic stripe representing bile
- A hyperechoic line representing stone
- A posterior acoustic shadow

Cholecystitis

Cholecystitis is inflammation of the gallbladder caused by obstruction of the draining ducts. Most commonly, this inflammation is caused by gallstones, but it can also be caused by sludge or tumors. The danger of this inflammation is that obstructed bile is highly susceptible to infection; thus, cholecystitis is usually treated and cured by surgery to remove the gallbladder (cholecystectomy) [7]. Common sonographic findings include gallbladder wall thickening (Figure 7.17), pericholecystic fluid (Figure 7.18), or multiple findings (Figure 7.19). Keep in mind that the presence of ascites can lead to sonographic findings of pericholecystic fluid as well as a thickened gallbladder wall (Figure 7.20).

Ralls *et al.* demonstrated that finding gallstones and a sonographic Murphy sign on bedside ultrasound had a positive predictive value of 92.2% for diagnosing cholecystitis [1]. Negative findings (no stones, no sonographic Murphy) were associated with a negative predictive value of 95.2%. This is important because it gives literature support to the goal-directed study idea and removes some of the diagnostic insensitivity of the common bile duct and anterior gallbladder wall signs. A more recent study by Summers

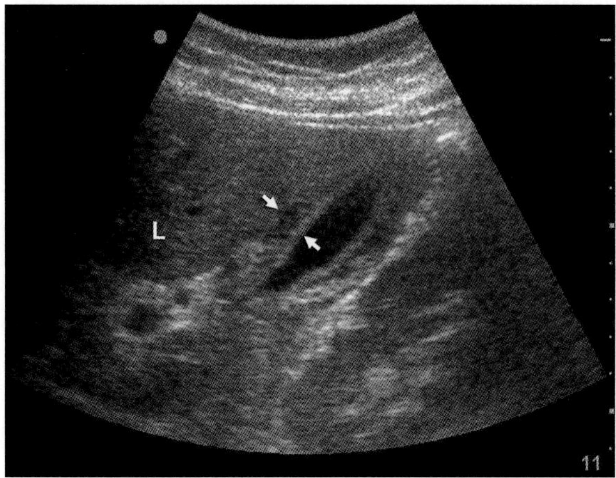

Figure 7.17

Thickened gallbladder wall (measured between arrows) within liver (L).

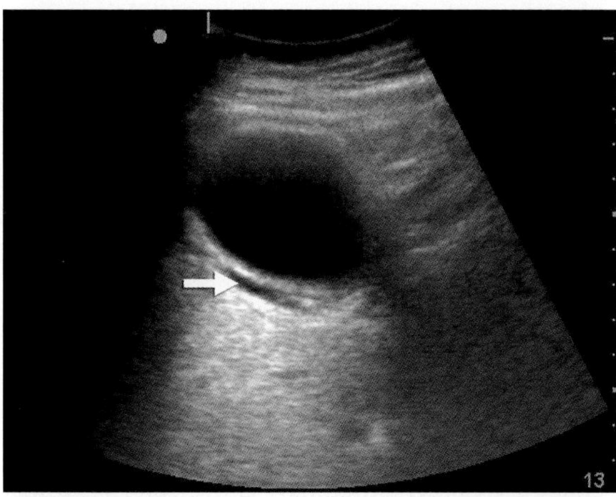

Figure 7.18

Pericholecystic fluid (arrow) visible behind gallbladder.

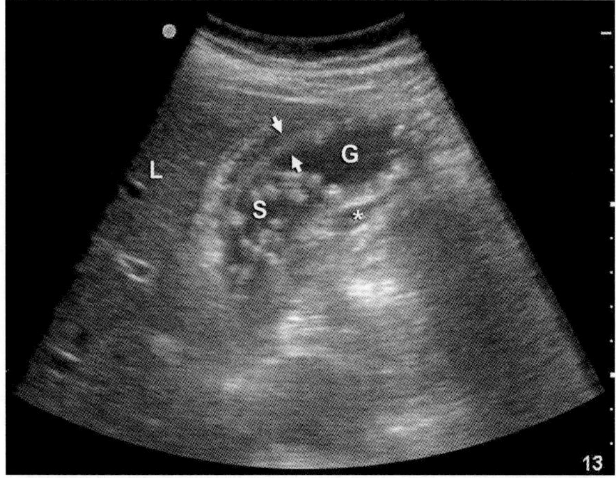

Figure 7.19

Acute cholecystitis. Note liver (L), gallbladder (G) with thickened wall (arrows), stones (S), and pericholecystic fluid (*).

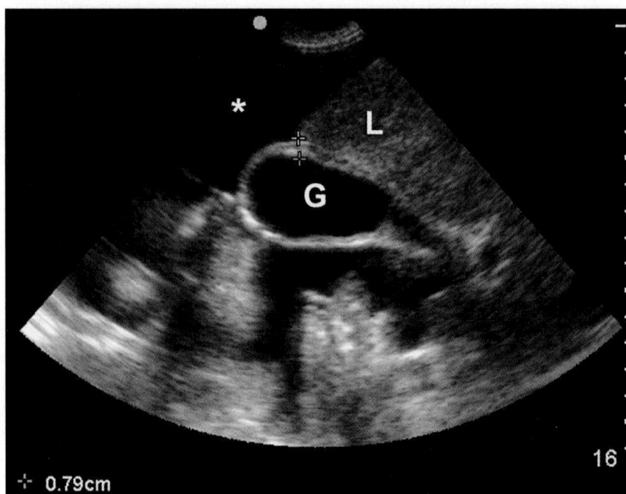

Figure 7.20
Gallbladder (G) with thickened wall (calipers) and ascites (*). Liver (L) visible at right of screen.

and colleagues demonstrated emergency department ultrasound to have similar test characteristics to radiology department sonography for the detection of acute cholecystitis [8].

Chronic cholelithiasis is usually accompanied with chronic cholecystitis. The wall of the gallbladder may become thickened and fibrotic, which may prevent the gallbladder from contracting and expanding normally.

There are many common variants and additional abnormalities that may be visualized during an ultrasound examination of the gallbladder – most of which are beyond the scope of this text. One abnormality that deserves mention is biliary sludge (Figure 7.21). Biliary sludge may be detected as a dependent layer of variable non-shadowing echogenicity in the gallbladder. It is frequently detected in states associated with biliary stasis, such as limited oral intake. It has also been known to cause biliary obstruction and cholecystitis.

Acute acalculous cholecystitis

Acute acalculous cholecystitis is the presence of an inflamed gallbladder in the absence of a gallstone obstructing the cystic or common bile duct. It typically occurs in the setting of a critically ill patient (e.g., severe burns, trauma, lengthy postoperative care, prolonged intensive care) and accounts for 5% of cholecystectomies. Because abdominal pain, fever, and leukocytosis are relatively common in these patients, the physician must have a high index of suspicion to make the diagnosis. The etiology is believed to have an ischemic basis, and a gangrenous gallbladder may result. This condition has an increased rate of complications and mortality [7].

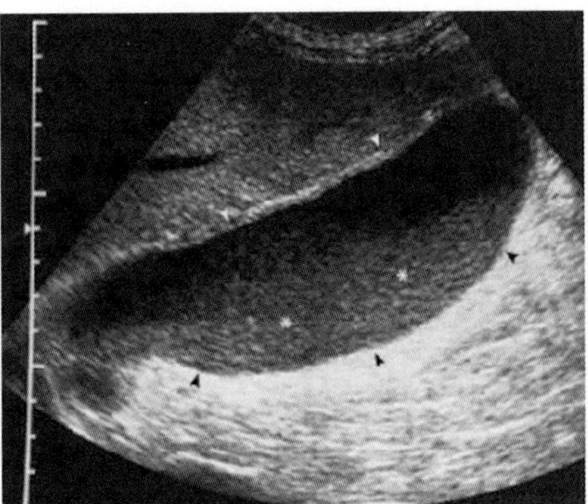

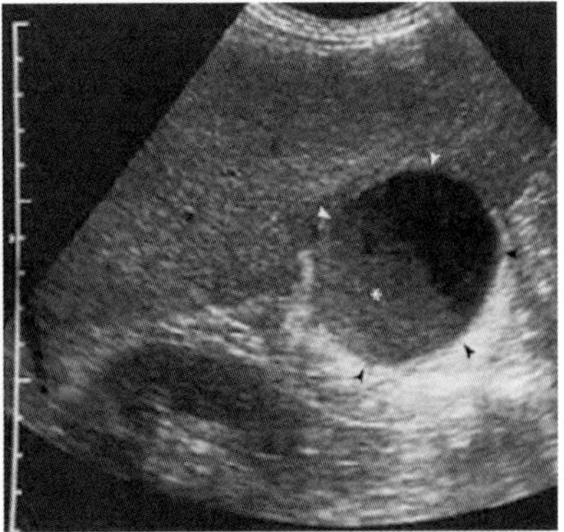

Figure 7.21
Longitudinal (*left*) and transverse (*right*) views of gallbladder containing sludge (*).

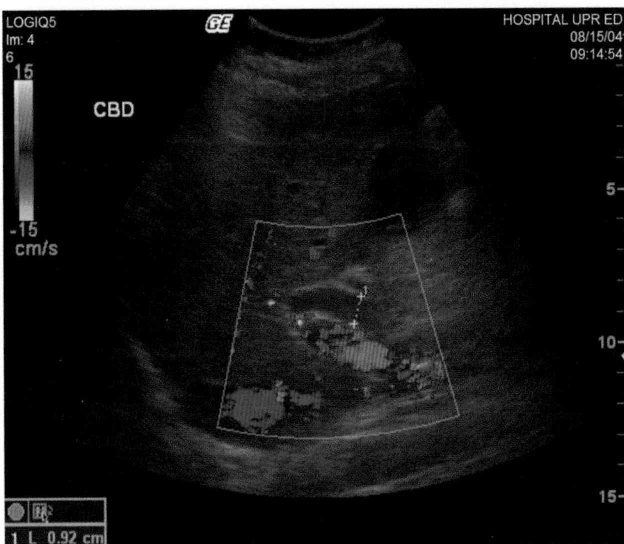

Figure 7.22
Color Doppler helps identify dilated common bile duct. Courtesy of Dr. Manuel Colon, Hospital of the University of Puerto Rico, Carolina, PR.

Ultrasound findings of acalculous cholecystitis would be the same for cholecystitis, except for the absence of gallstone shadowing. A sonographic Murphy sign, thickened gallbladder wall, dilated bile ducts (Figures 7.22 and 7.23), and pericholecystic fluid are all ultrasound evidence used to help make the diagnosis in these patients.

An uncommon subtype known as acute emphysematous cholecystitis is generally caused by infection with clostridial organisms and occlusion of the cystic artery associated with atherosclerotic vascular disease and, often, diabetes. These patients will have air in the

(A)

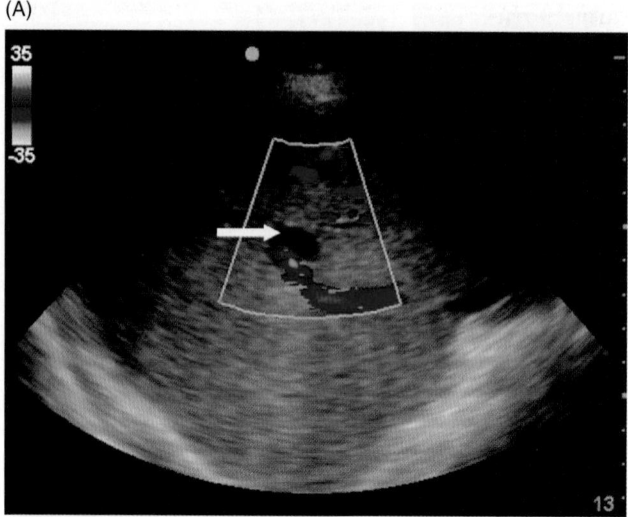

(B)

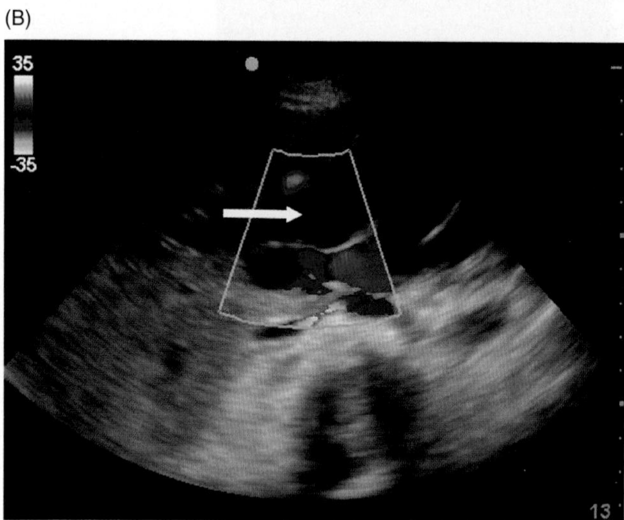

Figure 7.23

(*A*) Dilated bile duct (arrow) visible within liver parenchyma. Note the lack of color Doppler flow within the CBD compared to the vessels. (*B*) Significant intrahepatic ductal dilatation with tortuous bile ducts visible (arrow). Again the lack of flow within the ducts is highlighted using color Doppler.

gallbladder wall, and the image will show speckled scattering of the ultrasound waves with distal reverberation artifacts. These patients are often clinically very sick, and this diagnosis carries a much higher mortality rate [9].

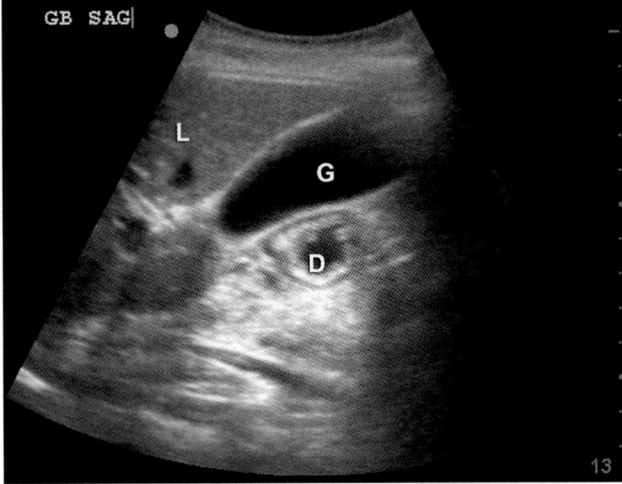

Figure 7.24
Gallbladder (G) is seen within liver parenchyma (L). The duodenum (D) is visible posterior to the gallbladder in this image.

Mimics

There are several common mimics which are important to discuss. The duodenum is often mistaken for gallbladder by the novice sonographer. Since a normal duodenum can appear similar to an abnormal gallbladder, this is important to distinguish. Differentiating the two relies upon an understanding of anatomy and the typical sonographic appearance of a cystic structure versus bowel. Figure 7.24 demonstrates gallbladder and duodenum in the same image, and Table 7.3 offers a list of features helpful in distinguishing the two structures.

First, the gallbladder wall is fibrous and typically acts as a bright reflector. Even in the setting of wall edema with cholecystitis, there are bright areas of wall between areas of edema. The wall of the duodenum is dark, like most bowel wall. The duodenum courses near the liver but is never surrounded by

Table 7.3 How to distinguish gallbladder from duodenum

Gallbladder	Duodenum
Bright wall	Dark wall
Surrounded by liver	Next to liver
Middle hepatic ligament	Not present
Static	Peristalsis
Contained	Tubular
Connects to portal vein	Does not

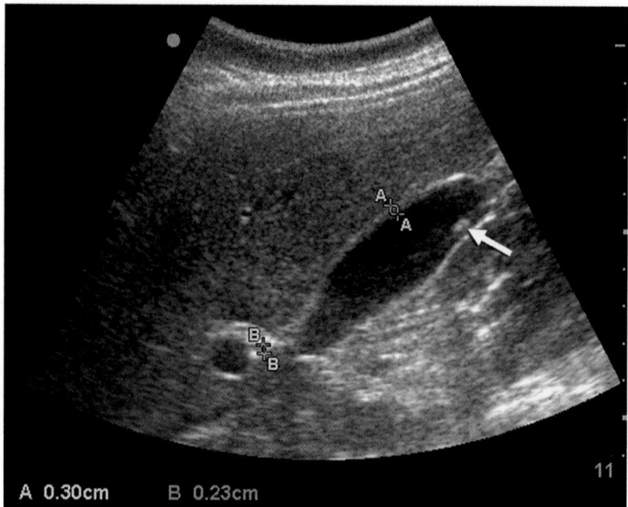

Figure 7.25
Gallbladder polyp (arrow). In this image a normal gallbladder wall (caliper A) and common bile duct (caliper B) are visible as well.

it like the gallbladder. The middle hepatic ligament connects the portal vein to the gallbladder; no connection exists to the duodenum. Observing the duodenum over time should reveal peristalsis; this will not occur in the gallbladder. The gallbladder is "finite," and clear boundaries can be visualized by scanning through from top to bottom, left to right. In contrast, the duodenum leads to the stomach proximally and jejunum distally. On ultrasound, this creates an appearance of a structure which continues for some time in either direction, lacking the gallbladder's clear boundaries.

Another mimic to note is that polyps can be mistaken for gallstones. Note that polyps should not create acoustic shadows (Figure 7.25) and they do not move as the patient moves. Changing position will cause gravity to act on gallstones, whereas polyps will remain fixed in position. Although the lack of gallstones may be reassuring in a patient with acute abdominal pain, remember that polyps may represent malignancy and require close follow-up regardless of the acute clinical course.

Sample clinical protocol

Figure 7.26 demonstrates how bedside sonography can be incorporated into the evaluation of patients with possible biliary disease. Application of similar protocols varies widely. In some centers, surgeons will operate based on an appropriate clinical picture and bedside ultrasound. In other centers, a normal bedside ultrasound may direct the clinician to perform a CT scan as a first-line study in undifferentiated abdominal pain. It is important to adopt an algorithm which is compatible with the emergency physician and consultant practice at your own institution.

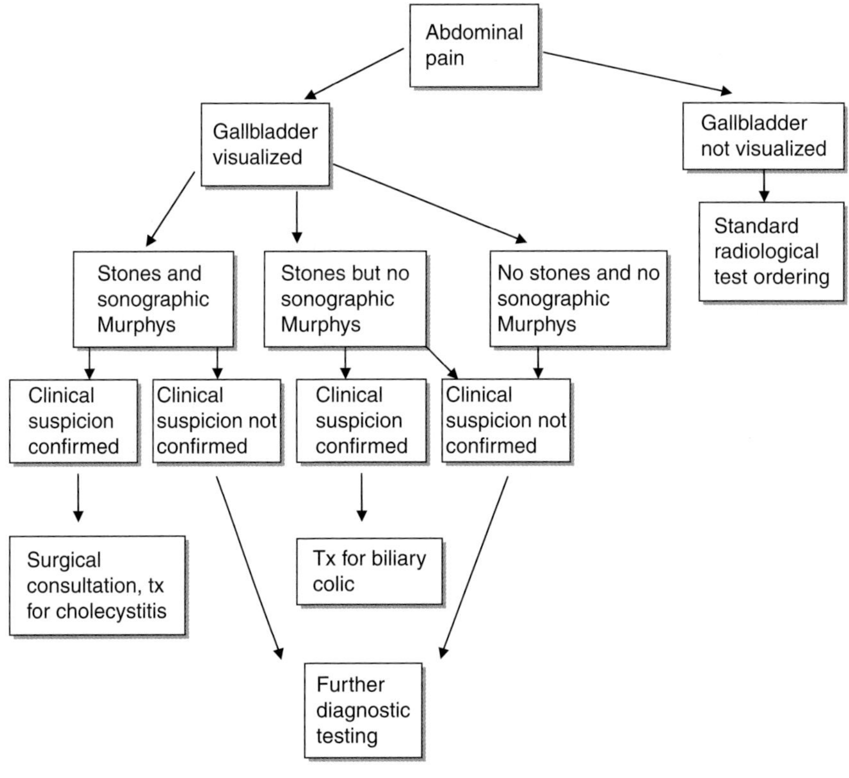

Figure 7.26
Sample clinical protocol for the evaluation of possible acute cholecystitis.

Literature review

Reference	Methods	Results	Notes
Ralls *et al.* 1985 [1]	Compared results for focused gallbladder US exam (look for stones and/or sonographic Murphy sign) and full gallbladder US exam (including CBD, pericholecystic fluid, gallbladder wall thickness).	PPV of focused exam for cholecystitis 92.2%. NPV of focused exam was 95%.	Provided radiology literature support for performing focused US gallbladder exam without compromising diagnostic accuracy.
Johnston & Kaplan 1993 [7]	Evaluated prevalence and incidence data in biliary disease.	10%–15% adult population with gallstones. No symptoms after 15 years – unlikely to develop symptoms.	Provided data for defining prevalence and incidence of disease.

Reference	Methods	Results	Notes
		10%–18% risk of symptoms over 5–15 years. 900 000 cholecystectomies a year at cost of $5 billion.	
Durston *et al.* 2001 [10]	Randomized patients to emergency department (ED) US vs. standard of care (no ED US) in undifferentiated abdominal pain.	With introduction of ED sonography, diagnostic accuracy for biliary disease improved from 28% to 70%. Decrease in return visits for pain – 1.67 vs. 1.25. Decrease in complications from stones – 6.8% vs. 1.7%.	Outcomes evaluation after introduction of ED sonography for the evaluation of undifferentiated abdominal pain.
Kendall & Shimp 2001 [11]	Compared test characteristics of emergency physician (EP)-performed and formal radiology biliary US.	Cholelithiasis diagnostic sensitivity 96%, specificity 88%. Time to EP-performed study <10 min.	Further define accurate test characteristics of EP-performed study. Suggest time savings as well.
Rosen *et al.* 2001 [12]	Compared sensitivity and specificity of EP-performed vs. formal radiology biliary US for diagnosis of cholecystitis.	EP sensitivity 91%, specificity 66%. Formal US sensitivity 69%, specificity 95%.	First study to note increased sensitivity of EP-performed biliary US for diagnosing cholecystitis over formal study. Suggests linkage with care physician knowledge of pretest probability.
Blaivas *et al.* 1999 [13]	Compared length of stay (LOS) in patients who had EP-performed gallbladder US vs. those who had radiology-performed gallbladder US. Retrospective study.	Median LOS 7% less in patients with EP-performed US. Median LOS "after hours" 15% less in patients with EP-performed US.	Time savings for patients with EP-performed US.
Gaspari *et al.* 2009 [14]	Compared proportion of adequate images and agreement with expert over-read in ED scans performed by credentialed vs. non-credentialed EPs.	Credentialed EPs performed technically complete scans 80% of the time; over 90% rated as excellent or good image quality.	Image quality, interpretation, and proportion of scans with a complete image set all increased after 25 scans.

References

1. Ralls PW, Colletti PM, Lapin SA, *et al.* Real-time sonography in suspected acute cholecystitis: prospective evaluation of primary and secondary signs. *Radiology* 1985; **155**: 767–71.
2. Shea JA, Berlin JA, Escarce JJ, *et al.* Revised estimates of diagnostic test sensitivity and specificity in suspected biliary tract disease. *Arch Int Med* 1994; **154**: 2573–81.
3. Finberg HJ, Birnholz JC. Ultrasound evaluation of the gallbladder wall. *Radiology* 1979; **133**: 693–8.
4. Engel JM, Deitch EA, Sikkema W. Gallbladder wall thickness: sonographic accuracy and relation to disease. *AJR Am J Roentgenol* 1980; **134**: 907–9.
5. Parulekar SG. Ultrasound evaluation of common bile duct size. *Radiology* 1979; **133**: 703–7.
6. MacDonald FR, Cooperberg PL, Cohen MM. The WES triad: a specific sonographic sign of gallstones in the contracted gallbladder. *Gastrointest Radiol* 1981; **6**: 39–41.
7. Johnston DE, Kaplan MM. Pathogenesis and treatment of gallstones. *N Engl J Med* 1993; **328**: 412–21.
8. Summers SM, Scruggs W, Menchine MD, *et al.* A prospective evaluation of emergency department bedside ultrasonography for the detection of acute cholecystitis. *Ann Emerg Med* 2010; **56**: 114–22.
9. Blaquiere RM, Dewbury KC. The ultrasound diagnosis of emphysematous cholecystitis. *Br J Radiol* 1982; **55**: 114–16.
10. Durston W, Carl ML, Guerra W, *et al.* Comparison of quality and cost-effectiveness in the evaluation of symptomatic cholelithiasis with different approaches to ultrasound availability in the ED. *Am J Emerg Med* 2001; **19**: 260–9.
11. Kendall JL, Shimp RJ. Performance and interpretation of focused right upper quadrant ultrasound by emergency physicians. *J Emerg Med* 2001; **21**: 7–13.
12. Rosen CL, Brown DF, Chang Y, *et al.* Ultrasonography by emergency physicians in patients with suspected cholecystitis. *Am J Emerg Med* 2001; **19**: 32–6.
13. Blaivas M, Harwood RA, Lambert MJ. Decreasing length of stay with emergency ultrasound examination of the gallbladder. *Acad Emerg Med* 1999; **6**: 1020–3.
14. Gaspari RJ, Dickman E, Blehar D. Learning curve of bedside ultrasound of the gallbladder. *J Emerg Med* 2009; **37**: 51–6.

8 Ultrasound of the deep venous system

Introduction

Evaluation for deep vein thrombosis (DVT) can be one of the most useful exams for emergency and critical care physicians. There are approximately 250 000 new diagnoses of DVT and 50 000 deaths from thromboembolic disease annually [1,2]. The estimated rate of propagation from DVT to pulmonary embolism ranges from 10% to 50% [1,2]. Because the incidence of DVT is so high and because this disease is so prevalent in critical and acute care settings, the ability to rule in or rule out DVT at the bedside is a particularly powerful tool. The simplified compression technique described in this chapter evaluates for DVT at two anatomic sites of the lower extremity venous system. This protocol has been evaluated in multiple randomized controlled studies and has become a well-accepted protocol used for decision making in conjunction with clinical pretest probability assessments [3–17].

Calf vein assessment is not described in this chapter. There exists some controversy over the clinical relevance of isolated calf vein DVT and the need to emergently assess for this entity [18]. Many radiology departments and vascular laboratories do not routinely assess for DVT distal to the popliteal vein. Proponents of whole-leg ultrasonography note that it can detect calf vein DVT and obviate the need for a follow-up study at a later point (which is the general recommendation after a normal two-point sonogram). Others point to the risks of anticoagulating a distal DVT whose natural clinical course has been demonstrated to be spontaneous resolution more than 50% of the time. In 2008, a randomized study of whole-leg sonography versus two-point compression sonography in patients with a positive D-dimer found the two diagnostic strategies to be equivalent in the evaluation of suspected DVT [19]. There was no difference between the two groups in the rate of venous thromboembolism (VTE) at three months.

Focused questions for DVT ultrasound

The questions for DVT ultrasound are as follows:

1. Does the common femoral vein fully compress?
2. Does the popliteal vein fully compress?

Anatomy

The anatomy of the lower extremity should be reviewed so that the DVT compression ultrasound exam can be performed properly. The iliac vein becomes the common femoral vein (CFV) as it leaves the pelvis. The most

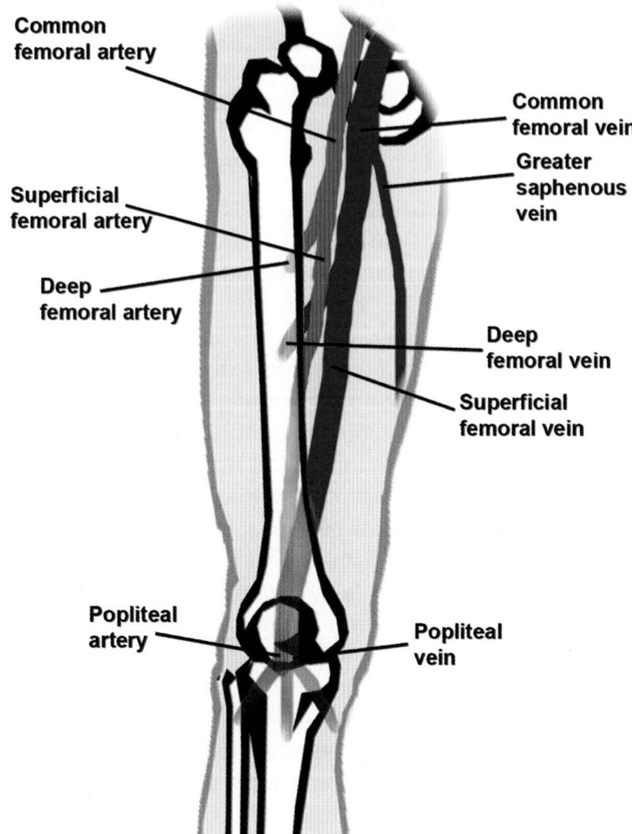

Figure 8.1
Deep vascular anatomy of the lower extremity.

proximal tributary of the CFV is the greater saphenous vein (GSV) (Figure 8.1). The common femoral then splits into the superficial and deep femoral in the proximal thigh – both of these vessels are part of the deep venous system despite their names. At the knee, the superficial femoral becomes the popliteal vein running in the posterior fossa of the knee joint and is joined by its tributaries, the tibial vein and peroneal vein.

It is not surprising that clots, as shown by venography studies, seem to cluster at the branch points of the venous system. One common explanation is that the increased turbulent flow at these branch points produces increased wear and tear on the vessel walls, thus making these areas predisposed to clot formation.

Data from these venography studies support the use of the simplified compression technique because identification of clot in the popliteal vein or CFV should identify any DVTs identified by venography (Figure 8.2); there were no cases in these initial studies where a DVT did not involve either the popliteal vein or the CFV, or both.

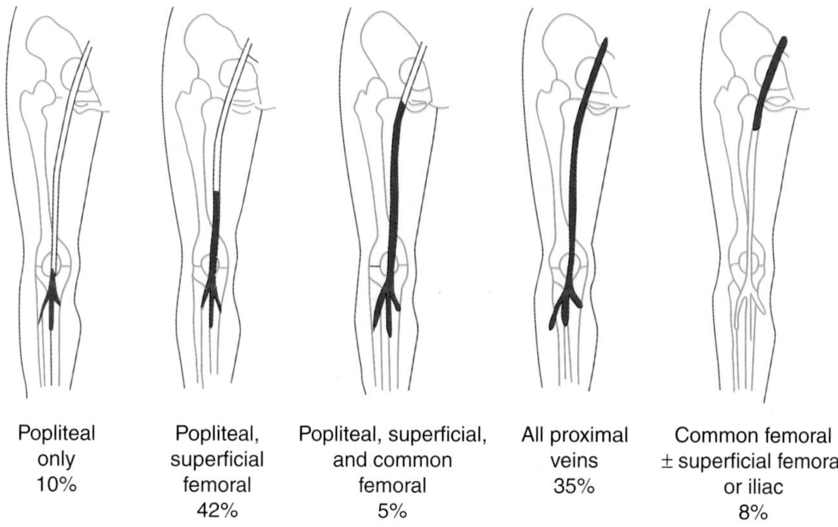

Figure 8.2

Proportion of DVT cases with clot at each location. Note that all clots in this series involve either the popliteal vein or the femoral vein, or both. Figure created from data presented in Cogo A, Lensing AW, Prandoni P, *et al.* Distribution of thrombosis in patients with symptomatic deep vein thrombosis. Implications for simplifying the diagnostic process with compression ultrasound. *Arch Intern Med.* 1993 Dec 27; 153(24): 2777–80.

Although the anatomy around the femoral triangle is described in more detail in Chapter 15, it is also reviewed here. Figure 8.3 shows a transverse view of the femoral triangle, just inferior to the inguinal canal. At this level, the CFV is distinct from the GSV, which separates to take a more superficial and medial course as it moves distally. The common femoral artery (CFA) at this level has not yet bifurcated.

Figure 8.4 shows the probe slightly distal to the femoral triangle. Here the CFV has bifurcated into the superficial femoral vein (SFV) and deep femoral vein (not visualized at this level). The CFA has now bifurcated into the superficial femoral artery (SFA) and deep femoral artery (DFA).

The popliteal vein (PV) and popliteal artery (PA) are found in the popliteal fossa (Figure 8.5). In general, the PV is superficial to the PA. There is occasional anatomic variability, so the artery may be anterior to the vein in rare cases. This can be distinguished by using adjunctive methods such as spectral and color Doppler and compression.

Technique

Probe selection

For the evaluation of DVT, a high-frequency linear-array probe is best. In larger patients or in patients with lower extremity edema, lower-frequency

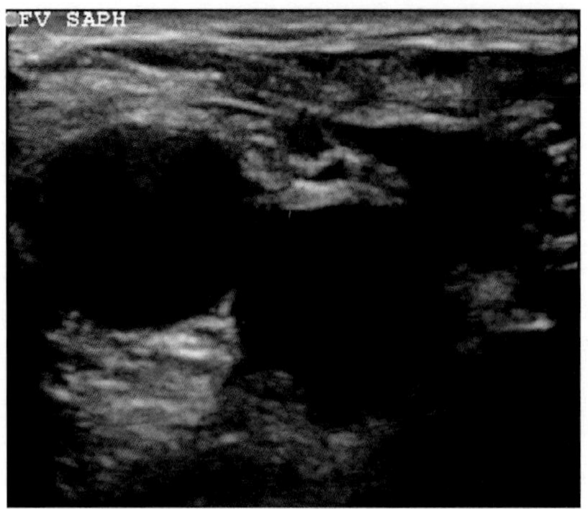

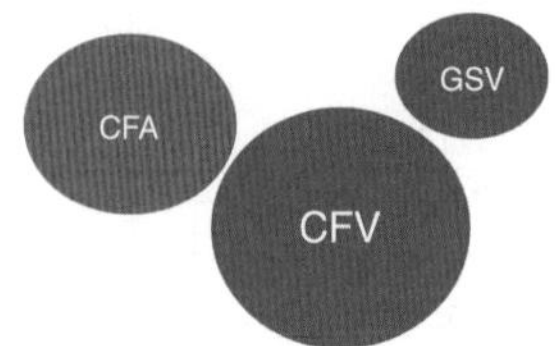

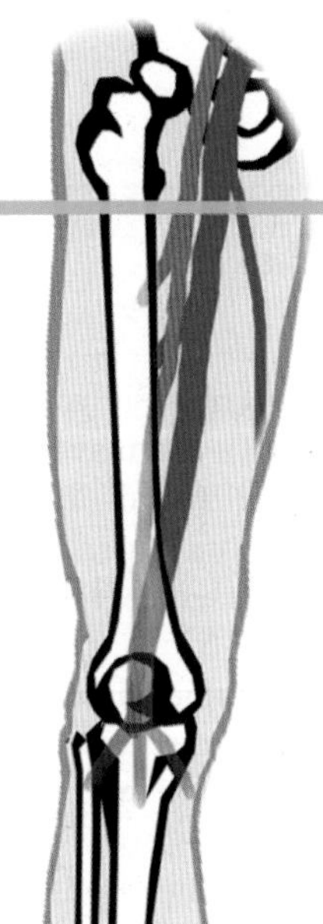

Figure 8.3
Common femoral vein.

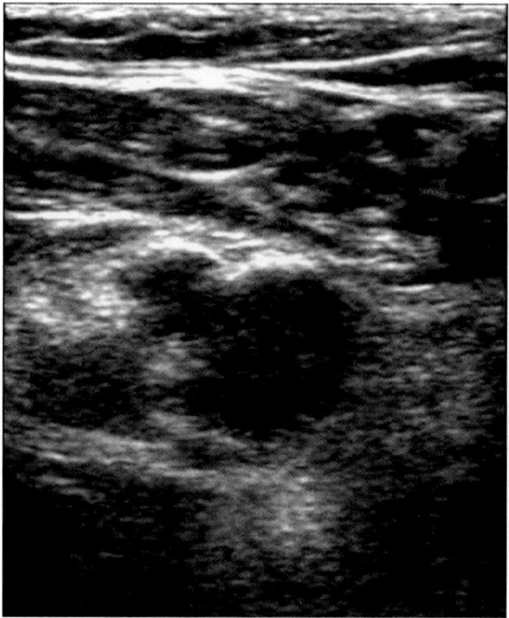

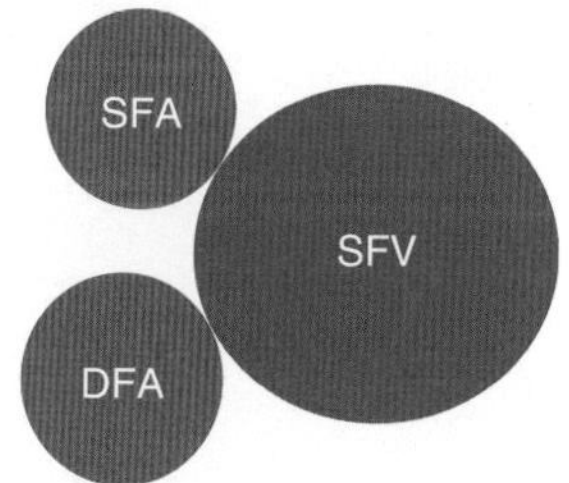

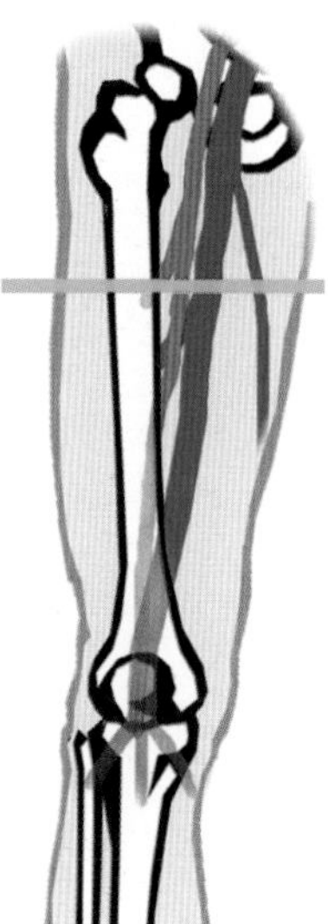

Figure 8.4
Superficial femoral vein.

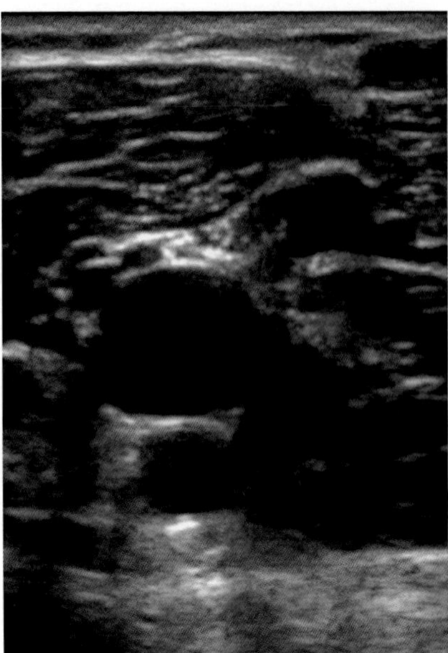

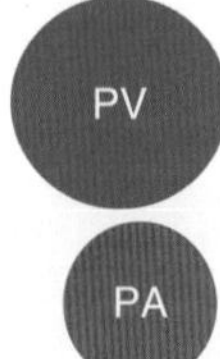

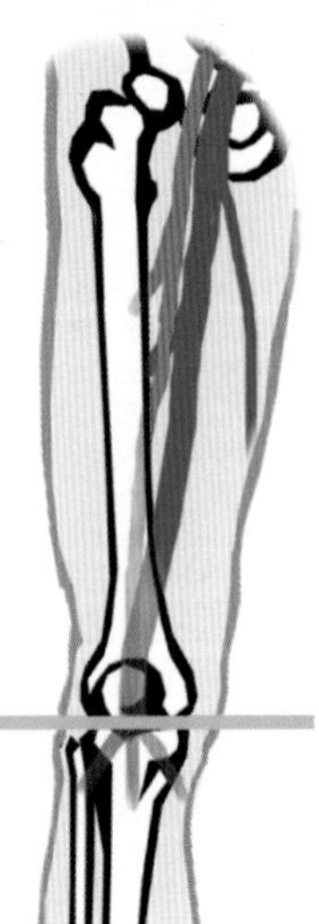

Figure 8.5
Popliteal vein.

probes allow for better penetration of the sound beams; however, the image can usually be obtained with the high-frequency linear probe (5–12 MHz).

Views

At least two "regions" are necessary for a complete screening exam:

1. Common femoral vein demonstrating compression of vessel. This usually involves visualizing both the common femoral and greater saphenous veins as seen in Figure 8.3. Some authors have argued that it is prudent to compress both the common femoral and greater saphenous veins and then to slide distal to the femoral triangle to compress the superficial femoral vein as well.
2. Popliteal vein demonstrating compression of vessel. Again it is prudent to evaluate the popliteal vein through the entire popliteal fossa.

In Figures 8.6 and 8.7, probe positioning for femoral vein and popliteal vein visualization is demonstrated. The probe marker should be directed toward the patient's right side.

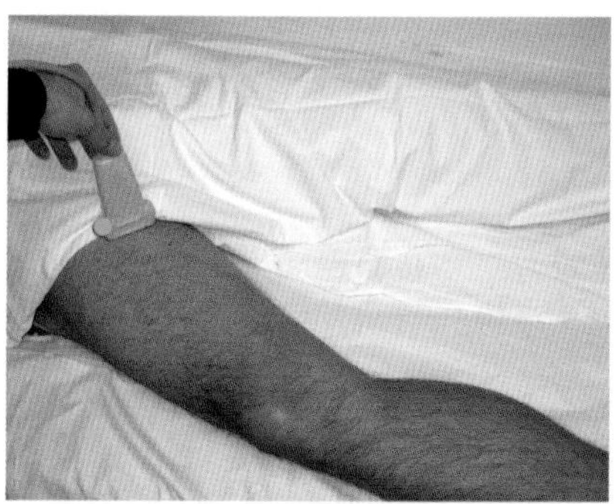

Figure 8.6

Probe position for common femoral vein. Probe marker (green dot) should face the patient's right side.

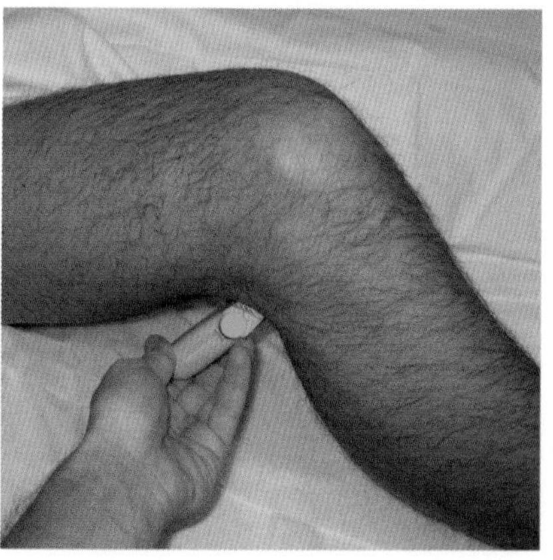

Figure 8.7

Probe position for popliteal vein. Probe marker (green dot) should face the patient's right side.

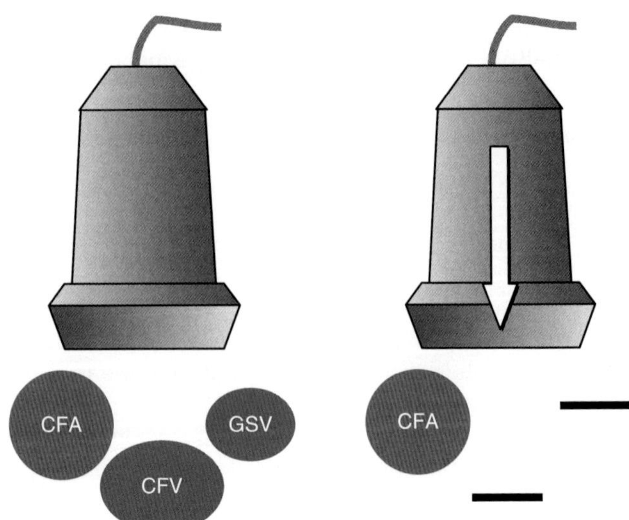

Figure 8.8
Compression technique.

If the veins are collapsible to a thin line with external pressure applied (Figure 8.8), the vein is presumed to be patent and there is no clot present. If the vein does not collapse with external pressure, there is presumed to be clot within the lumen of the vessel preventing complete collapse.

There are a few structures that can be mistaken for a non-compressible vessel and that are worth mentioning. Lymph nodes can look like clot within a hypoechoic vessel as they have a ring of hypoechoic fluid surrounding the node. However, they are easy to distinguish because if the probe is turned longitudinally, it will become obvious that the object is circular and not tubular. Baker's cysts can cause the same phenomenon in the popliteal fossa, but again dynamic scanning in longitudinal and transverse planes should remove any doubt. Pseudoaneurysms and groin hematomas can also be misleading, and caution should be exercised in clinical situations where these diagnoses are being considered. This is where color Doppler can often be helpful [10].

Scanning tips

- Proper patient positioning can greatly improve image quality.
  - Have the patient externally rotate his or her leg to better visualize the common femoral vein.
  - For the popliteal vein, have the patient hang his or her leg over the edge of the bed to distend the vessels, or perform the scan with the patient in a prone position.
- Be sure the veins fully compress. A normal vein will completely disappear when compressed enough. If the walls do not touch, consider DVT.
- Make sure to apply pressure evenly. The probe should be perpendicular to the skin. If pressure is being applied at an angle, the vessel may appear not to collapse because of unevenly distributed pressure.

Normal images

Figures 8.9–8.11 show normal ultrasound images of venous anatomy.

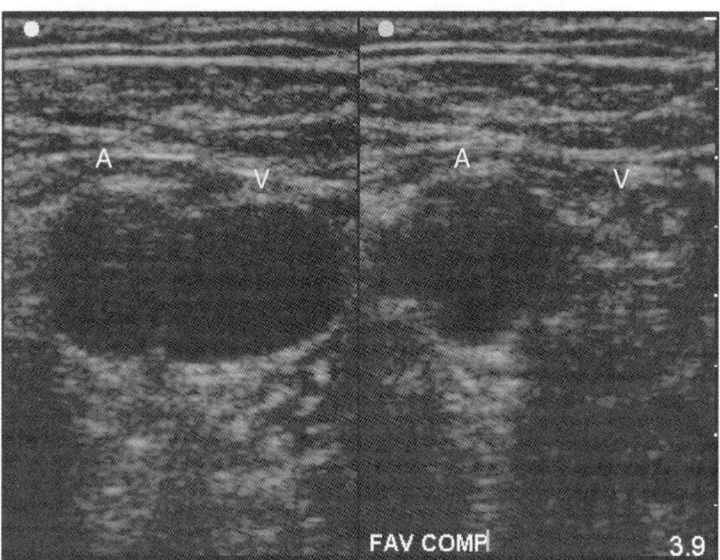

Figure 8.9
Common femoral artery (A) and vein (V), with compression (*right*).

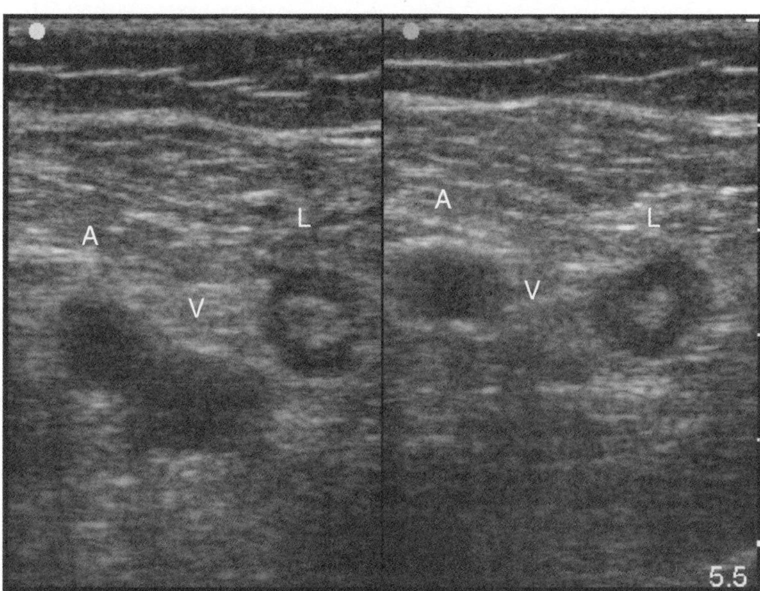

Figure 8.10
Common femoral artery (A), vein (V), and enlarged lymph node (L), with compression (*right*).

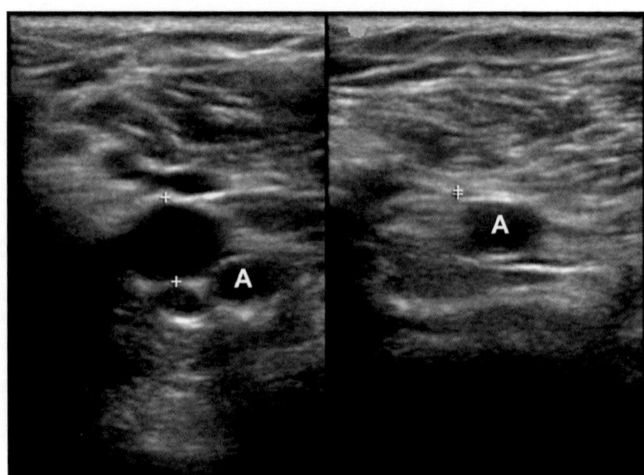

Figure 8.11
Popliteal artery (A) and vein (calipers). Compression demonstrated (*right*).

Abnormal images

Figures 8.12–8.16 show ultrasound images of venous anatomy with clot present.

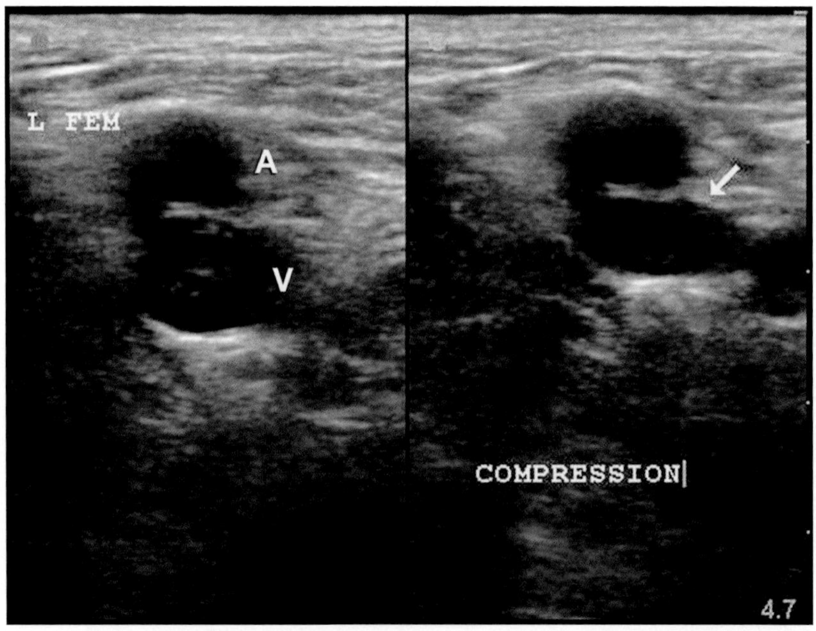

Figure 8.12
Common femoral artery (A) and vein (V), with compression (*right*). Note the hyperechoic material within the vein, as well as the lack of compressibility of the vessel (arrow).

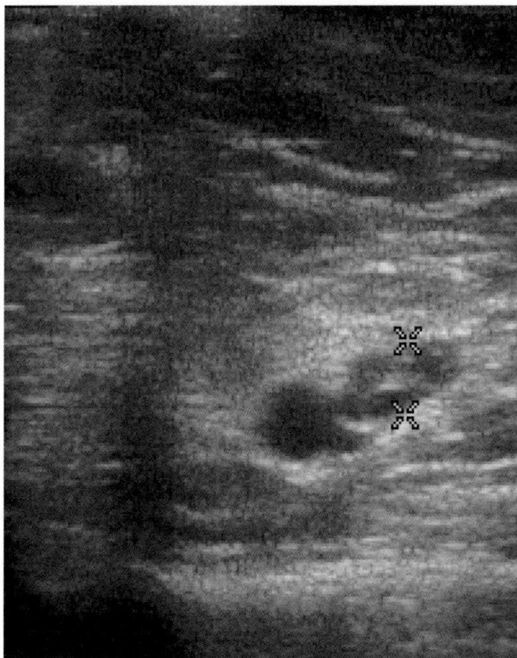

Figure 8.13

Popliteal artery and vein. The vein is marked with calipers. Note the lack of compressibility and echogenic material within the lumen.

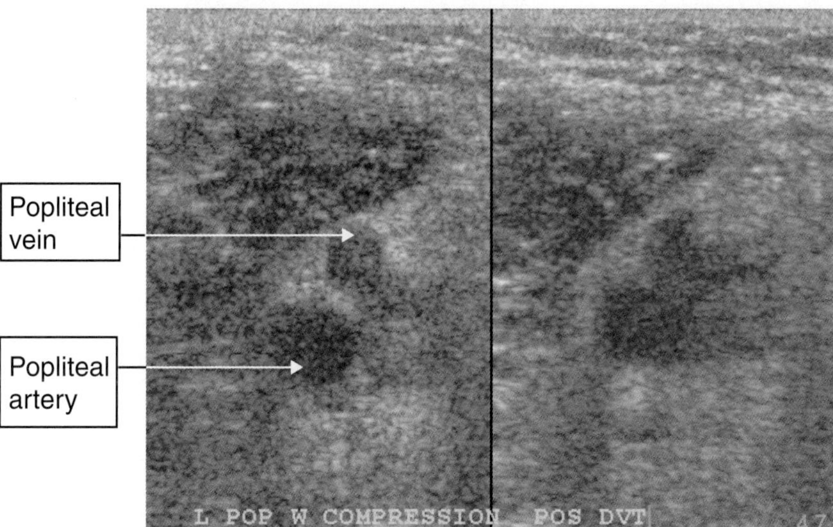

Figure 8.14

Popliteal vein with DVT; no change in vein caliber with compression (*right*).

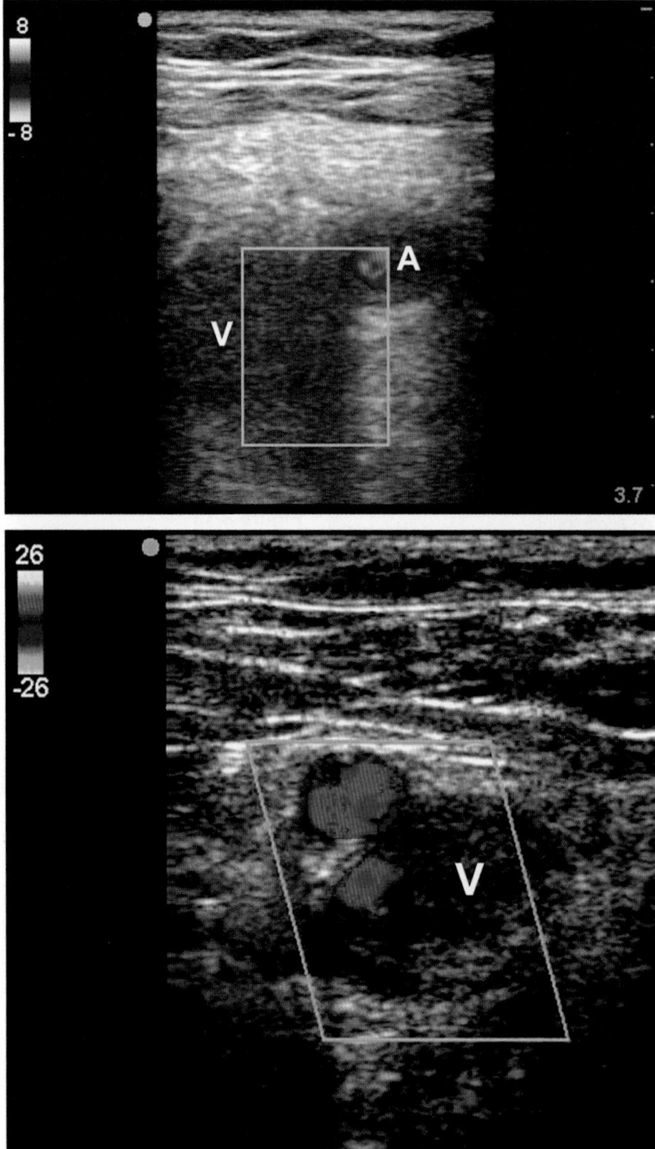

Figure 8.15

Common femoral vein (V) incompressible in these two cases. Doppler demonstrates flow within arteries (red) but not veins, confirming DVT.

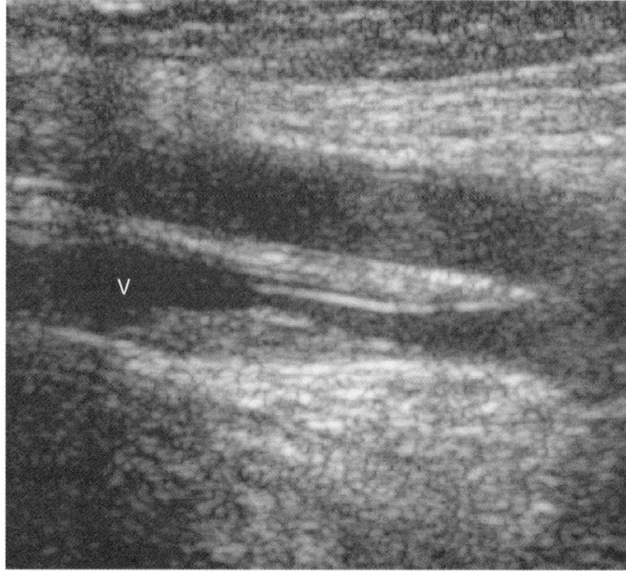

Figure 8.16
This longitudinal image of the common femoral vein (V) demonstrates echogenic material within the lumen. Note that the thrombus does not occlude the entire vessel diameter. This could represent a chronic DVT, where some recannulation has begun to take place.

Sample clinical protocol

When used in conjunction with D-dimer testing, bedside ultrasound is sensitive enough to exclude DVT when the study is normal and specific enough to begin treatment when clot is demonstrated [12,19]. The protocol shown in Figure 8.17 illustrates how this concept can be applied to a patient care algorithm. The specific type of D-dimer assay as well as the experience level of the bedside sonographers must be considered when employing protocols such as this.

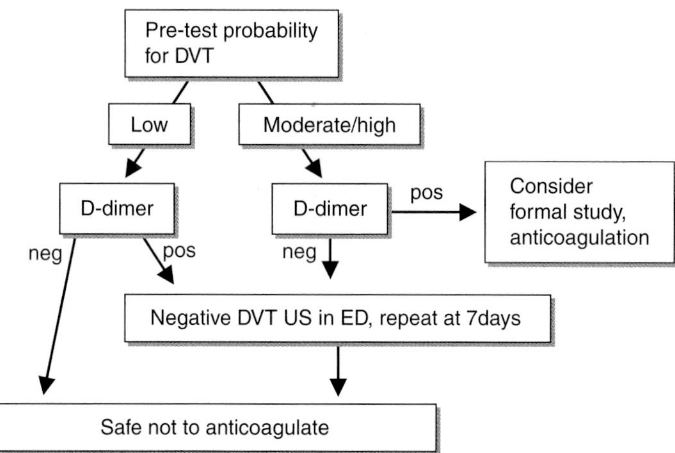

Figure 8.17
Clinical protocol for the evaluation of possible DVT.

Advanced techniques

Upper extremity DVT involving the internal jugular, subclavian, or axillary veins can impact patients who are hypercoagulable or have indwelling central venous or percutaneous inserted central catheters (PICC). The test characteristics of upper extremity DVT assessment using bedside ultrasound have not been described. However, it is reasonable to assume that clot would cause a lack of vessel compressibility just as with lower extremity DVT. Therefore upper extremity assessment may be more useful in confirming the presence of DVT than excluding the diagnosis. In addition, using compression to assess for vessel patency is recommended prior to attempts at central venous cannulation (see Chapter 15). Figure 8.18 demonstrates thrombus within the internal jugular vein. Undiagnosed, this process could make internal jugular vein cannulation dangerous and likely impossible.

Although not frequently employed by emergency physicians, assessing augmentation and respiratory variation using pulsed-wave Doppler is a common practice among radiologists. In cases where a stronger clinical suspicion for DVT may lead one to pursue a more involved bedside study, the following techniques may be employed. Both techniques involve the use of Doppler to visualize flow differences in the veins.

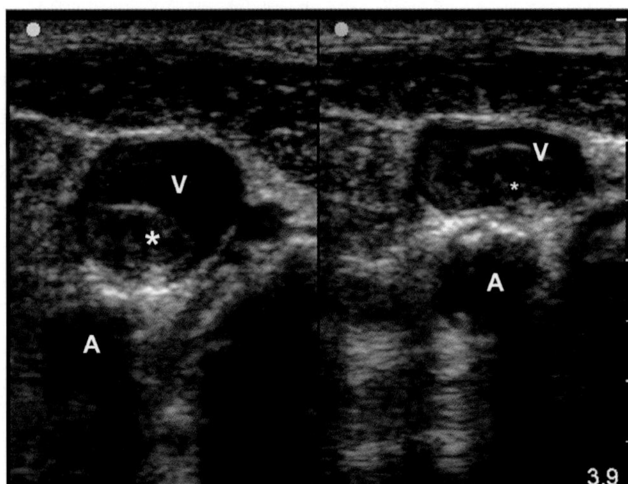

Figure 8.18
Thrombus (*) within internal jugular vein (V). With pressure (*right*), neither the vein nor the carotid artery (A) compress.

Augmentation

To assess augmented venous return, compress the soft tissue of the calf at some point distal to the standard probe position on the leg. With the Doppler over the vein, note any changes in flow as the distal vein is compressed. In a normal vein, distal compression causes a rapid, temporary increase in venous return. This implies an unobstructed path for blood flow *distal* to the probe,

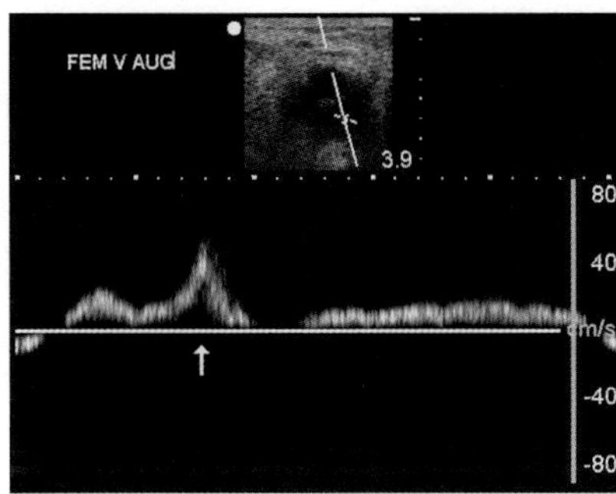

Figure 8.19
Augmentation (arrow).

from the point of compression. In Figure 8.19, note the rapid increase in flow velocity on the scale at the bottom of the screen. The arrow indicates the augmentation.

Respiratory variation

To assess respiratory variation, note any changes in flow during respiration with the Doppler over the vein. In a normal vein, changes in intra-abdominal and intrathoracic pressures during the respiratory cycle cause cyclic variations in venous return. This implies an unobstructed path for blood flow *proximal* to the probe, toward the iliac veins and inferior vena cava. In Figure 8.20, note the gradual variations in flow velocity on the scale at the bottom of the screen.

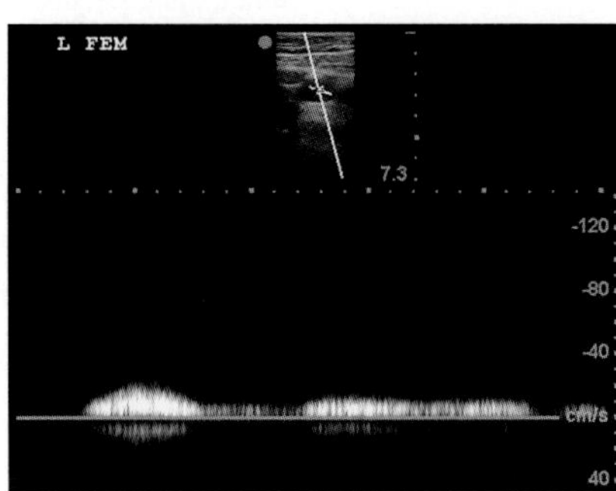

Figure 8.20
Respiratory variation.

Literature review

Reference	Methods	Results	Notes
Blaivas *et al.* 2000 [10]	Prospective comparison of bedside compression technique with duplex sonography by radiology.	98% correlation between bedside and formal studies; mean scan time < 4 min per patient.	Bedside exam accurate, augmentation not helpful.

Reference	Methods	Results	Notes
Burnside *et al.* 2008 [17]	Systematic review of 6 studies: Blaivas *et al.* 2000 [10] Frazee *et al.* 2001 [12] Jang *et al.* 2004 [13] Theodoro *et al.* 2004 [14] Jacoby *et al.* 2007 [15] Magazzini *et al.* 2007 [16] All were emergency physician (EP)-performed US followed by radiology US.	936 patients total, 132 DVTs. Sensitivity 95%, specificity 96%.	Pooled data may be limited by small sample sizes, most studies by highly skilled EP sonographers and lack of reporting on DVT location.
Cogo *et al.* 1998 [11]	Prospective evaluation of compression US, anticoagulation withheld if normal.	0.7% complication rate during follow-up period using clinical algorithm for anticoagulation.	It is safe to defer anticoagulation when compression US is normal.
Bernardi *et al.* 2008 [19]	Randomized study of 2-point compression vs. whole-leg sonography in patients with positive D-dimer.	2098 patients randomized. Higher prevalence of DVT in whole-leg group due to detection of calf DVT, but same rate of symptomatic venous thromboembolism and outcomes at 3 months.	Rate of proximal DVT detection same with both strategies: no higher yield with whole-leg vs. 2 point compression. Raises question of need for anticoagulation in isolated calf DVT.

New directions

There are several ways in which the use of bedside sonography for VTE is evolving. One is the increased use of non-invasive means to exclude or confirm the diagnosis of VTE. Rather than focusing on the test characteristics of compression sonography alone, there is growing evidence for the utility of combining DVT sonography with D-dimer and clinical risk scores to more efficiently evaluate for DVT.

Several studies cited in this chapter describe algorithms for the evaluation of DVT and PE using D-dimer and sonography. One study demonstrated that a negative D-dimer ruled out 31% of 918 cases and sonography demonstrated thrombus in 17% [20]. Thus, almost half of suspected VTE cases could be managed without the use of ionizing radiation or intravenous contrast, and potentially more rapidly as well. This makes bedside testing an attractive option in the assessment of this common pathology.

The articles cited in this chapter demonstrate reasonable accuracy of point-of-care sonography performed by non-radiologists. A recent study showed near-100% sensitivity and specificity in 199 subjects assessed by a group of emergency physicians with heterogeneous sonography experience [21]. In this study, each physician underwent a mere 10-minute session on DVT assessment prior to enrolling patients. Thus, the limits on variables such as machine capability and operator experience remain ripe for study.

References

1. Anderson FA, Wheeler HB, Goldberg RJ, *et al.* A population-based perspective of the hospital incidence and case-fatality rates of deep vein thrombosis and pulmonary embolism. The Worcester DVT Study. *Arch Int Med* 1991; **151**: 933–8.
2. Gillum RF. Pulmonary embolism and thrombophlebitis in the United States, 1970–1985. *Am Heart J* 1987; **114**: 1262–4.
3. Lensing AW, Doris CI, McGrath FP, *et al.* A comparison of compression ultrasound with color Doppler ultrasound for the diagnosis of symptomless postoperative deep vein thrombosis. *Arch Intern Med* 1997; **157**: 765–8.
4. Lensing AW, Prandoni P, Brandjes D, *et al.* Detection of deep vein thrombosis by real-time B-mode ultrasonography. *N Engl J Med* 1989; **320**: 342–5.
5. Poppiti R, Papanicolaou G, Perese S, Weaver FA. Limited B-mode venous imaging versus complete color-flow duplex venous scanning for detection of proximal deep venous thrombosis. *J Vasc Surg* 1995; **22**: 553–7.
6. Frederick MG, Hertzberg BS, Kliewer MA, *et al.* Can the US examination for lower extremity deep vein thrombosis be abbreviated? A prospective study of 755 examinations. *Radiology* 1996; **199**: 45–7.
7. Birdwell BG, Raskob GE, Whitsett TL, *et al.* The clinical validity of normal compression ultrasonography in outpatients suspected of having deep venous thrombosis. *Ann Intern Med* 1998; **128**: 1–7.
8. Trottier SJ, Todi S, Veremakis C. Validation of an inexpensive B-mode ultrasound device for detection of deep vein thrombosis. *Chest* 1996; **110**: 1547–50.
9. Heijboer H, Buller HR, Lensing A, *et al.* A comparison of real-time compression ultrasonography with impedance plethysmography for the diagnosis of deep vein thrombosis in symptomatic outpatients. *N Engl J Med* 1993; **329**: 1365–9.
10. Blaivas M, Lambert MJ, Harwood RA, Wood JP, Konicki J. Lower-extremity Doppler for deep venous thrombosis: can emergency physicians be accurate and fast? *Acad Emerg Med* 2000; **7**: 120–6.
11. Cogo A, Lensing AW, Koopman MM, *et al.* Compression ultrasonography for diagnostic management of patients with clinically suspected deep vein thrombosis: prospective cohort study. *BMJ* 1998; **316**: 17–20.
12. Frazee BW, Snoey ER, Levitt A. Emergency department compression ultrasound to diagnose proximal deep vein thrombosis. *J Emerg Med* 2001; **20**: 107–12.
13. Jang T, Docherty M, Aubin C, Polites G. Resident-performed compression ultrasonography for the detection of proximal deep vein thrombosis: fast and accurate. *Acad Emerg Med* 2004; **11**: 319–22.

14. Theodoro D, Blaivas M, Duggal S, Snyder G, Lucas M. Real-time B-mode ultrasound in the ED saves time in the diagnosis of deep vein thrombosis (DVT). *Am J Emerg Med* 2004; **22**: 197–200.
15. Jacoby J, Cesta M, Axelband J, *et al.* Can emergency medicine residents detect acute deep venous thrombosis with a limited, two-site ultrasound examination? *J Emerg Med* 2007; **32**: 197–200.
16. Magazzini S, Vanni S, Toccafondi S, *et al.* Duplex ultrasound in the emergency department for the diagnostic management of clinically suspected deep vein thrombosis. *Acad Emerg Med* 2007; **14**: 216–20.
17. Burnside PR, Brown MD, Kline JA. Systematic review of emergency physician-performed ultrasonography for lower-extremity deep vein thrombosis. *Acad Emerg Med* 2008; **15**: 493–8.
18. Righini M, Paris S, Le Gal G, *et al.* Clinical relevance of distal deep vein thrombosis: review of literature data. *Thromb Haemost* 2006; **95**: 56–64.
19. Bernardi E, Camporese G, Buller H, *et al.* Serial 2-point ultrasonography plus D-dimer vs whole-leg color-coded Doppler ultrasonography for diagnosing suspected symptomatic deep vein thrombosis: a randomized controlled trial. *JAMA* 2008; **300**: 1653–9.
20. Perrier A, Desmarais S, Miron MJ, *et al.* Non-invasive diagnosis of venous thromboembolism in outpatients. *Lancet* 1999; **353**: 190–5.
21. Crisp JG, Lovato LM, Jang TB. Compression ultrasonography of the lower extremity with portable vascular ultrasonography can accurately detect deep venous thrombosis in the emergency department. *Ann Emerg Med* 2010; **56**: 601–10.

9 Respiratory ultrasound

Introduction

Over the last five years, research describing the use of ultrasound for respiratory conditions has proliferated, and new and exciting ways to diagnose and manage the dyspneic patient using ultrasound continue to be identified. Thoracic ultrasound is reviewed for a variety of applications throughout this book. The role of thoracic ultrasound in the diagnosis of pneumothorax and hemothorax is covered in Chapter 2, and the safety benefit of ultrasound when performing procedures such as thoracentesis is presented in Chapter 16.

This chapter, therefore, will focus on the role of ultrasound in airway management and the role of thoracic ultrasound in the diagnosis of pulmonary edema or extravascular lung water (EVLW). The terminology that has been developed by pioneers in thoracic ultrasound for identifying EVLW and the concepts behind it are described, because they are crucial to the diagnostic use of ultrasound for all thoracic applications.

The two most basic concepts of thoracic ultrasound – A-lines and B-lines – are described here. There are many other potential applications for thoracic ultrasound, and indeed German, French and Danish physicians routinely use ultrasound to diagnose consolidations, infarctions and inflammatory thoracic conditions. For more detailed descriptions of these applications and others used in the evaluation of the dyspneic patient, sonographers are encouraged to read Dr. Daniel A. Lichtenstein's book, *General Ultrasound in the Critically Ill* [1]. Thoracic ultrasound is an area of extensive research, and the potential for guiding the management of patients with lung disease is enormous. Specific pediatric applications will be discussed in Chapter 13.

Focused questions for respiratory ultrasound

The questions for airway ultrasound are as follows:

1. Where is the cricothyroid membrane?
2. Is the intubation successful?

The questions for chest ultrasound are as follows:

1. Are A-lines present?
2. Are B-lines present?

Anatomy

Airway

When using ultrasound to identify anatomy in the neck, it is important to start midline and to visualize the hyperechoic tracheal rings in both a longitudinal and a transverse plane (Figure 9.1). The cricothyroid membrane can be seen in the longitudinal plane as the most superior dark space above the most proximal tracheal ring. Its appearance has been described as "sandwich-like," as the dark spaces above and below the membrane are longer than those in between the bright dense cartilage of the tracheal rings (Figure 9.2).

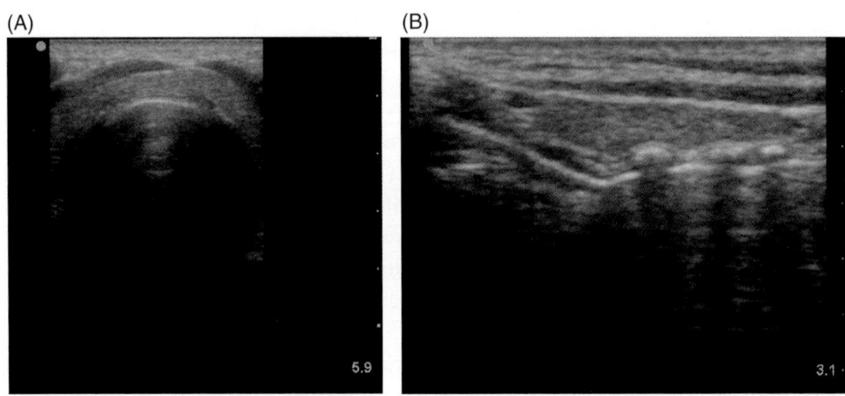

Figure 9.1
(*A*) Transverse and (*B*) longitudinal views of the trachea.

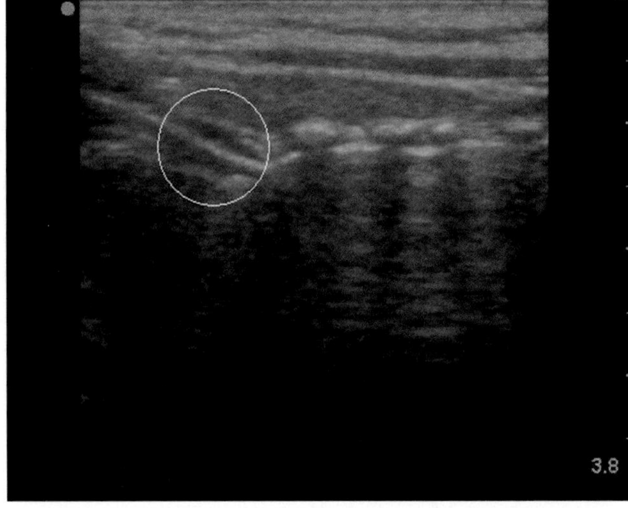

Figure 9.2
Longitudinal view of the cricothyroid membrane.

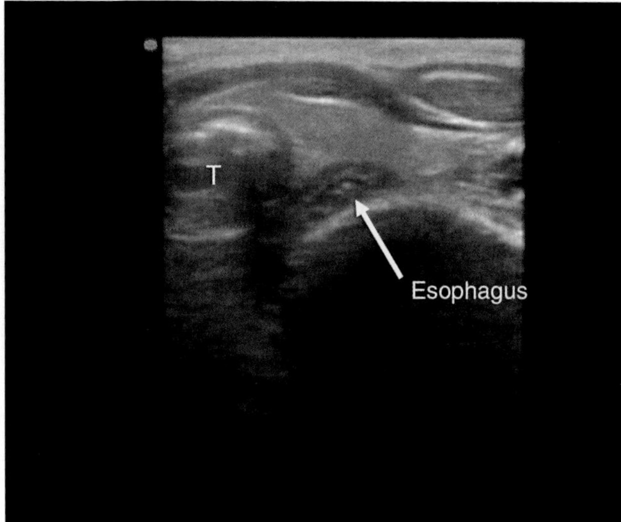

Figure 9.3
View of the esophagus just lateral to the trachea (T).

In addition, by applying Doppler, the arteries and veins that supply the thyroid tissue can be identified. In emergency situations, seeing these vessels can help you avoid them. More importantly, an emergent cricothyrotomy is attempted when swelling or hemorrhage in the neck distorts normal anatomy. Ultrasound can identify these fluid collections and help find the tracheal ring landmarks if they have been pushed from their normal anatomic position. Finally, the esophagus is usually visualized as a collapsed hyperdense structure just to the left of the trachea. The layers of esophageal mucosa can be seen to the right of the tracheal shadow in Figure 9.3. If the probe is held transverse over the mid trachea, the reflective shadow of the endotracheal tube can be visualized passing through the trachea. If it is seen entering the esophagus laterally, this can be immediately corrected without insufflation or other confirmatory testing required. Intubation can also be confirmed by correlating lung sliding to mechanical ventilation [2]. Normal *bilateral* lung sliding after intubation indicates correct endotracheal tube placement.

Chest

When using ultrasound to make diagnoses in lung pathology, it is important to recall some of the basic principles described in Chapter 1. One of the reasons that the normal lung is so difficult to image with ultrasound is that air is not a good transducer of sound waves. Air molecules tend to scatter sound waves in infinite directions, making it difficult for the transducer to receive any organized information from the returning sound wave. This property can actually be helpful in chest ultrasound, because a well-aerated and normal lung will not show much at all except for the horizontal reverberation artifact between the skin and the pleura that occurs when sound is

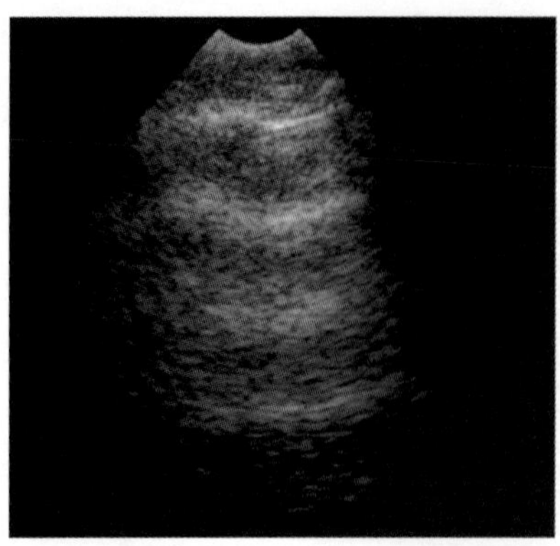
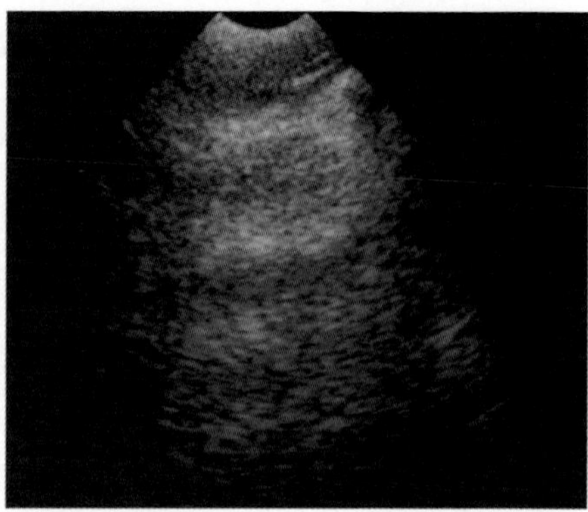

Figure 9.4
A-lines. Note that the reverberations are horizontally oriented.

scattered distal to the pleura and not reflected back to the ultrasound probe. These reverberation artifacts have been termed *A-lines* (Figure 9.4), and their presence signals the presence of normal aerated lung [1].

This is particularly helpful, because the absence of A-lines indicates that something has changed in the lung physiology so that lung tissue is now transmitting sound waves in a different pattern. The most common change is when the interstitium of the lung begins to fill with fluid. This occurs with pulmonary edema, infection, contusion, and many other pathologic states. Instead of being scattered, sound is now transmitted through the abnormal interstitium. Where previously there was thin alveolar wall tissue surrounded by air, now the interstitium is filled with fluid, and this tissue is conducive to sound-wave transmission. Sound waves get trapped in the fluid-filled interstitium of pulmonary tissue and create artifacts called *B-lines* (Figure 9.5) [1,3,4]. The important feature to note in looking for extravascular lung water or pulmonary edema is that the bright B-line extends all the way to the edge of the sonographic window and moves with respiratory motion (i.e., with pleural sliding). Moreover, sonographic B-lines tend to appear on ultrasound much earlier than radiographic B-lines appear on chest radiography and before symptoms develop [1,5]. In addition, as more fluid collects, more sonographic B-lines appear and they can start to coalesce. Instead of dark shadows, the lung becomes bright white. Research suggests that the number of B-lines correlates directly with the amount of interstial fluid [1,5–8]. These discoveries have suggested all kinds of new clinical applications, and research is rapidly expanding the use of chest sonography.

Lichtenstein has further subdivided this phenomenon, based on careful study of the pattern of these artifacts in different pulmonary pathologic states. For this introduction, however, an understanding of the basic difference between A-lines and B-lines and what that signifies for changes in lung physiology will suffice.

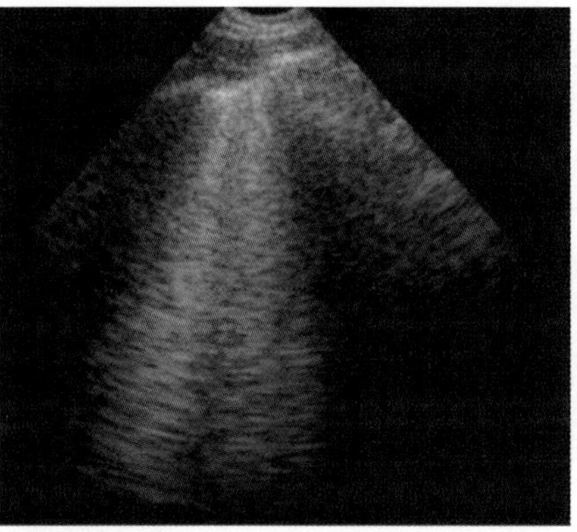
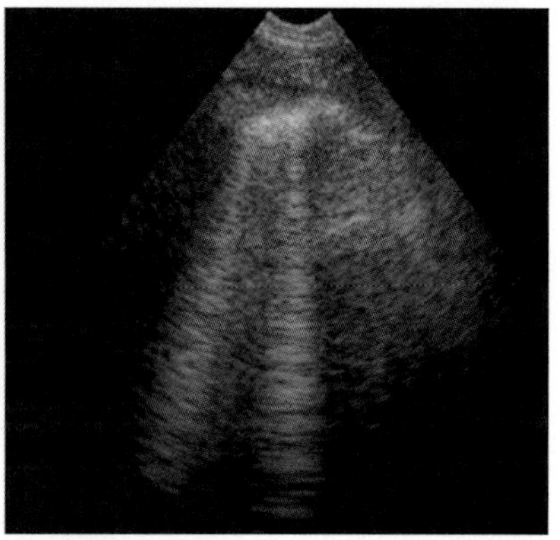

Figure 9.5
B-lines. Note the vertical orientation of the reverberations.

Technique

Probe selection

Airway

The linear high-frequency probe is most often used when looking at the more superficial structures of the neck. The high resolution this probe offers is essential when trying to identify the cricothyroid membrane.

Chest

The curvilinear or phased-array 2–5 MHz probe is most often used in chest ultrasound to ensure that the sound waves penetrate through the chest wall tissue and into the lung parenchyma. Higher-frequency linear probes can be used, but because their penetration is limited, their use should be restricted to evaluating at the pleura. In addition, research looking at ultrasound's diagnostic test characteristics for extravascular lung water has been performed largely with lower-frequency probes. Therefore it is strongly recommended that sonographers follow this technique, as the test characteristics for higher-frequency probes have not been well defined.

Views

Airway

Initially the probe is held transversely with the probe marker to the patient's right to identify the tracheal rings and to find the midline. The probe can then be rotated to the longitudinal or sagittal plane with the probe marker to the patient's head and the probe position on the neck can be gently moved superiorly until the cricothyroid membrane is visualized.

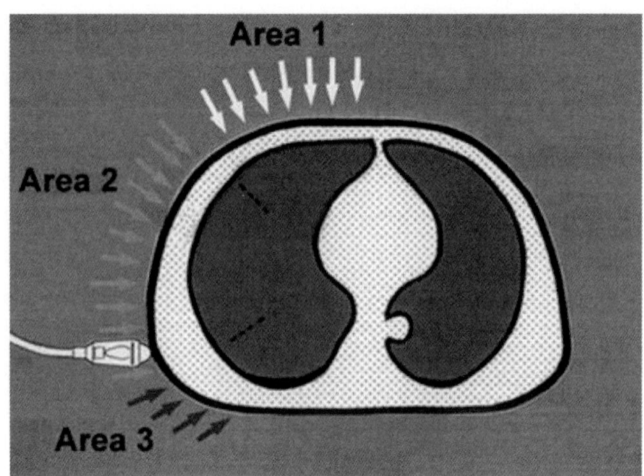

Figure 9.6

Chest sonography zones. Reproduced with permission from Lichtenstein DA, Lascols N, Meziere G, Gepner A. Ultrasound diagnosis of alveolar consolidation in the critically ill. *Intensive Care Med* 2004; **30**: 276–81.

Chest

Lichtenstein describes nine zones of the chest [1,3]. The anterior segment (area 1 in Figure 9.6) is bound by the sternum, clavicle, and anterior axillary line, and can be divided into four zones. The lateral segment (area 2) is bound by the anterior and posterior axillary lines and is divided into two zones, and the posterior segment (area 3) is bound by the posterior axillary line and the vertebral column and is divided into three zones. In the supine patient, consolidative fluid will be more obvious in the posterior segments, while air will be more apparent in the anterior segments. However, interstitial fluid most often distributes evenly [1,7,11].

Newer and more abbreviated scanning protocols have been developed to faciliate application in more acute and emergent patient evaluations. Volpicelli has described an eight-zone scanning protocol (four zones for each hemithorax) and has defined a positive scan as two positive zones (more than three B-lines visualized per zone) in each hemithorax (Figure 9.7) [4,10]. Lichtenstein himself has published an abbreviated scanning protocol for the more acutely dyspneic patient. The "BLUE" protocol requires that the sonographer scan patients sitting upright and evaluate both anterior hemithoraces looking for "predominant" B-line patterns. If this is present, the scan is positive [11].

Obviously these three scanning protocols range from more objective, quantitative protocols to more subjective and qualitative protocols. The preferred protocol depends on the clinical setting. Patients in the intensive care unit who are being scanned serially may need more quantitative evaluations, while patients in the emergency department may need quicker, more qualitative evaluations. Further research and work in international consensus conferences is currently under way to better refine the scanning protocol for

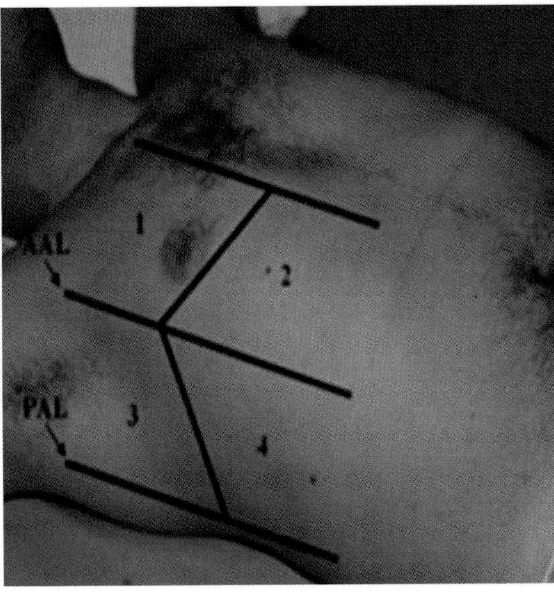

Figure 9.7
Volpicelli's sonography zones.

extravascular lung water, but the concept and the correlation of B-lines with interstitial edema has been well established.

Scanning tips

Trouble with the airway images

Unable to see the tracheal ring?

- Try sliding or fanning the probe to the left or right. Sometimes the trachea (especially in emergent airway situations) is not midline.
- Adjust the depth (increase). If the depth is too shallow it can sometimes be hard to get a handle on the anatomy.

Trouble with the chest images

No A-lines or B-lines?

- Try imaging in different planes or segments of the chest wall. It is important to at least look in anterior and lateral segments. Some machines use significant "post processing" to help clarify anatomic images and erase artifacts. This can cause significant degredation in the ability to use ultrasound for thoracic applications, and so asking if post-processing techniques can be turned off or minimized may be important when picking a machine if you plan to use it for thoracic imaging.

Unclear image?

- If the patient has a pneumothorax with subcutaneous air, images can be difficult to obtain, so attempt to circumvent the subcutaneous air with different patient and probe positioning if possible.

Normal images

Figures 9.1–9.4 are examples of normal airway and lung ultrasound scans.

Abnormal images

Figure 9.5 shows the appearance of B-lines. Ultrasound can also be useful to assess lung water in a dynamic fashion [5,9,10]. Figure 9.8 demonstrates

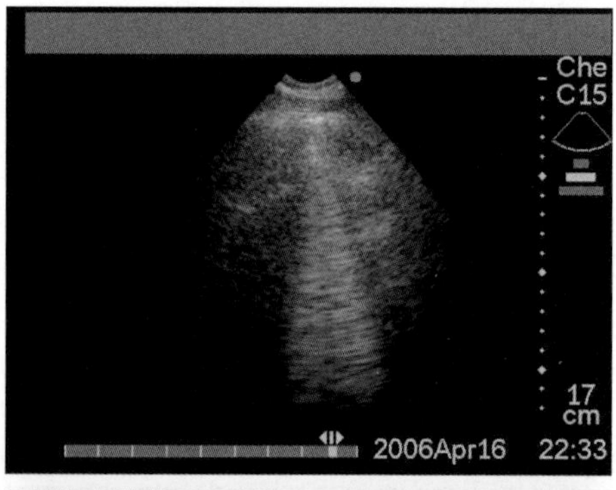

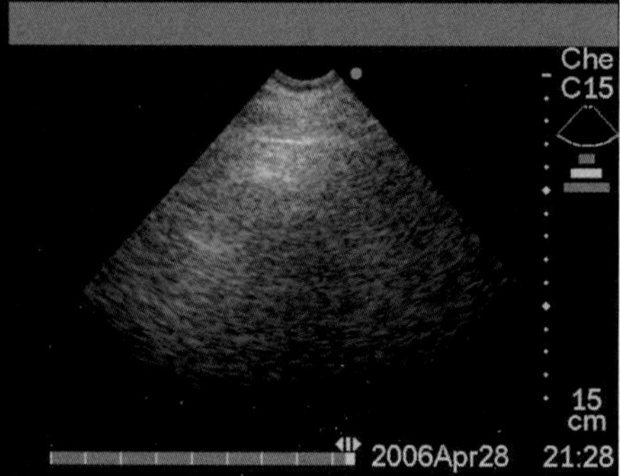

Figure 9.8

These images are from the same patient. The first image was taken when the patient was suffering from high-altitude pulmonary edema and was symptomatic with hypoxia. The second image was taken after treatment and after symptoms had resolved. When the second image was obtained, the patient had normal oxygenation. Courtesy of Dr. Peter Fagenholz, Massachusetts General Hospital, Boston, MA.

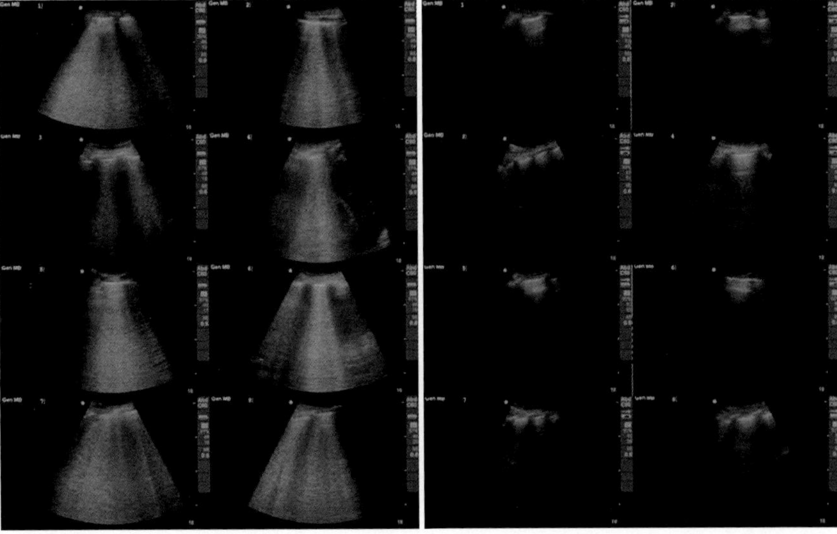

Figure 9.9
These images were taken from the same patient before (*left*) and after (*right*) using continuous positive airway pressure to treat acute decompensated heart failure. The second group of eight images were obtained about one hour after the first. Courtesy of Dr. Andrew Liteplo, Massachusetts General Hospital, Boston, MA.

the appearance (top) and resolution (bottom) of B-lines in high-altitude pulmonary edema. Figure 9.9 shows a similar pattern in a patient with acute heart failure.

Literature review

Reference	Methods	Results	Notes
Lichtenstein & Meziere 1998 [3]	66 patients with dyspnea evaluated for multiple comet tail artifacts (B-lines) as sign of pulmonary edema.	Sensitivity of 100% and specificity of 92% in the diagnosis of pulmonary edema when compared to COPD.	Evidence supporting the use of B-lines for diagnosing pulmonary edema.
Agricola *et al.* 2005 [6]	Correlation of B-lines with invasive measurements of pulmonary congestion and cardiac function.	Comparison of lung US and pulmonary artery wedge pressures showed good correlation ($r = 0.48$, $p = 0.001$).	First evidence showing lung US comparability to invasive measurements of pulmonary wedge pressure as gold standard.

Reference	Methods	Results	Notes
Liteplo *et al.* 2009 [7]	Observational study looking at lung US for diagnosing congestive heart failure (CHF) using Volpicelli scanning protocol.	Positive lung scan increased the likelihood ratio (LR) for CHF diagnosis by 3.88 while NT-proBNP only increased LR for CHF by 2.3.	Evidence that lung US is at least comparable to NT-proBNP for diagnosing CHF.
Frassi *et al.* 2007 [8]	290 patients with acute dyspnea and/ or chest pain syndrome were evaluated on hospital admission with lung US and followed for 16 months.	Patients with high initial B-line scores had a worse prognosis and higher event scores at 16 months than patients with low B-line scores. B-line scores outperformed other echocardiographic variables as a univariate predictor.	B-line scores provide prognostic information and risk stratification in patients with acute heart failure.
Volpicelli *et al.* 2008 [10]	Prospective study evaluating the time course to resolution for B-lines after treatment for CHF.	81 patients with diagnosis of acute heart failure showed clearing of their B-lines after treatment.	Lung US proposed as alternative to serial chest x-rays for following CHF resolution.
Lichtenstein *et al.* 2008 [11]	Observational study using an integrated US protocol to evaluate 260 patients with acute respiratory failure in the ICU.	Using the scanning protocol, the correct diagnosis was made by US in 90.5% of cases.	First integrated lung US scanning protocol used for diagnostic purposes in acute respiratory failure.

New directions

There are many exciting areas for expanding the use of this application. Prehospital use of chest ultrasound in assisting in the differentiation between congestive heart failure and chronic obstructive pulmonary disease could mean the early initiation of disease-specific therapy. In addition, the use of lung ultrasound in the assessment of EVLW could help with monitoring in critical care settings and could begin to replace the need for serial chest x-rays.

References

1. Lichtenstein DA (ed.). *General Ultrasound in the Critically Ill*. New York, NY: Springer; 2004.
2. Weaver B, Lyon M, Blaivas M. Confirmation of endotracheal tube placement after intubation using the ultrasound sliding lung sign. *Acad Emerg Med* 2006; **13**: 239–44.

3. Lichtenstein D, Meziere G. A lung ultrasound sign allowing bedside distinction between pulmonary edema and COPD: the comet-tail artifact. *Intensive Care Med* 1998; **24**: 1331–4.
4. Volpicelli G, Mussa A, Garofalo G, *et al.* Bedside lung ultrasound in the assessment of alveolar-interstitial syndrome. *Am J Emerg Med* 2006; **24**: 689–96.
5. Noble VE, Murray AF, Capp R, *et al.* Ultrasound assessment for extravascular lung water in patients undergoing hemodialysis: time course for resolution. *Chest* 2009; **135**: 1433–9.
6. Agricola E, Bove, T, Oppizzi M, *et al.* "Ultrasound comet-tail images": a marker of pulmonary edema. A comparative study with wedge pressure and extravascular lung water. *Chest* 2005; **127**: 1690–5.
7. Liteplo AS, Marill KA, Villen T, *et al.* Emergency thoracic ultrasound in the differentiation of the etiology of shortness of breath (ETUDES): sonographic B-lines and N-terminal pro-brain-type natriuretic peptide in diagnosing congestive heart failure. *Acad Emerg Med* 2009; **16**: 201–10.
8. Frassi F, Gargani L, Tesorio P, *et al.* Prognostic value of extravascular lung water assessed with ultrasound lung comets by chest sonography in patients with dyspnea and/or chest pain. *J Cardiac Fail* 2007; **13**: 830–5.
9. Fagenholz PF, Gutman JA, Murray AF, *et al.* Chest ultrasonography for the diagnosis and monitoring of high-altitude pulmonary edema. *Chest* 2007; **131**: 1013–18.
10. Volpicelli G, Caramello V, Cardinale L, *et al.* Bedside ultrasound of the lung for the monitoring of acute decompensated heart failure. *Am J Emerg Med* 2008; **26**: 585–91.
11. Lichtenstein DA, Meziere GA. Relevance of lung ultrasound in the diagnosis of acute respiratory failure: the BLUE protocol. *Chest* 2008; **134**: 117–25.

10 Ocular ultrasound

Introduction

Ocular ultrasound as used by the emergency or critical care physician has several applications. The diagnosis of lens disruption and/or retinal detachment can be made with ultrasound, and this has been well described in the ophthalmology and radiology literature [1,2]. Ultrasound can also diagnose the presence of ocular foreign bodies [1–3]. However, more recently, other research directions for ocular ultrasound have included the use of ultrasound to measure the optic nerve sheath diameter. Here, the concept is based on the idea that increased intracranial pressure (ICP) is reflected through the nerve sheath, causing edema and swelling. Since increases in ICP are transmitted by the cerebrospinal fluid (CSF) down the perineural subarachnoid space of the optic nerve, this expansion of the nerve sheath can be measured by ultrasound [4–6]. In many ways, this technique parallels the concept of papilledema as a marker for increased ICP. However, optic nerve ultrasonography is arguably easier to perform and more quantifiable than the presence or absence of papilledema. It is this interest in ultrasound's potential to measure ICP non-invasively that has sparked much research.

Many ocular ultrasound studies have been done to try to define normal optic nerve diameter ranges and where enlargement becomes pathologic and correlates with increased ICP. Although research is ongoing, to date most researchers have found that both pediatric and adult ocular nerve sheath diameters > 5 mm correlate well with evidence of increased ICP as measured by degree of hydrocephalus, intrathecal infusions where lumbar pressures were measured, or CT evidence of increased ICP [7–10]. In addition, more recent studies have correlated optic nerve sheath diameter > 5 mm with invasive ICP measurements as a gold standard [11–14]. Although much research is still needed to better define the clinical utility of this technique, the literature support to date and the need for non-invasive techniques to assess ICP allow researchers to be optimistic about the future of this application.

Focused questions for ocular ultrasound

The questions for ocular ultrasound are as follows:

1. Is the optic nerve sheath diameter > 5 mm?
2. Is there other obvious ocular pathology (lens dislocation, retinal detachment, foreign body)?

Anatomy

When viewed on ultrasound, several ocular anatomic features are worth noting. The globe is seen as a dark fluid-filled structure, because the vitreous is largely fluid and so will appear dark on ultrasound (Figures 10.1 and 10.2).

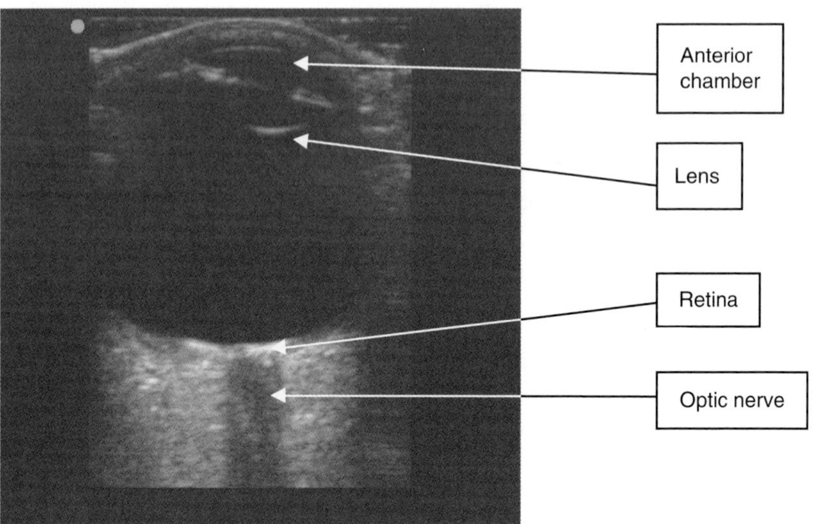

Figure 10.1
Normal ultrasound of the eye.

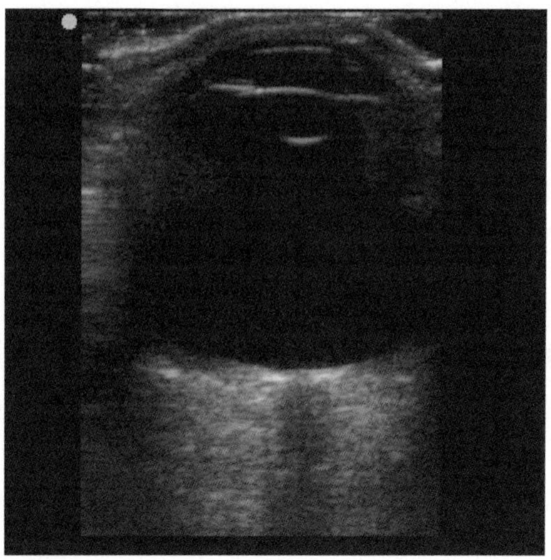

Figure 10.2
Normal ultrasound of the eye.

The anterior chamber is often seen in cross-section as a separate fluid-filled structure just anterior to the hyperechoic line of the lens. The retina is not seen unless it is detached from the posterior aspect of the globe. Ultrasound is used in ophthalmology for many advanced diagnostic applications, but these two structures (lens and retina) are easily assessed by the emergency physician. Ultrasound findings of abnormal lens or retinal position may help facilitate referral or consultation for formal evaluation and expedite identification of ocular pathology [3].

For ocular nerve sheath measurements, the dark shadow of the optic nerve sheath should be identified posterior to the retina. The perineural sheath travels from the brain to each orbit, and contains CSF in continuous communication with intracranial CSF. Therefore, increased ICP is transmitted to the optic nerve, causing edema and swelling of the nerve sheath. Pathology studies have shown that 3 mm posterior to the retina, the nerve sheath is particularly porous and thus is postulated to be most responsive to these transmitted pressures [6]. Therefore, when measuring the diameter of the nerve sheath to assess ICP, the convention is that the sheath diameter should be measured 3 mm posterior to the retinal rim. There is still some controversy as to whether this shadow is actually the true optic nerve sheath or the shadow from the optic disc, given that the edges of the shadow appear crisp and straight in a way that suggests a non-anatomic image [15,16]. However, whether this is the optic disc shadow or truly the optic nerve sheath, there is growing evidence showing correlation with invasive measures. As there are obvious clinical benefits to having a non-invasive way to measure ICP, this application continues to receive attention.

Technique

Probe selection

Because the structures being imaged here are so superficial, the linear high-frequency probe should be used. Several ultrasound companies make probes specifically for ocular ultrasound that have a very small footprint and an even higher frequency than the standard vascular range (> 10 MHz, as opposed to the standard 7–10 MHz). However, this special probe is not necessary for acquiring adequate images for the diagnostic applications described here (although the higher the frequency, the more detailed the image).

There is literature describing a coronal technique in which a small-footprint probe is placed in the temporal window over the temporal bone [14,15]. The eye is directed toward the probe and a cross-section of the sheath and the nerve is observed. There is evidence that this technique shows improved inter-rater reliability and does not have the same challenge of imaging through the lens which may distort distal imaging [14,15]. However, this technique has not been correlated with invasive measurements or non-invasive surrogates for increased ICP, and as normal images appear to be smaller than those obtained with the linear probe, the nomogram for normal and abnormal images has not been defined. Moreover, this technique is optimized when a patient can direct his or her gaze toward the probe; this is not always possible in patients with increased ICP, and so it may not be a feasible alternative.

Views

When imaging the eye, it is prudent to apply a clear film adhesive strip or Tegaderm over the closed lid of the eye before applying the gel, to prevent contamination of the conjunctiva. In addition, it should be obvious that this exam is contraindicated in anyone with open ocular trauma or periorbital wounds, or in anyone in whom applied pressure could cause further injury. To perform the exam, the linear probe is rested gently on the orbital rim, with the gel providing the interface with the globe itself. Caution should be used when applying pressure on the globe from the probe. Occasionally, patients can have a vagal-type response to the increased pressure being applied to the globe (oculocardiac reflex). In rare cases, this stimulus can be enough to cause bradycardia and syncope.

As with all imaging, it is standard to acquire images in two planes, transverse and longitudinal, to ensure true diameters are being measured.

Scanning tips

No nerve sheath shadow seen?

- For the nerve sheath shadow to be seen, the ultrasound beam or plane needs to transect the nerve, which enters the orbit at a slight angle. With gentle rocking of the probe or moving slightly to the lateral edge of the globe, the nerve sheath will usually come into view.

Unclear image?

- Often, because of the variation in the curve of the orbital rim, more gel is needed to increase the interface of the probe with the surface of the eye.

Normal images

Figures 10.3 and 10.4 demonstrate measurement of the optic nerve sheath diameter.

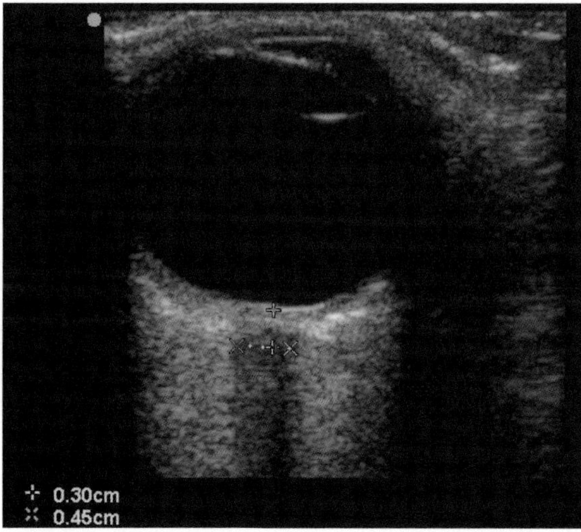

Figure 10.3

Normal optic nerve sheath measurement. Sheath diameter 3 mm posterior to retina = 4.5 mm.

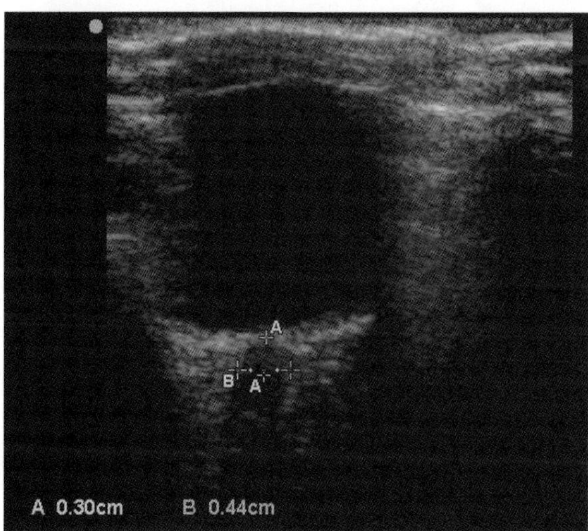

Figure 10.4

Normal optic nerve sheath measurement. Sheath diameter = 4.4 mm.

Abnormal images

A dilated optic nerve sheath (Figure 10.5) correlates with elevated ICP [7–14]. The retina is not well visualized unless there is a retinal detachment. It is then seen in relief as a thin hyperechoic line (Figure 10.6) surrounded by anechoic fluid above (vitreous) and below (often blood). Lens dislocation can also be readily seen, as in Figure 10.7.

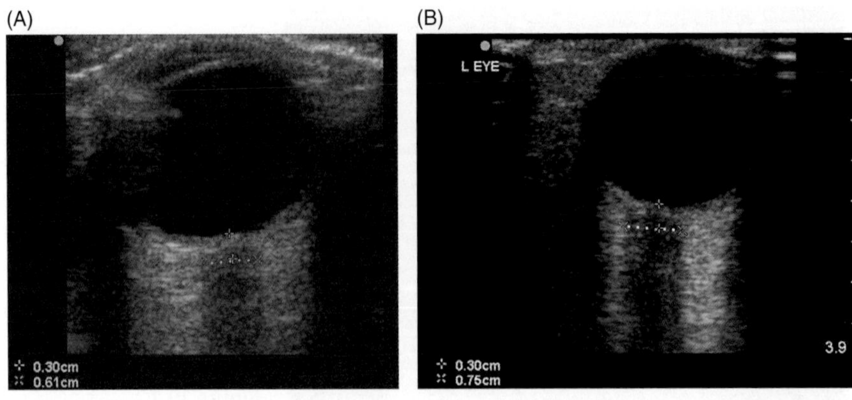

Figure 10.5

Dilated optic nerve. Sheath diameter = (*A*) 6.1 mm and (*B*) 7.5 mm.

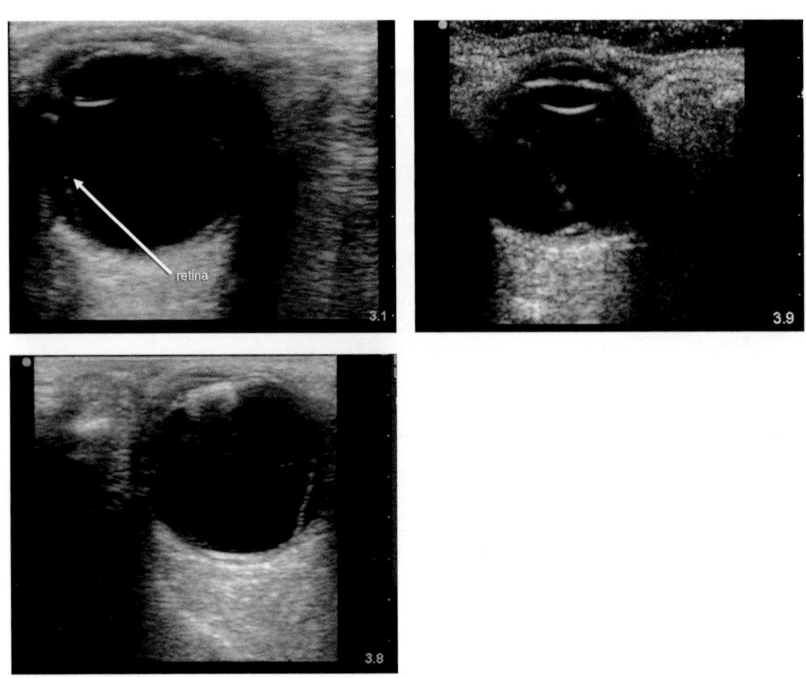

Figure 10.6

Three images of retinal detachment.

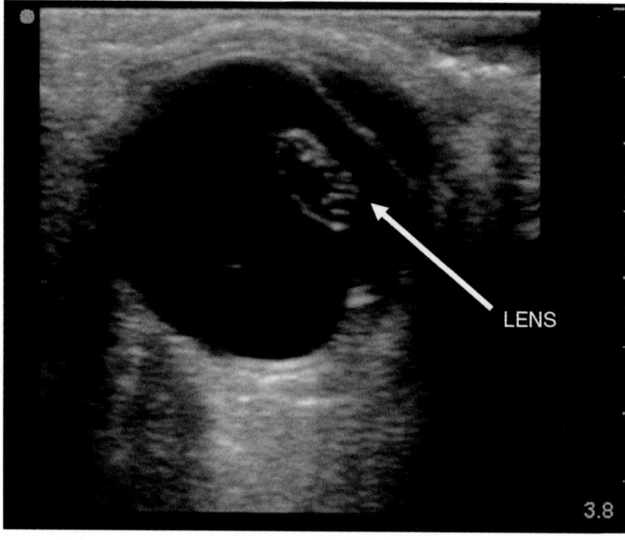

Figure 10.7
Lens dislocation.

Literature review

Reference	Methods	Results	Notes
Galetta *et al.* 1989 [4]	Pre- and postlumbar puncture sonography of optic nerve sheath in a patient with pseudotumor cerebri.	Decrease in size of optic nerve sheath with removal of cerebrospinal fluid (CSF) during lumbar puncture.	Proof of concept that optic nerve sheath size correlates with elevated intracranial pressure (ICP).
Newman *et al.* 2002 [7]	Children with VP shunts in place who were suspected of having elevated ICP had optic nerve sheath diameter (ONSD) measurements taken with US.	Measurements > 4.5 mm correlated with evidence of hydrocephalus and increased ICP.	By using normal controls, attempt to establish absolute ONSD value that correlates with elevated ICP.
Kimberly *et al.* 2008 [12]	Measured ONSD in patients with intraventricular drains. Developed ROC curve for ONSD measurement and ICP > 20 cm H_2O.	Using an ROC curve, the authors systematically confirmed the commonly used threshold of ONSD > 5 mm to detect ICP > 20 cm H_2O.	Directly correlates ventriculostomy measurements of ICP with US ONSD measurements and provides further support for the use of ONSD measurements as a non-invasive test for elevated ICP.

Reference	Methods	Results	Notes
Blaivas *et al.* 2002 [3]	Patients with eye complaints presenting to the emergency department had ocular US performed in addition to usual standard of care evaluation.	26/61 patients had ocular pathology identified on US that facilitated ophthalmology referral or further testing.	Bedside US is useful in the diagnosis of multiple ocular complaints and in identifying a variety of ocular pathology.

New directions

There are many exciting areas for expanding the use of this application. Prehospital or remote medical providers could use this technique to determine who should be evacuated to centers with neurosurgical capabilities. Different scanning techniques for measuring the optic nerve show potential for having increased inter-rater reliability and therefore increased clinical utility. Finally, automated volume sweeps could correlate nerve sheath volume with ICP, and this could be a more reproducible technique. As research continues, the accuracy of the test and the potential for this non-invasive ICP monitoring technique in critical care settings can be further evaluated.

References

1. Bedi DG, Gombos DS, Ng CS, Singh S. Sonography of the eye. *AJR Am J Roentgenol* 2006; **187**: 1061–72.
2. Baum G, Greenwood I. The application of ultrasonic locating techniques to ophthalmology. II. Ultrasonic slit lamp in the ultrasonic visualization of soft tissues. *Arch Ophthalmol* 1958; **60**: 263–79.
3. Blaivas M, Theodoro D, Sierzenski PR. A study of bedside ocular ultrasonography in the emergency department. *Acad Emerg Med* 2002; **9**: 791–9.
4. Galetta S, Byrne SF, Smith JL. Echographic correlation of optic nerve sheath size and cerebrospinal fluid pressure. *J Clin Neuroopthalmol* 1989; **9**: 79–82.
5. Liu D, Kahn M. Measurement and relationship of subarachnoid pressure of the optic nerve to intracranial pressures in fresh cadavers. *Am J Opthalmol* 1993; **116**: 548–56.
6. Hansen HC, Helmke K. The subarachnoid space surrounding the optic nerves: an ultrasound study of the optic nerve sheath. *Surg Radiol Anat* 1996; **18**: 323–8.
7. Newman WD, Hollman AS, Dutton GN, Carachi R. Measurement of optic nerve sheath diameter by ultrasound: a means of detecting acute raised intracranial pressure in hydrocephalus. *Br J Ophthalmol* 2002; **86**: 1109–13.

8. Blaivas M, Theodoro D, Sierzenski PR. Elevated intracranial pressure detected by bedside emergency ultrasonography of the optic nerve sheath. *Acad Emerg Med* 2003; **10**: 376–81.
9. Hansen H, Helmke K. Validation of the optic nerve sheath response to changing cerebrospinal fluid pressure: ultrasound findings during intrathecal infusion tests. *J Neurosurg* 1997; **87**: 34–40.
10. Neulander M, Tayal VS, Blaivas M, Norton J, Saunders T. Use of emergency department sonographic measurement of optic nerve sheath diameter to detect CT findings of increased intracranial pressure in adult head injury patients. *Acad Emerg Med* 2005; **12**: S1139.
11. Geeraerts T, Launey Y, Martin L, *et al.* Ultrasonography of the optic nerve sheath may be useful for detecting raised intracranial pressure after severe brain injury. *Intensive Care Med* 2007; **33**: 1704–11.
12. Kimberly HH, Shah S, Marill K, Noble V. Correlation of optic nerve sheath diameter with direct measurement of intracranial pressure. *Acad Emerg Med* 2008; **15**: 201–4.
13. Soldatos T, Karakitsos D, Chatzimichail K, *et al.* Optic nerve sonography in the diagnostic evaluation of adult brain injury. *Crit Care* 2008; **12**: R67.
14. Shah S, Kimberly HH, Marill KA, Noble VE. Ultrasound techniques to measure the optic nerve: is a specialized probe necessary? *Med Sci Mon* 2009; **15**(5): MT63–8.
15. Blehar DJ, Gaspari RJ, Montoya A, Calderon R. Correlation of visual axis and coronal axis measurements of optic nerve sheath diameter. *J Ultrasound Med* 2008; **2**: 407–11.
16. Ballantyne SA, O'Neill G, Hamilton R, Hollman AS. Observer variation in the sonographic measurement of optic nerve sheath diameter in normal adults. *Eur J Ultrasound* 2002; **15**: 145–9.

11 Soft tissue and musculoskeletal ultrasound

Introduction

Interest in soft tissue and musculoskeletal ultrasound has grown rapidly over the past five years – not just among emergency physicians but among rheumatologists, orthopedists, primary care physicians, podiatrists, and many others as well. Clinicians have taken notice as evidence mounts of the ability of ultrasound to improve their diagnostic capabilities, not only by making anatomy plain at the bedside but also, more importantly, by evaluating function dynamically. This chapter will provide a brief overview of soft tissue and musculoskeletal ultrasound, but for those who are interested entire courses and textboooks dedicated to this topic are available. As pressure to decrease the use of expensive diagnostic imaging such as magnetic resonance imaging (MRI) increases, the use of diagnostic ultrasound for musculoskeletal complaints will likely continue to grow.

Soft tissue

While the differentiation between abscess and cellulitis would seem to be clinically apparent, research has shown that clinicians are not as accurate in making this distinction as they think using clinical exam parameters alone [1,2]. Ultrasound is readily able to make this distinction. In this way, painful drainage procedures can be avoided in those who have no drainable collection, and return visits can be avoided in those who were not adequately treated with incision and drainage. In addition, ultrasound can highlight sonographic features that should make a clinician more suspicious of aggressive infectious processes such as necrotizing fasciitis and Fournier's gangrene [3,4]. These include layering fluid along the fascial plane and "dirty shadows" or white shadows indicating the presence of air within the area of inflammation. Finally, once an abscess is identified, ultrasound can make the drainage procedure more accurate and identify surrounding vessels and nerves so that complications can be avoided. Procedural guidance will be discussed further in Chapter 16.

Bone and tendons

Although long bone fractures are often detected clinically, the sensitivity of the physical exam is insufficient to exclude pathology. In addition, the management of fractures varies considerably, based on characteristics undetectable by physical exam alone (displacement, angulation, comminution). Thus, clinicians often rely on plain x-ray (as well as CT and MRI) to characterize fractures in patients with extremity trauma. In addition, identifying orthopedic injuries that involve tendon injuries versus those where tendon function is intact is essential but can be difficult in the setting of an acute injury. Visualizing the tendon throughout passive and active range of motion can facilitate the identification and diagnosis of tendon disruption – and expedite consultation, referral, and/or treatment.

Therefore, bedside ultrasound's role in the evaluation of orthopedic injuries is threefold. First, in a select group of injuries, diagnosis and treatment may be more rapid by using ultrasound rather than other modalities. There is some evidence that ultrasound is superior to plain x-ray in selected fractures (sternal, rib) [5–7]. In addition, there are some clinical scenarios where bedside diagnoses can expedite traction, anesthesia, and other maneuvers such as alignment through closed reduction [8,9]. Second, advanced imaging modalities are not always available. In some emergency departments, even plain x-rays take a significant amount of time to be performed, especially when performed serially in reduction procedures. In austere environments, portable bedside ultrasound technology may be all that is available, given the setup costs and bulk of x-ray, CT, and MRI machines. Third, increasing awareness of radiation exposure parameters continues to challenge assumptions about "safe" levels of exposure, and x-ray radiation is relatively contraindicated in some patients, especially children. Radiation exposure can be minimized using ultrasound as an alternative diagnostic tool, and ultrasound can be especially helpful in monitoring reductions.

Focused questions for soft tissue and musculoskeletal ultrasound

The questions for soft tissue ultrasound are as follows:

1. Is there any fluid collection?
2. Are there signs of fasciitis?
3. Is there a foreign body?

The questions for musculoskeletal ultrasound are as follows:

1. Is there an interruption in the bony cortex?
2. Can a degree of angulation or displacement be assessed?
3. Is the tendon injured?

Anatomy

As described previously, subcutaneous tissue and muscle are readily visualized with ultrasound because they transmit sound well. Bone acts as a bright

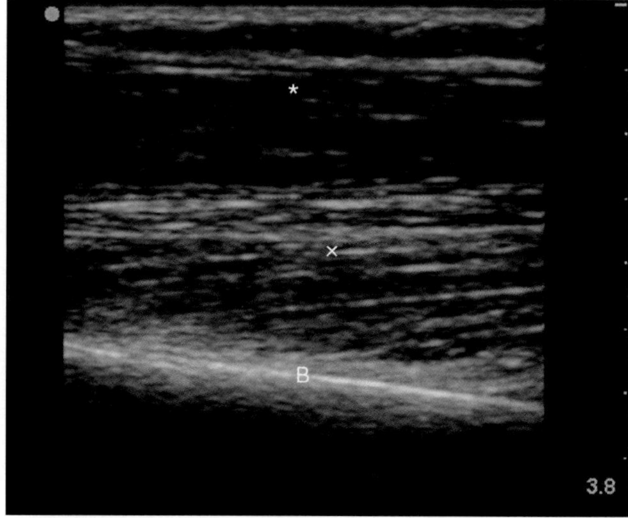

Figure 11.1
Image demonstrating the normal ultrasound appearance of soft tissue and musculoskeletal layers. Note the hypoechoic subcutaneous tissue layer (*) separated from the linear striations of the muscle (×) by a dense bright fascial line and the bright hyperechoic reflection of the bone (B).

reflector, yielding a strong echogenic signal and distal shadowing. The different soft tissue and musculoskeletal layers, including the epidermis, dermis, subcutaneous tissue, fascia, muscle, and bone, all have characteristic ultrasound features and are distinguishable as shown in Figure 11.1.

Technique

Probe selection

Use a high-frequency linear probe to best assess the superficial soft tissue and gain the highest resolution for imaging bony structures. However, if there is substantial soft tissue present, lower-frequency probes can be used.

Views

At least two views are useful (longitudinal and transverse) for all soft tissue and musculoskeletal applications.

Soft tissue

Scan with the linear probe from an area of normal tissue, fanning through the area of abnormal tissue entirely. Observe "cobblestoning" or fluid tracking throughout the subcutaneous tissue in areas of cellulitis or edema (Figure 11.2) and look at the fascial plane to evaluate whether there is fluid tracking along the fascia (Figure 11.3). If a fluid collection is seen, use Doppler flow to ensure that the anechoic space is not a vessel and to identify nearby

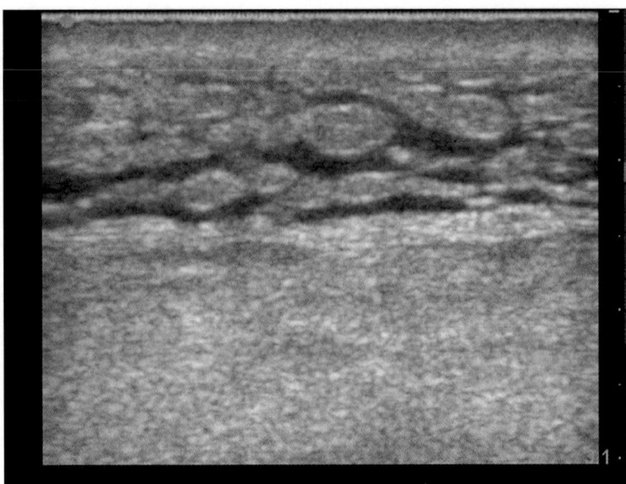

Figure 11.2
Cobblestoning.

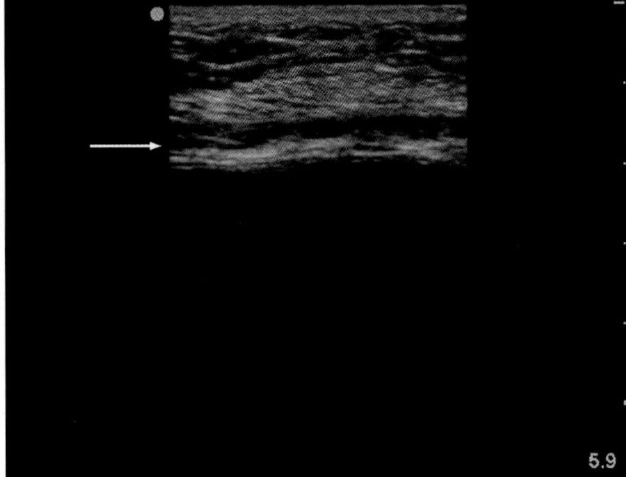

Figure 11.3
Dark fluid lining the fascial plane.

vessels that may complicate incision and drainage (Figure 11.4). Often, because abscesses are filled not with clear fluid but with debris, the echotexture of abscesses can be more heterogeneous and have increased gray-scale tones compared to simple fluid (Figure 11.5). If it is difficult to see the outline of the collection because of this increased gray-scale, gentle pressure can be applied and the "squish sign" or movement of purulent material within the abscess can be seen in real time. Make sure to warn the patient before attempting this maneuver, however, since it has the potential to be painful.

Musculoskeletal

Scan along the entire extremity to be assessed – from its proximal to distal articulation. Begin in a longitudinal plane, and note the depth of soft tissue

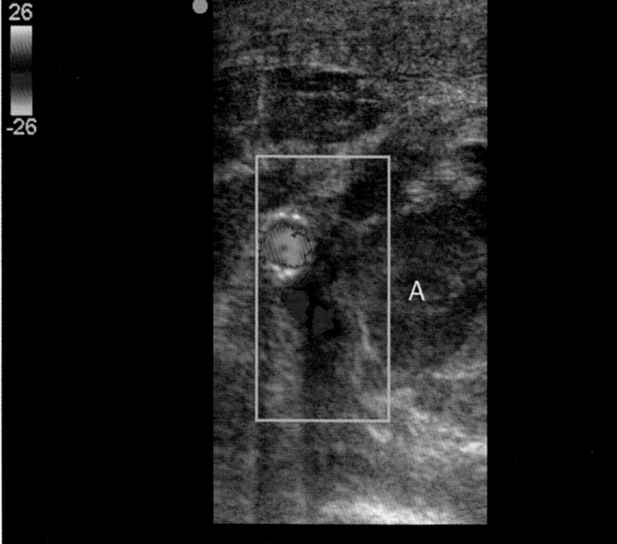

Figure 11.4
Image demonstrating the proximity of vessels to a large abscess (A) and the clinical benefit of using Doppler prior to incision and drainage.

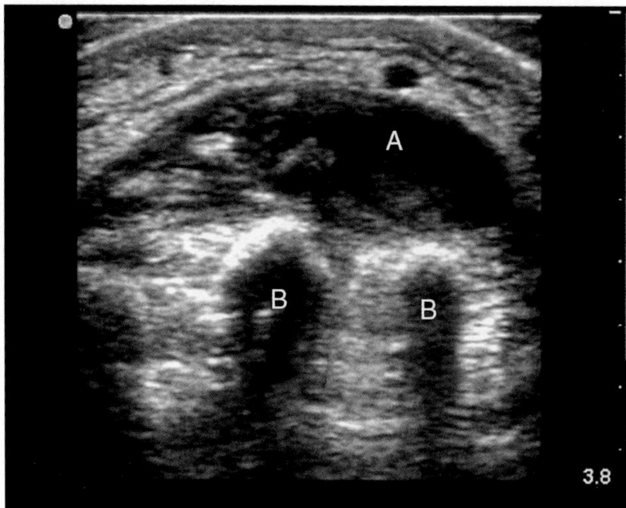

Figure 11.5
The echotexture of an abscess (A) is often mixed, showing the debris and cellular material present in a purulent collection. B marks the bony shadows of the metacarpals.

and the intact cortex (with distal shadowing). As the site of suspected fracture is approached, soft tissue swelling or hematoma, as well as a more obvious break in the cortex, may be noted. Although the longitudinal view is often more useful, transverse views may also demonstrate these findings and give information as to the degree of angulation or displacement. When evaluating the tendons, the longitudinal plane is better. Line up the probe in a position parallel to the length of the tendon. Occasionally a standoff pad or water

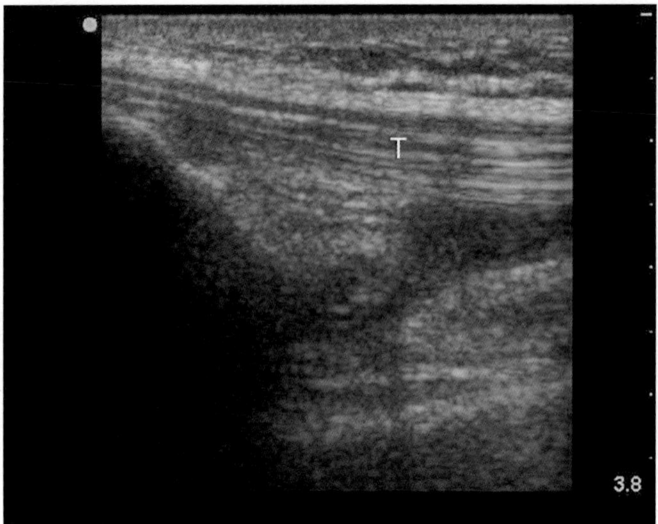

Figure 11.6
A normal tendon (T).

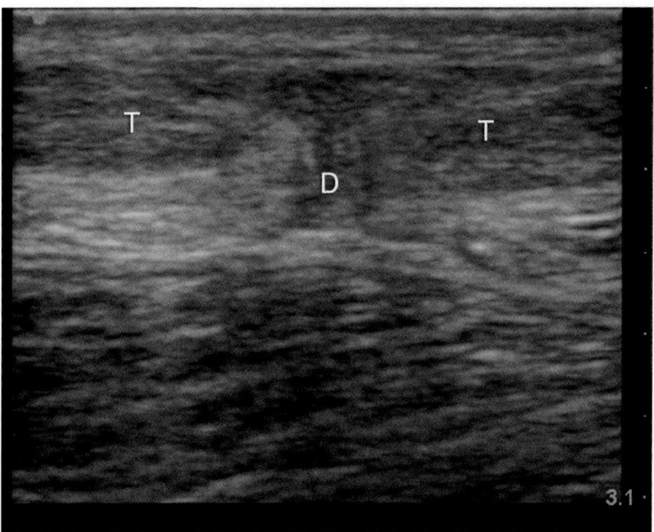

Figure 11.7
A disrupted tendon. The break, with darker hemorrhage, shows as a disruption (D) of the normal linear, fibrillar pattern of the tendon (T).

bath (see Chapter 16) will be necessary for very superficial structures. Then observe the linear, fibrillar tendon (Figure 11.6) throughout passive and active range of motion. Disruption in the tendon will cause the defect to widen with flexion and/or extension (Figure 11.7).

Scanning tips

Bone or tendon too superficial?

- Try using a water bath or standoff pad to bring the structures of interest further from the ultrasound beam.

Can't find break or disruption?

- It is helpful to have the patient point to the area of maximal tenderness and look there.

Anatomy appears strange?

- Perform ultrasound on the contralateral side to compare the anatomy side by side.

Not sure the fluid collection is an abscess?

- Always use color Doppler to help distinguish fluid collections from vessels.

Normal images

Figures 11.8–11.10 demonstrate normal soft tissue, tendon, and bony anatomy.

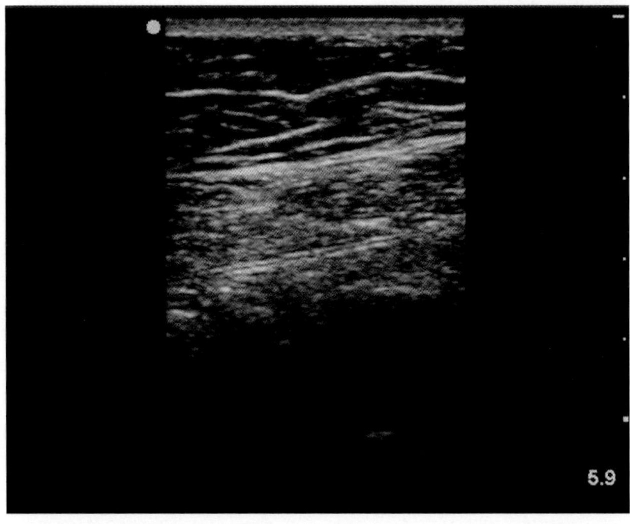

Figure 11.8
Normal soft tissue.

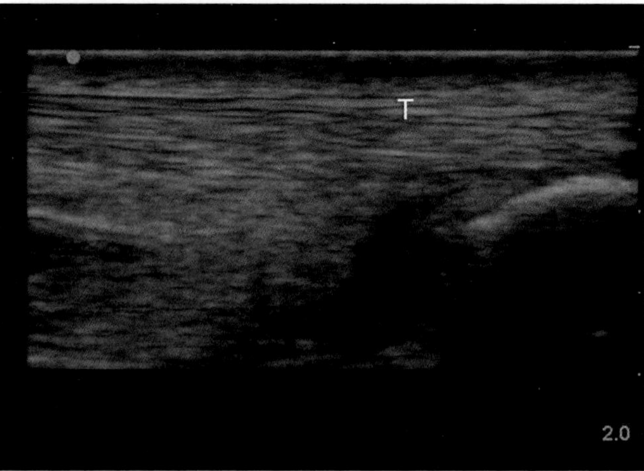

Figure 11.9
Normal tendon (T).

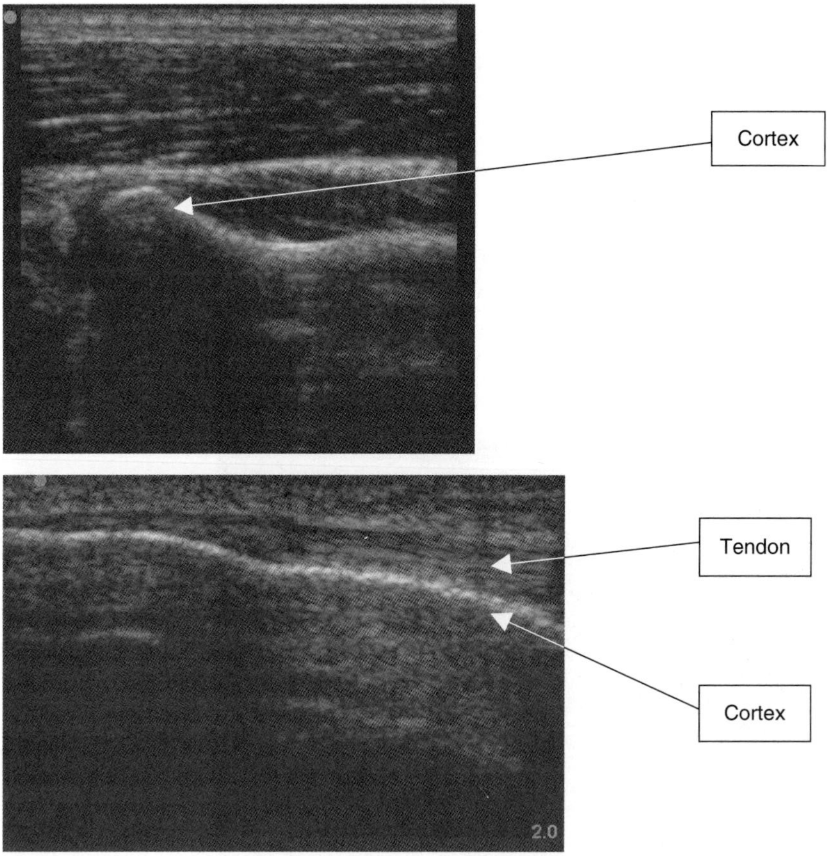

Cortex

Tendon

Cortex

2.0

Figure 11.10
Normal cortex: smooth and uninterrupted bright white line.

Abnormal images

Figures 11.11–11.14 demonstrate abnormal soft tissue and tendon anatomy, and show the interruption in cortex seen with a fracture.

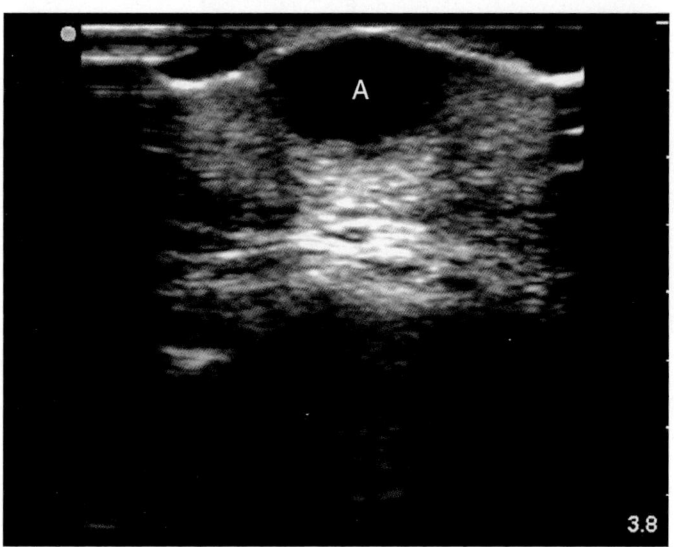

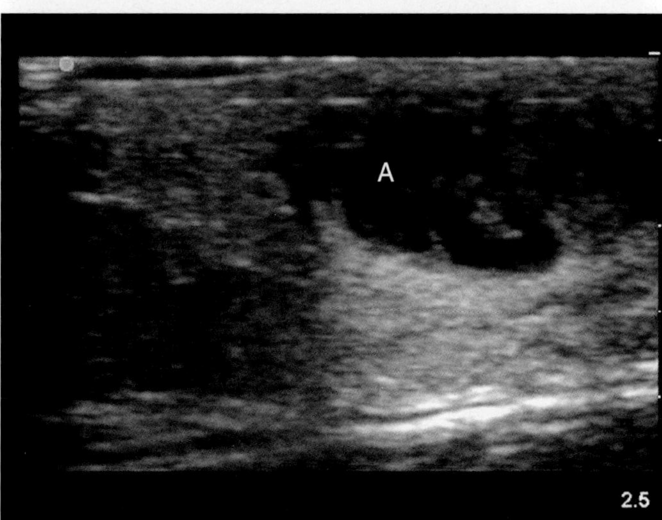

Figure 11.11

Abscess (A), showing posterior acoustic enhancement. This is because the density of the fluid-filled abscess is less than that of the surrounding tissue, so the sound waves are attenuated less as they pass through the abscess cavity. This finding of posterior acoustic enhancement can be helpful when the abscess cavity is isoechoic due to debris, making it easier to distinguish an abscess.

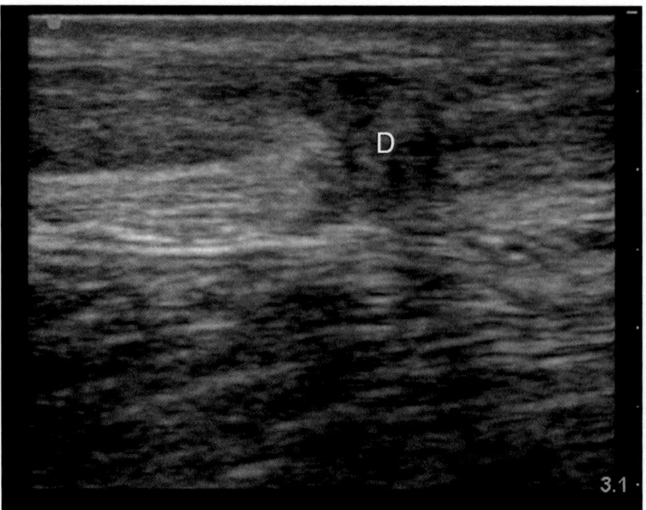

Figure 11.12
Disrupted tendon (D).

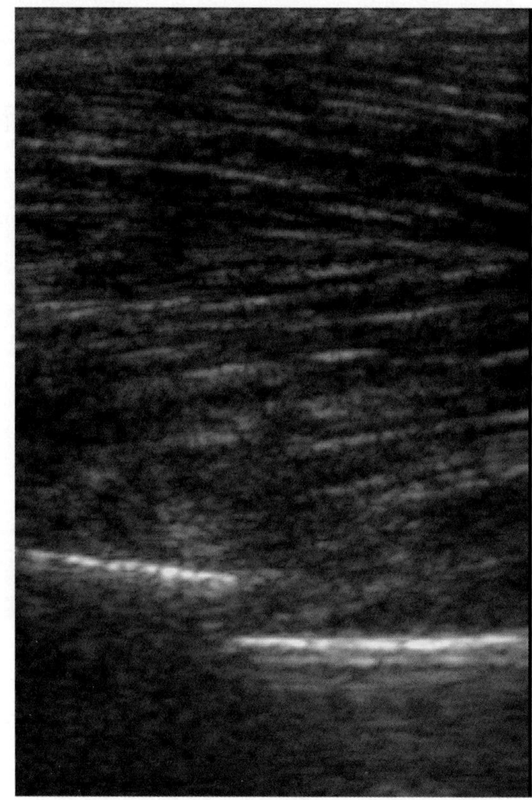

Figure 11.13
A fibula fracture with soft tissue swelling. Note the cortical disruption (broken bright white line).

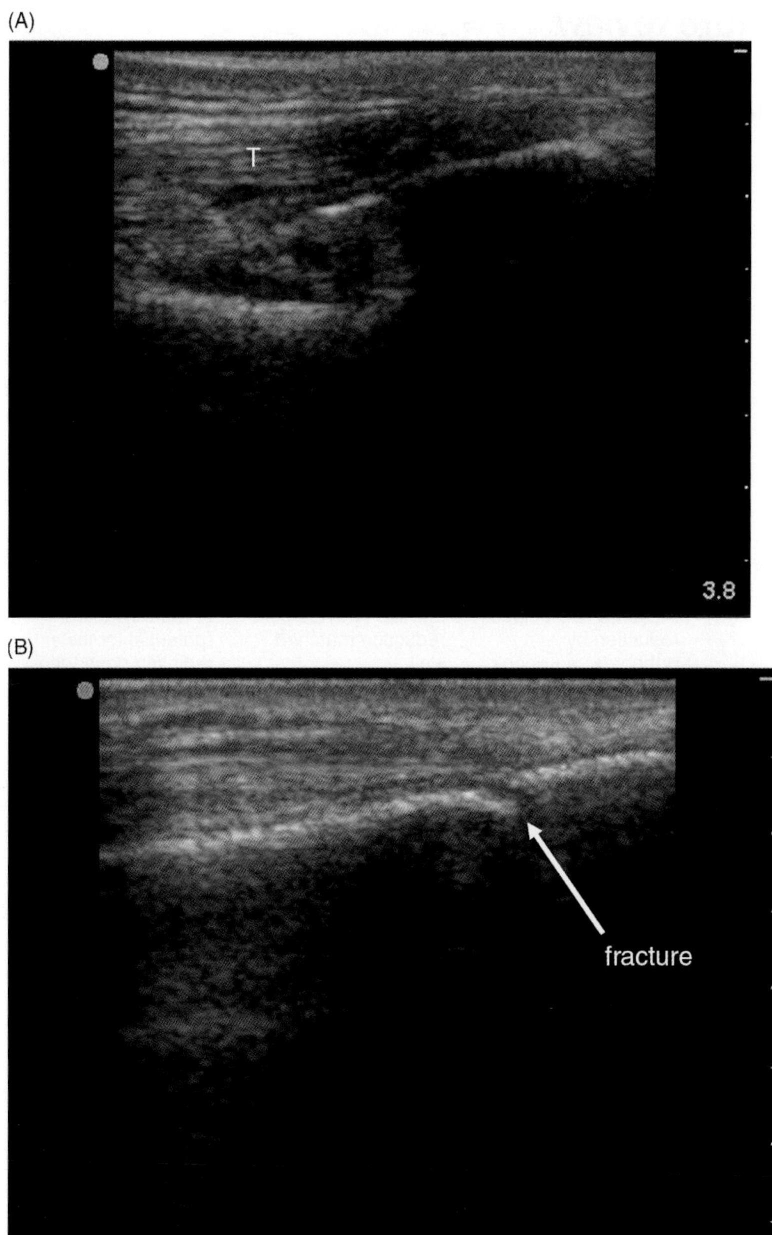

Figure 11.14
Fractured radius: (*A*) before and (*B*) after reduction. Note intact tendon (T).

Literature review

Reference	Methods	Results	Notes
Tayal *et al.* 2006 [2]	Prospective evaluation of clinician assessment for presence or not of abscess in patients with soft tissue infections before and after US.	US changed management in 56% of cases – 39/82 patients had a drainage procedure performed and 32/44 patients had a drainge procedure averted or further testing ordered.	First study to show the impact on clinical decision making of soft tissue US performed by emergency physicians.
Dulchavsky *et al.* 2002 [9]	95 patients with extremity trauma evaluated with US by orthopedic cast technicians.	Specificity for all fracture types was 100%; sensitivity varied by location (83–92% long bones, 50% hand/foot).	Non-physicians with minimal US training can accurately diagnose long bone fracture; test not sufficiently sensitive.
Chern *et al.* 2002 [8]	27 patients with displaced distal radius fractures. US guided reduction by orthopedic surgeons in emergency department.	Adequate reduction in all cases, radiographic and US findings post reduction matched well.	US may be useful in aiding reduction of radius fractures (potential for lower radiation dose than x-ray techniques).
Griffith *et al.* 1999 [7]	Compared US with x-ray in the diagnosis of rib fractures.	US superior to plain x-ray in diagnosing rib fractures.	Open door for further study, given gold standard outperformed by new modality.

New directions

The use of elastography to help characterize the severity or even type of infection is something that in the future may help clinicians decide who will require intravenous versus oral antibiotics. Moreover, there may be soft tissue ultrasound findings that could help identify infections caused by methicillin-resistant or other organisms that are clinically important because they require different treatment approaches. These are areas of active research.

For musculoskeletal evaluations, ultrasound may actually be an improvement over standard of care for fractures. As mentioned, the diagnosis of rib and sternal fractures by ultrasound has been shown to be more accurate than plain films [5–7]. Moreover, if tendon injuries can correctly and effectively be identified by ultrasound there may be cost savings that would propel this to a first-line diagnostic test in the acute setting. Comparative effectiveness studies will need to be done, but the potential is there.

References

1. Squire BT, Fox JC, Anderson C. ABSCESS: applied bedside sonography for convenient evaluation of superficial soft tissue infections. *Acad Emerg Med* 2005; **12**: 601–6.
2. Tayal VS, Hasan N, Norton HJ, Tomaszewski CA. The effect of soft-tissue ultrasound on the management of cellulitis in the emergency department. *Acad Emerg Med* 2006; **13**: 384–8.
3. Chau CLF, Griffith JF. Musculoskeletal infections: ultrasound appearances. *Clin Radiol* 2005; **60**: 149–59.
4. Bartolotta TV, Midiri M, Caruso G, Iovane A. [Necrotizing fasciitis of the scrotum (Fournier's gangrene): ultrasound findings] [Italian]. *Radiologica Medica* 2000; **100**: 510–12.
5. Mariacher-Gehler S, Michel BA. Sonography: a simple way to visualize rib fractures. *AJR Am J Roentgenol* 1994; **165**: 1268.
6. Steiner GM, Sprigg A. The value of ultrasound in the assessment of bone. *Br J Radiol* 1992; **65**: 589–93.
7. Griffith JF, Rainer TH, Ching ASC, *et al.* Sonography compared with radiography in revealing acute rib fracture. *AJR Am J Roentgenol* 1999; **173**: 1603–9.
8. Chern TC, Jou IM, Lai KA, *et al.* Sonography for monitoring closed reduction of displaced extra-articular distal radial fractures. *J Bone Joint Surg Am* 2002; **84-A**: 194–203.
9. Dulchavsky SA, Henry SE, Moed BR, *et al.* Advanced ultrasonic diagnosis of extremity trauma: the FASTER examination. *J Trauma* 2002; **53**: 28–32.
10. Marshburn TH, Legome E, Sargsyan A, *et al.* Goal-directed ultrasound in the detection of long bone fractures. *J Trauma* 2004; **57**: 329–32.
11. Gaspari R, Blehar D, Mendoza M, *et al.* Use of ultrasound elastography for skin and subcutaneous abscesses. *J Ultrasound Med* 2009; **28**: 855–60.

12 Gastrointestinal ultrasound

Introduction

For years – maybe decades – gastrointestinal ultrasound has developed under the auspices of radiology departments. Specialized protocols for the ultrasound diagnosis of many gastrointestinal pathologic processes and disease states have evolved over time. There has been little interest on the part of emergency and critical care clinicians to learn these applications, however, and little desire on the part of radiologists to advocate for gastrointestinal ultrasound, because frankly computed tomography (CT) is easier to obtain, is viewed as more accurate and less operator-dependent, and is perceived as standard of care. The focus on resource utilization, cost, and radiation exposure may change this, and indeed – especially as a screening test – there may be a substantial role for utilizing ultrasound in several common gastrointestinal conditions. This chapter will review some of the most promising applications.

Appendicitis

The ultrasound diagnosis of appendicitis is certainly not new, and ultrasound is most often the first-line test in pediatrics (Figure 12.1) [1]. Using ultrasound as a screening test in adults suspected of having the disease has fallen out of favor with the increased accuracy and ease in obtaining "appy protocol" CT scans [2]. However, with increased focus on cost and radiation exposure, perhaps utilizing ultrasound to rule in positive cases and reserving CT for non-diagnostic ultrasounds maybe a more effective strategy [3,4]. The challenge is that the reported diagnostic accuracy of ultrasound for acute appendicitis varies greatly, with sensitivity ranges from 44% to 94% and specificity ranges from 47% to 95%. In addition, almost all of this research has looked only at scans performed by radiologists or ultrasound technologists [5] and not point-of-care provider ultrasounds.

Hernia

Often hernias are clinically obvious and the decision to go to the operating room is based on:

1. the ability to reduce the hernia
2. the suspicion of incarceration or strangulation

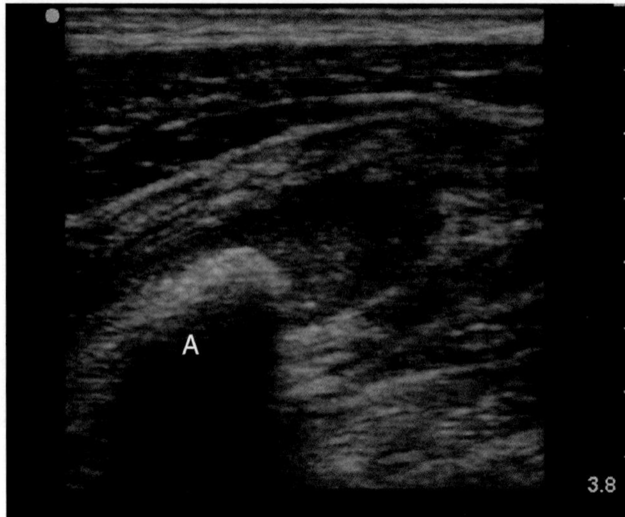

Figure 12.1
Appendicitis with shadowing appendicolith (A).

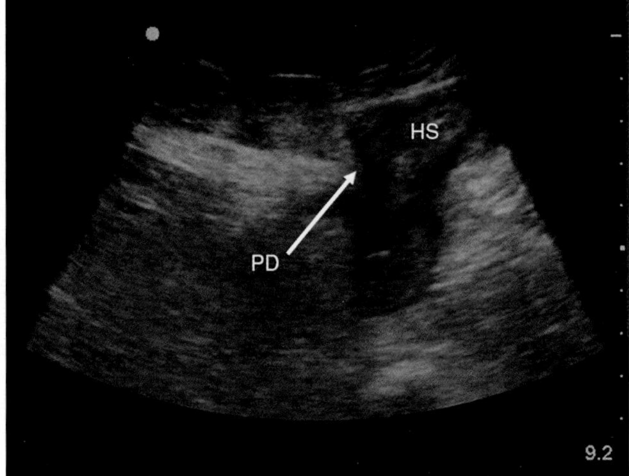

Figure 12.2
Hernia. Edematous bowel wall or hernia sac (HS) pouching out through peritoneal defect (PD).

While these seem like simple decision points, it is often not so straightforward. Patients with high body mass indexes (BMI) or with multiple scars as a result of repeated abdominal surgeries can be quite challenging. Studies have shown how ultrasound can assist in clinical decision making in these difficult patients [6,7], and pertinent ultrasound characteristics have been evaluated for their accuracy in making the diagnosis of an incarcerated hernia (Figure 12.2) [8]. The findings that are included in most published scanning

Table 12.1 Ultrasound characteristics evaluated in hernia scanning protocols

Abdominal wall defect
Hernia content (bowel vs. fatty tissue)
Presence or absence of free fluid in hernia sac
Wall thickness of herniated bowel loop
Presence or absence of fluid in herniated bowel loop
Diameter of small bowel in the abdomen
Presence or absence of color Doppler signals in hernia contents
Presence or absence of peristalsis in herniated bowel loop

protocols are listed in Table 12.1. Some authors have noted, however, that Doppler signal and peristalsis are less reliable findings of incarceration in patients with hernia [8].

Small bowel obstruction

Like hernia presentations, the clinical presentation for small bowel obstruction is characterized by abdominal pain accompanied by nausea and vomiting as well as decreased flatus. Plain films of the abdomen are used to identify dilated bowel loops that indicate the presence of obstruction, and this usually leads to the obtaining of CT images to help better define a patient's anatomy. However, ultrasound may have the potential to be the first-line screening test for small bowel obstruction, as it can be performed at the bedside and has been shown to have a sensitivity of 83% and a specificity of 100%, which is an improvement over plain radiography with published test characteristics in the 70% range [9]. Several studies have identified ultrasound characteristics that can be used to grade obstruction and indeed give a higher degree of detail regarding bowel wall edema, peristalsis and extraluminal fluid (Figure 12.3) [10,11]. Moreover, occasionally causes for obstruction can be identified (e.g., intussusception). In fact, the role of ultrasound is well established in the evaluation of suspected intussusception, with published sensitivity and specificity rates of 98–100% and 88–100%, respectively, and general acceptance of ultrasound as a first-line diagnostic test (12). Sonographically the intussuscipiens (receiving loop) contains the intussusceptum (donor loop) and looks like a large (usually >5 cm) folded mass of layered bowel. On the transverse scan this has been described as a "target" or "doughnut" sign (Figure 12.4). Intussusception is discussed in more detail in Chapter 13.

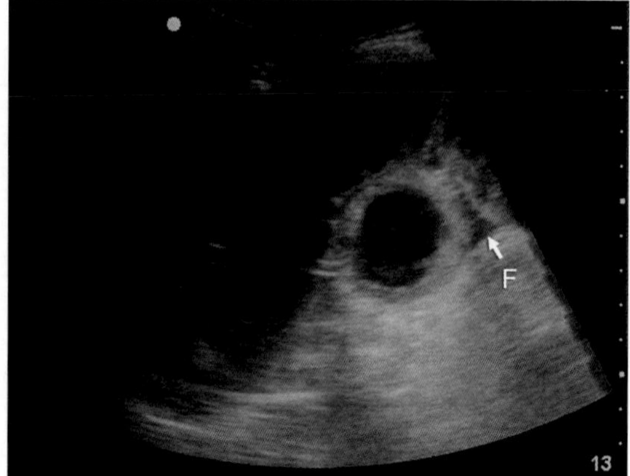

Figure 12.3

Small bowel obstruction, showing dilated bowel loops and some extraluminal free fluid (F).

(A)

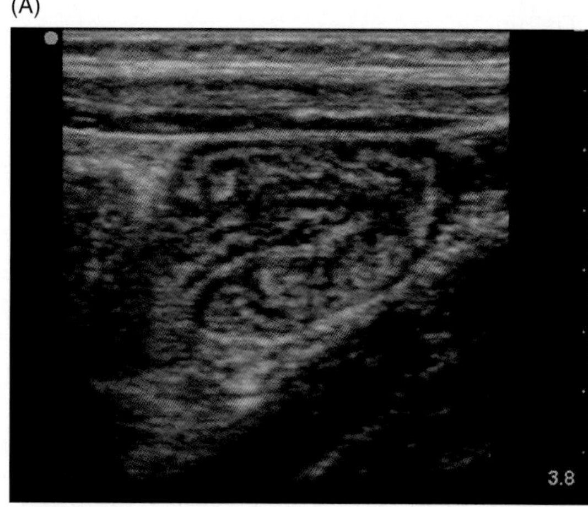

(B)

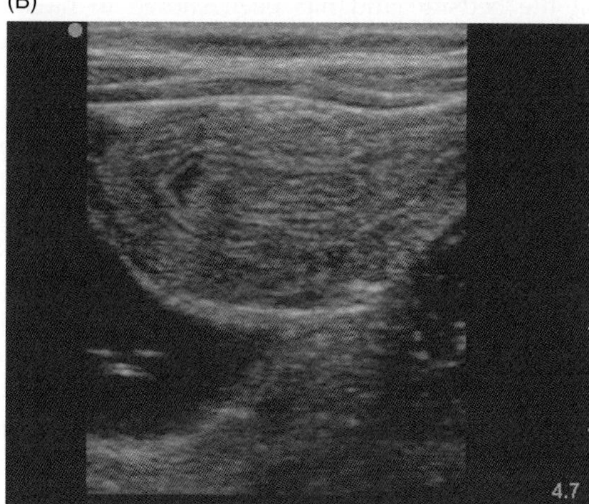

Figure 12.4

Longitudinal and transverse view of intussusception: (*A*) telescoped bowel in long axis; (*B*) the transverse "target sign."

Perforated viscus/free air

Air is not well visualized with ultrasound, and therefore it would seem unusual to look for "free" air with ultrasound in the setting of suspected perforated viscus. However, extraluminal or intraluminal gas can be seen, as the abrupt density difference between bowel mucosa and air causes a change in impedence that leads to a bright echogenic reverberation (see Chapter 1) or "ring-down" artifact. This can also be seen when air lines the peritoneum. This "dirty shadowing" or "ring-down" should prompt further investigation or imaging, but it is highly suggestive of extraluminal air (Figure 12.5) [13], and could be a powerful screening tool in patients with acute peritonitis.

(A)

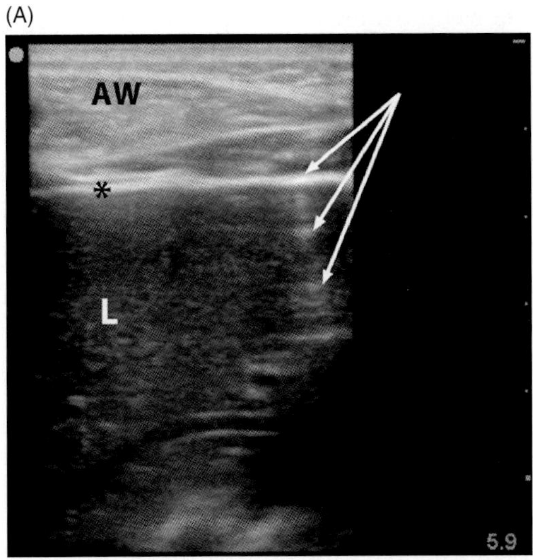

(B)

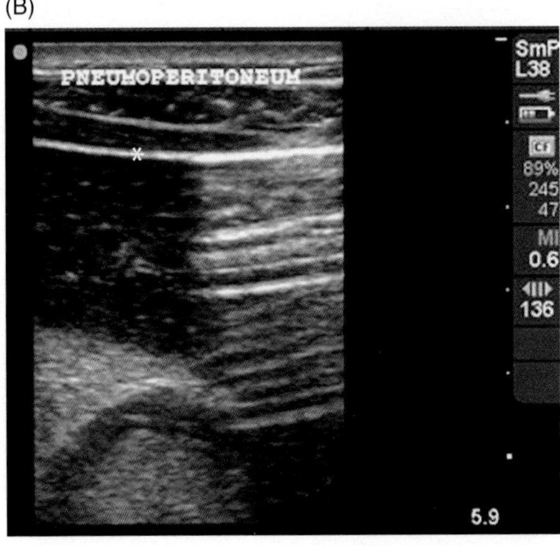

Figure 12.5

Peritoneal free air with reverberation or "ring-down" artifact. (*A*) Abdominal wall (AW), liver (L), and peritoneal lining (*), with arrows showing the reverberation artifact. Image used with permission from Hoffmann B (ed.). *Ultrasound Guide for Emergency Physicians*, www.sonoguide.com, courtesy of Dr. Beatrice Hoffmann. (*B*) More extensive reverberation artifact (*). Image courtesy of Dr. Hamid Shokoohi, George Washington University Medical Center, Washington DC.

Focused questions for gastrointestinal ultrasound

The questions for the ultrasound diagnosis of appendicitis are as follows:

1. Is there a dilated (> 6 mm) appendix visualized and is it compressible?
2. Is there an appendicolith?
3. Is there extraluminal fluid?

The questions for the ultrasound evaluation of hernia are as follows:

1. Is there a defect in the peritoneal lining?
2. Is there dilated, thickened bowel proximal to the hernia?
3. Is there extramural free fluid within the hernia sac?
4. Is there pendulous (back and forth) movement of the intraluminal contents?

The questions for the ultrasound evaluation of small bowel obstruction are as follows:

1. Is the small bowel dilated (> 25 mm jejunum, > 15 cm ileum)?
2. Is there extraluminal fluid?
3. Is the bowel wall thickened (> 3 mm)?
4. Is there evidence of peristalsis?

The questions for the ultrasound evaluation of perforated viscus are as follows:

1. Is there extraluminal air shadowing or a ring-down artifact?

Anatomy

Small bowel is made up of four layers: the mucosa, submucosa, muscularis, and serosa. These layers are readily identifiable by ultrasound – both when the bowel is collapsed and when it is dilated and full of fluid (Figure 12.6). By holding the probe in place, peristalsis and occasionally white shadow indicating the interface between fluid and solid bowel contents or air can be seen. As the bowel starts to dilate, the wall becomes more edematous and the different bowel wall layers become even more visible (Figure 12.7). As the distended bowel becomes ischemic, edema will start to extravasate from the wall itself and extraluminal fluid will start to accumulate. Finally, in the case of obstruction, normal peristaltic movements will first increase and then slow to a stop. At this stage, the bowel contents can be visualized moving slowly back and forward in what has been described as a "pendulous" motion.

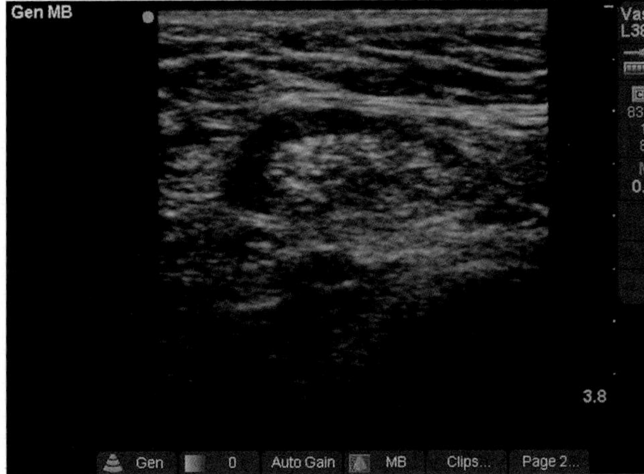

Figure 12.6
Normal small bowel with mucosal layers seen.

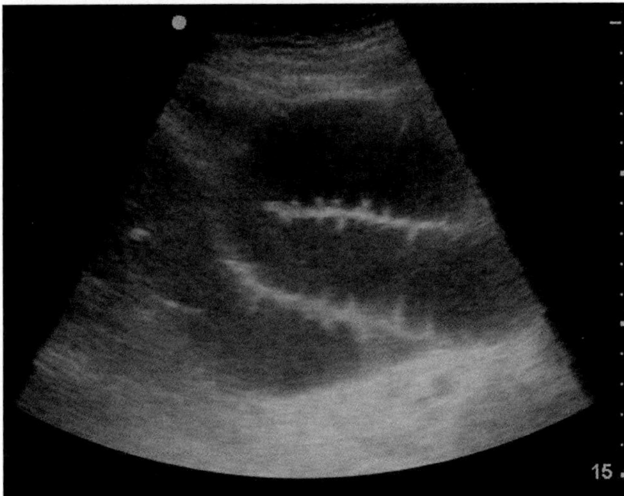

Figure 12.7
Dilated bowel loops.

Technique

Probe selection

Usually the area of interest is fairly superficial in appendicitis and hernia identification. Using a high-frequency linear probe gives more detail and better visualization of the peritoneal defect and bowel wall layers. However, if there is substantial soft tissue present, lower-frequency probes should be used to visualize beyond the peritoneum.

Views

Scanning protocols have been developed for complete evaluation of the abdomen and gastrointestinal system. In the acute or emergent setting, a good place to start is to ask the patient to point to the area of maximal pain and to begin the evaluation there.

For appendicitis, significant pressure must often be applied to try and "catch" the dilated appendix between the psoas muscle and the probe and

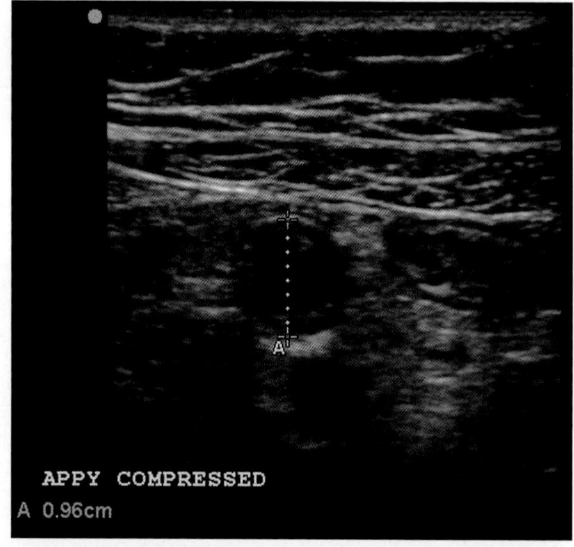

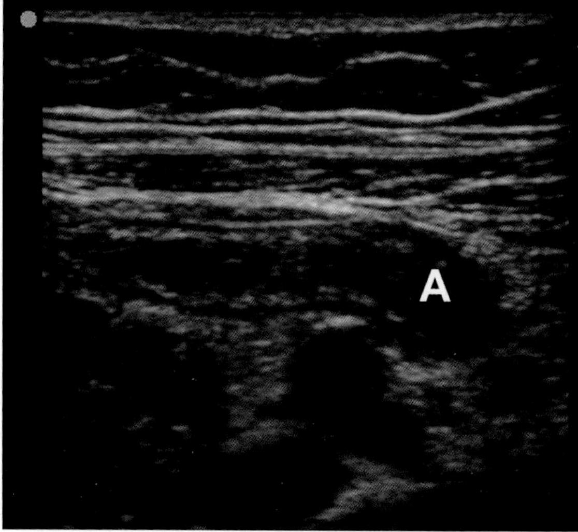

Figure 12.8

Transverse and longitudinal views of a dilated appendix (A) (D = 0.96 cm), consistent with appendicitis.

to push the small bowel out of the field of view. This can be painful, so adequate analgesia administered prior to the exam is suggested. Some authors have suggested a "mowing the lawn" technique, where the probe is swept back and forth over the abdomen with firm gentle pressure to evaluate the bowel in a systematic way. Once a dilated appendix is identified it is, as always, good practice to identify it in both the transverse and longitudinal view to establish a true diameter and to ensure it is truly a blind loop (Figure 12.8).

For hernia evaluation, the point of pain is often the area of the peritoneal defect, so evaluating this defect from several angles and recording bowel movement or its absence through the defect is important.

For small bowel obstruction, the same "mowing the lawn" technique is often utilized to ensure that a complete sense of the amount of small bowel dilatation is obtained, and whether or not a transition point or intussusceptum can be identified.

Scanning tips

No appendix identified?

- It is very difficult to visualize a normal appenidix, although occasionally a compressible, small (< 6 cm) appendix is seen. Seeing no appendix means either the patient does not have appendicitis or your ultrasound is non-diagnostic. Deciding to pursue alternative imaging depends on your clinical suspicion of disease.

Can't find a peritoneal defect?

- The challenge is to be systematic in your approach. Skipping areas means you could skip the area of defect. Occasionally in obese patients it helps to have someone hold the pannus back so you can systematically interrogate the peritoneum.

Anatomy appears strange?

- Remember that air-filled bowel is going to make it very difficult for the ultrasound to generate much of an image, and largely white shadows will be seen. Gentle consistent pressure or changing the patient's positioning can sometimes help to get you a better window.

Not sure what you are looking at?

- Always use color Doppler to help distinguish fluid collections from vessels.

Normal images

Figures 12.9 and 12.10 demonstrate normal bowel anatomy.

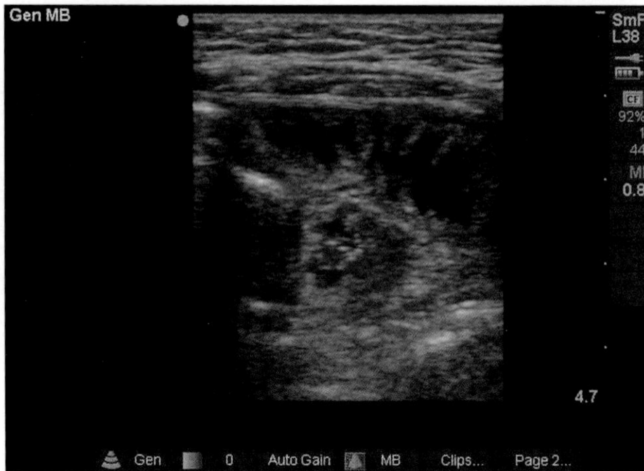

Figure 12.9
Normal bowel.

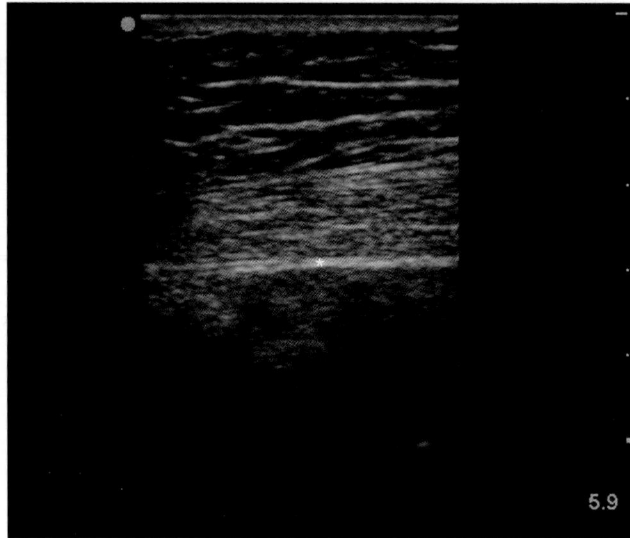

Figure 12.10
Intact peritoneum (*).

Abnormal images

Figures 12.11–12.15 demonstrate abnormal bowel and abdominal wall anatomy.

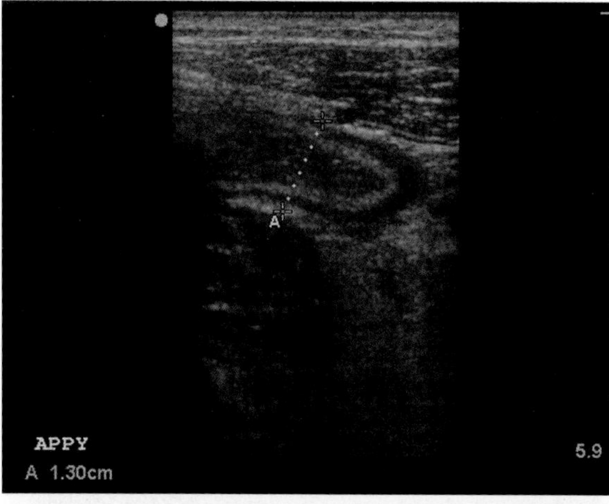

Figure 12.11

Appendicitis: long-axis view with diameter of 1.3 cm.

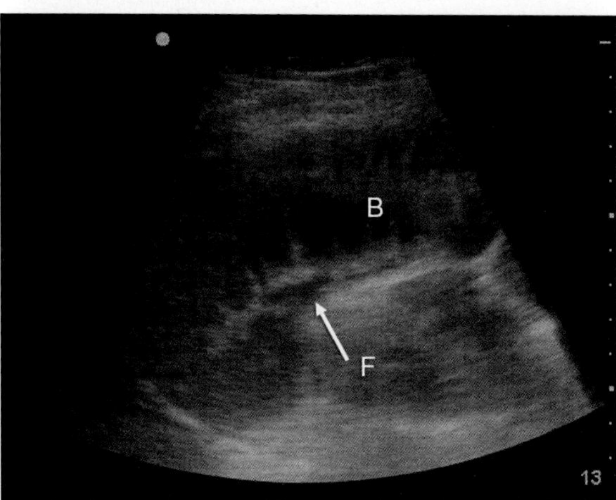

Figure 12.12

Small bowel obstruction with extraluminal free fluid (F) and dilated bowel loops (B).

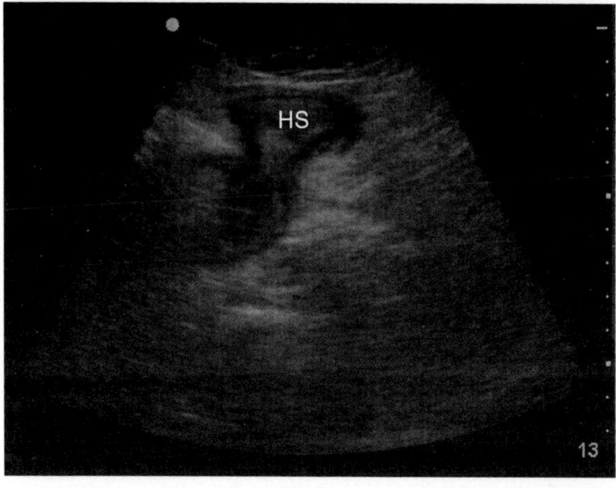

Figure 13.13

Abdominal wall hernia sac (HS).

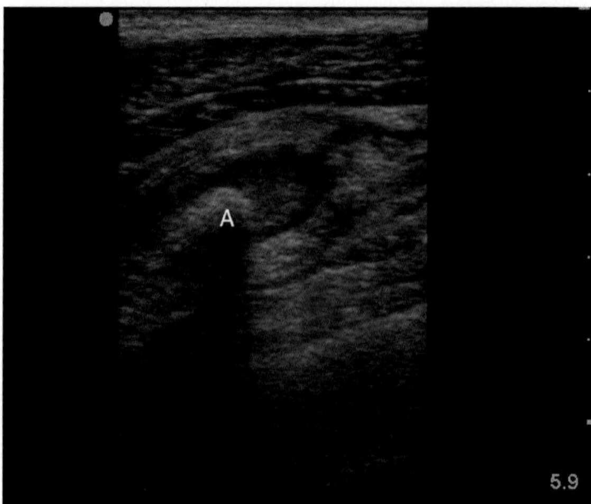

Figure 12.14
Appendicitis with appendicolith (A) and edematous bowel wall.

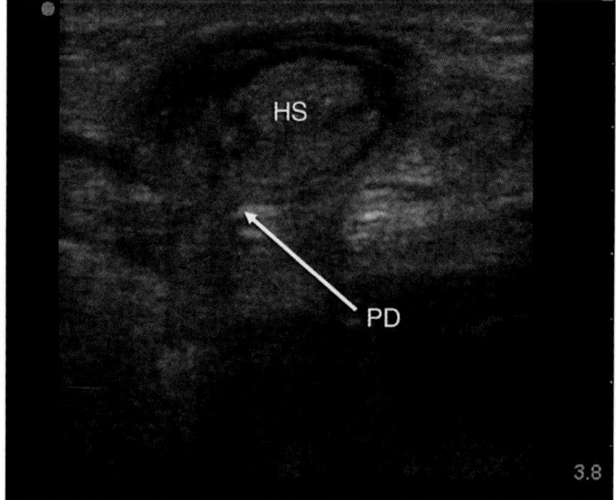

Figure 12.15
Hernia. HS, hernia sac; PD, peritoneal defect.

Literature review

Reference	Methods	Results	Notes
Ramarajan *et al.* 2009 [4]	680 patients with suspected appendicitis followed pathway of US followed by CT if ultrasound was equivocal. Outcomes were	407/680 patients followed pathway. 200/407 were managed without CT. Sensitivity was 99% and specificity 91% for pathway of US as screening test.	Outcome study looking at US as first-line test in suspected appendicitis. Retrospective, and unclear if CT use was reduced

Reference	Methods	Results	Notes
	correlated with US and CT findings.		compared to prior practice patterns, but helpful first step in evaluating if CT testing can be reduced.
Rettenbacher *et al.* 2001 [8]	Prospective US evaluation of 149 patients with hernia. US findings correlated with need for surgery.	Sonographic signs suggestive of incarceration included free fluid in hernia sac (91% of surgery cases) and bowel wall thickening (88% of surgery cases).	Defined US characteristics when evaluating hernia that predict incarceration.
Suri *et al.* 1999 [9]	32 patients with suspected intestinal obstruction had plain film, US, and CT performed and final diagnosis compared to imaging test results.	CT sensitivity 93%, specificity 100% for diagnosis of intestinal obstruction. US sensitivity 83% and specificity 100%. Plain films sensitivity 77% and specificity 50%.	While CT is more accurate, this study showed that US is superior to plain films, and that perhaps US should be used as first-line screening test.

New directions

Again, one of the major forces that will determine how patients are worked up diagnostically in the decades to come will likely be cost and a more conscientious approach to radiation exposure. Gastrointestinal complaints are most assuredly worked up more completely and with more accuracy by CT scanning. However, outcomes-based research looking at comparative effectiveness when clinicians use point-of-care ultrasound to screen for disease states may show not only that ultrasound can obviate some CT scans but perhaps that it can even be used to more closely monitor patients and replace many of the plain abdominal x-rays that are performed today.

References

1. Sivit CJ, Newman KD, Boenning DA, *et al.* Appendicitis: usefulness of US in diagnosis in a pediatric population. *Radiology* 1992; **185**: 549–52.
2. Anderson SW, Soto JA, Lucey BC, *et al.* Abdominal 64-MDCT for suspected appendicitis: the use of oral and IV contrast versus IV contrast material only. *AJR Am J Roentgenol* 2009; **193**: 1282–8.
3. Wong KK, Cheung TW, Tam PK. Diagnosing acute appendicitis: are we overusing radiologic investigations? *J Pediatr Surg* 2008; **43**: 2239–41.
4. Ramarajan N, Krishnamoorthi R, Barth R, *et al.* An interdisciplinary initiative to reduce radiation exposure: evaluation of appendicitis in

a pediatric emergency department with clinical assessment supported by a staged ultrasound and computed tomography pathway. *Acad Emerg Med* 2009; **16**: 1258–65.

5. Sivit CJ, Siegel MJ, Applegate KE, Newman KD. When appendicitis is suspected in children. *Radiographics* 2001; **21**: 247–62.
6. Young J, Gilbert AI, Graham MF. The use of ultrasound in the diagnosis of abdominal wall hernias. *Hernia* 2007; **11**: 347–51.
7. Bradley M, Morgan J, Pentlow B, Roe A. The positive predictive value of diagnostic ultrasound for occult herniae. *Ann R Coll Surg Engl* 2006; **88**: 165–7.
8. Rettenbacher T, Hollerweger A, Macheiner P, *et al.* Abdominal wall hernias: cross-sectional imaging signs of incarceration determined with sonography. *AJR Am J Roentgenol* 2001; **177**: 1061–7.
9. Suri S, Gupta S, Sudhakar PJ, *et al.* Comparative evaluation of plain films, ultrasound and CT in the diagnosis of intestinal obstruction. *Acta Radiol* 1999; **40**: 422–8.
10. Grassi R, Romano S, D'Amario F, *et al.* The relevance of free fluid between the intestinal loops detected by sonography in the clinical assessment of small bowel obstruction in adults. *Eur J Radiology* 2004; **50**: 5–14.
11. Schmutz GR, Benko A, Fournier L, *et al.* Small bowel obstruction: role and contribution of sonography. *Eur Radiol* 1997; **7**: 1054–8.
12. Verschelden P, Filiatrault D, Garel L, *et al.* Intussusception in children: reliability of ultrasound in diagnosis. A prospective study. *Radiology* 1992; **184**: 741–4.
13. Lee DH, Lim JH, Ko YT, Yoon Y. Sonographic detection of pneumoperitoneum in patients with acute abdomen. *AJR Am J Roentgenol* 1990; **154**: 107–9.

13 Pediatric ultrasound

Introduction

In the past five years, the number of publications looking at pediatric applications for bedside emergency or "point-of-care" ultrasound has increased exponentially. The growing interest in point-of-care ultrasound by pediatricians is logical, as pediatric patients are most at risk for exposure to repeated radiation [1]. The Alliance for Radiation Safety in Pediatric Imaging (also known as the Image Gently Alliance: www.pedrad.org) was formed to address the concern over radiation dosing in children. The American College of Radiology, American Institute of Ultrasound in Medicine, and dozens of other organizations have worked to reduce unnecessary radiation exposure for diagnostic and interventional radiology procedures, and as part of this effort interest in point-of-care ultrasound has increased.

Aside from lowering radiation exposure, ultrasound can be beneficial in other ways as well. Pediatric patients who require invasive procedures and/or diagnostic imaging where they must hold still can be especially challenging. Ultrasound can be performed while the pediatric patient is held by parents or trusted caregivers, thus avoiding unnecessary restraints and/or sedation. Moreover, given that physicians need to communicate with parents or caregivers with regard to a pediatric patient's illness, the visual instruction ultrasound provides can be used as a teaching tool to help illustrate pathophysiology.

This bulk of this chapter will review the indications that are most specific to pediatrics. However, it is important to note that the most common pediatric indications are often the most common in adults as well. Many pediatric acute care providers see enormous benefit in the use of bedside ultrasound for skin and soft tissue applications such as differentiating cellulitis from abscess or evaluating foreign bodies (described in Chapters 11 and 16). Pelvic ultrasound to assess first trimester pregnancy complications may be a very common use in the pediatric emergency department as well (see Chapter 4). A host of procedures benefit from ultrasound guidance: bladder catheterization, central and peripheral venous access, and arthrocentesis are just a few commonly encountered in the pediatric population (see Chapter 16). As ultrasound becomes incorporated into pediatric and pediatric critical care curriculums, whole textbooks will be devoted to pediatric applications. For this edition, a few specific pediatric applications most likely to be used in the acute setting will be reviewed – but stay tuned for more to come.

Abdominal applications

Appendicitis

The ultrasound diagnosis of appendicitis was reviewed in Chapter 12. The scanning technique and findings are essentially the same in adult and

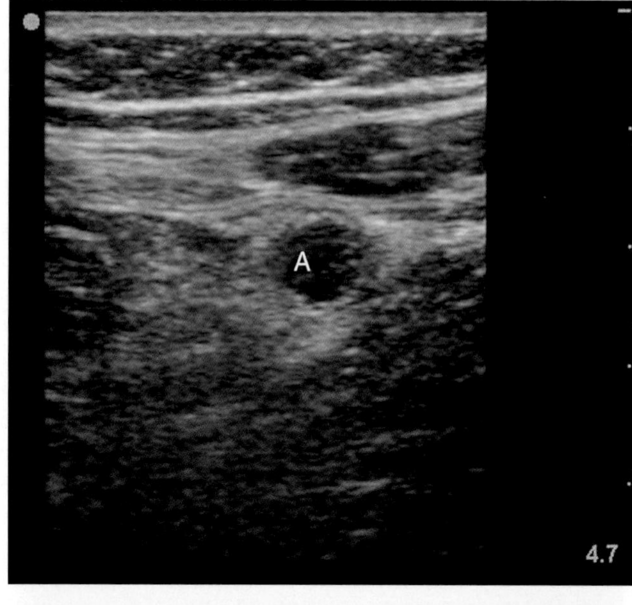

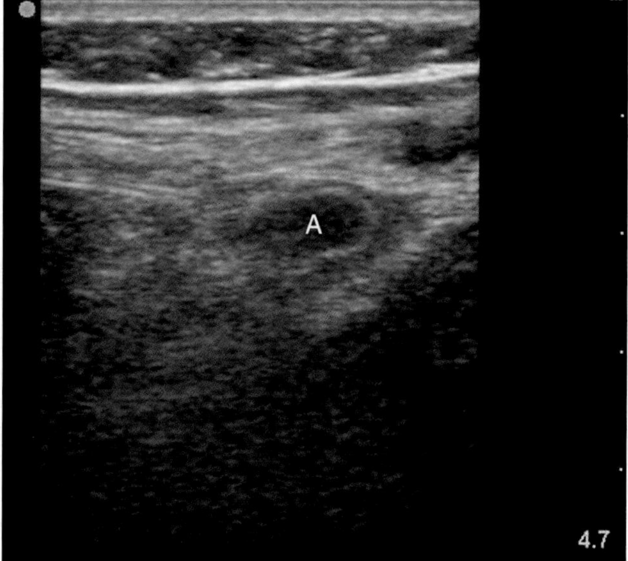

Figure 13.1
Appendicitis (A).

pediatric patients (Figure 13.1). Given the growing body of evidence highlighting concerns about radiation exposure in pediatric patients, and given the acceptable test characteristics of ultrasound for appendicitis, computed tomography (CT) should be reserved for those patients with non-diagnostic ultrasounds and high clinical suspicion for appendicitis.

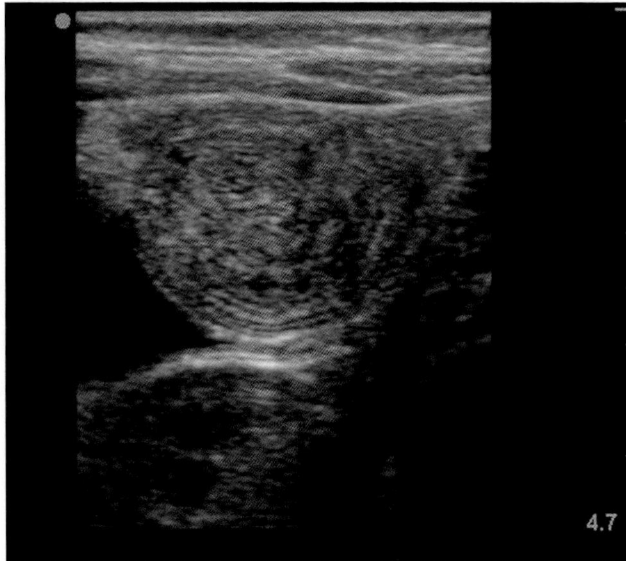

Figure 13.2
Intussusception.

Intussusception

As mentioned in Chapter 12, the role of ultrasound is well established in the evaluation of suspected intussusception, with published sensitivity and specificity rates of 98–100% and 88–100% respectively and general acceptance of ultrasound as a first-line diagnostic test [2]. Sonographically the intussuscipiens (receiving loop) contains the intussusceptum (donor loop) and looks like a large (usually $>$ 5 cm) folded mass of layered bowel. On the transverse scan this has been described as a "target" or "doughnut" sign (Figure 13.2). Occasionally, free peritoneal fluid can be seen surrounding the bowel loops. If large amounts of fluid or any evidence of free air are seen, perforation should be considered.

Pyloric stenosis

Pyloric stenosis likewise is a diagnosis that is usually made by ultrasound. While palpating an "olive-shaped mass" in the epigastrium can be considered sensitive and specific enough for diagnosis in the right clinical setting, diagnostic imaging is often required – and then ultrasound is the test of choice. The sonographic hallmark of pyloric stenosis is a thickened pyloric muscle greater than 4 mm with a canal length of 1.5 cm (Figure 13.3) [3]. Some authors use a lower transverse thickness cut-off of 3 mm to increase the test sensitivity [4]. Published accuracy numbers for ultrasound and pyloric stenosis approach 100% [5], although there are almost no studies looking at the characteristics of tests performed by pediatricians or emergency physicians.

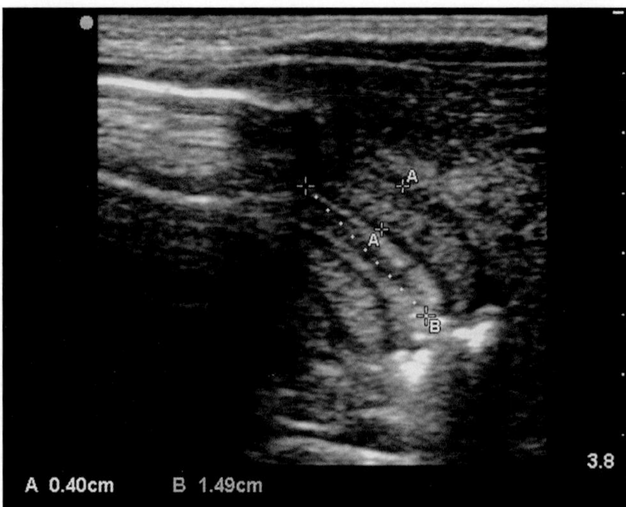

Figure 13.3
Pyloric stenosis.

Musculoskeletal applications

Extremity fracture identification and reduction

Not only is ultrasound a reliable method for diagnosing long bone fractures [6], but it is also useful in guiding reduction and so avoiding fluoroscopy or serial radiographs. There is a small but growing body of literature looking at ultrasound-guided fracture reductions by pediatricians and emergency physicians [7,8]. The technique and the views are no different in pediatric patients than they are in adults, and they can be reviewed in more detail in the section on fractures in Chapter 11 (Figure 13.4).

Skull fractures

There is also a small but growing body of literature looking at ultrasound and its accuracy in the diagnosis of skull fractures [9,10]. This is an interesting area of research because obviating the need for CT scanning could be of great value, given radiation exposure risks and concerns for sedation in pediatric patients with head injury. The literature to date suggests that screening with an ultrasound to rule out skull fractures could be a safe alternative for patients with minor head trauma. Those patients with a positive ultrasound could then be selectively sent for CT [10].

Hip effusions

Pediatric patients presenting with a limp or hip pain can be evaluated by clinicians for effusion using ultrasound. The focused question for ultrasound is to identify the presence or absence of an effusion. The significance of the effusion, however, and the indication for aspiration are still largely based

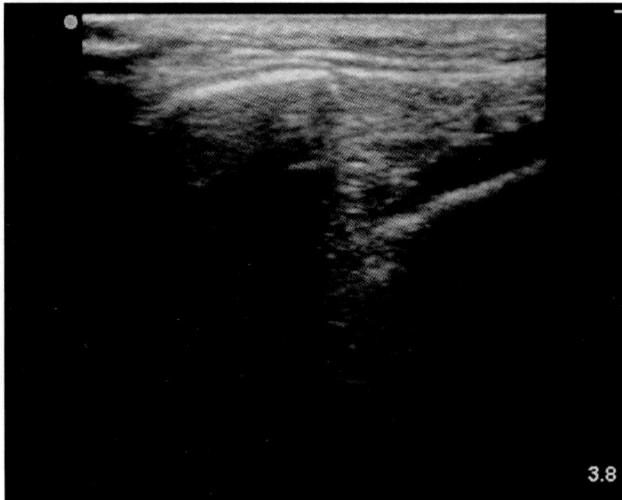

Figure 13.4
Fracture. Note the break in the otherwise smooth cortex.

on clinical history, laboratory values, and pain severity. While the absence of effusion effectively rules out septic arthritis, osteomyelitis is not well evaluated with ultrasound and may require further diagnostic imaging when indicated. Placing the hip in the extended and abducted position and scanning along the femoral neck seems to be the most efficacious scanning protocol [11]. There is also evidence that emergency physician practitioners have comparable accuracy when looking for effusions using radiology-performed studies as the gold standard, with a sensitivity of 0.8 (95% CI 0.51–0.95) and a specificity of 0.98 (95% CI 0.85–0.99) [12].

IVC evaluation for dehydration

Evaluating the collapsibility of the inferior vena cava (IVC) as a proxy for dehydration and central venous pressures will be discussed further in Chapter 14. While most of the research looking at this application has been done in adults, there is some literature to support its relevance in the evaluation of the dehydrated pediatric patient. Indeed, the ability of ultrasound to reliably diagnose moderate to severe dehydration across users and to monitor the response to fluid challenges may be one of the more efficacious applications in pediatric ultrasound. There are two standard imaging protocols: the longitudinal scan just distal to the right atrial junction and an IVC/aorta ratio protocol (Figure 13.5). The obvious benefit of the ratio in pediatrics is that the size of the aorta acts as a control for the age of the patient, and thus age-based IVC diameter sizes do not need to be memorized. IVC/aorta ratios have been shown to be significantly lower in patients before intravenous hydration (mean of 0.75 vs. 1.09 in hydrated patients) [13], and studies are ongoing to correlate this ratio with accepted clinical dehydration scores. One such study showed that the aorta/IVC ratio had a sensitivity of 93% and specificity of

(A)

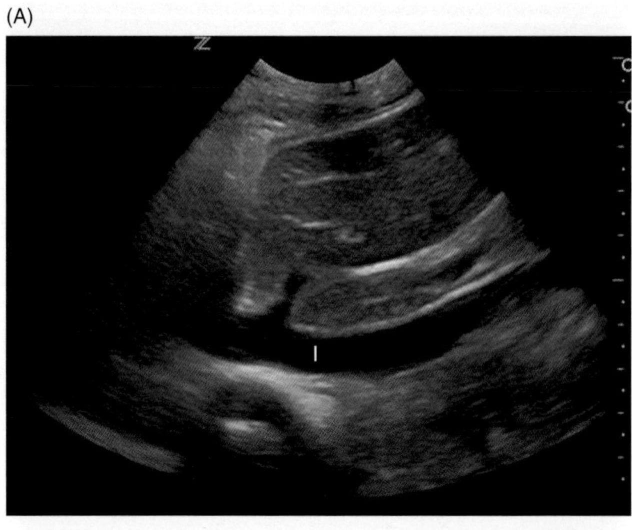

(B)

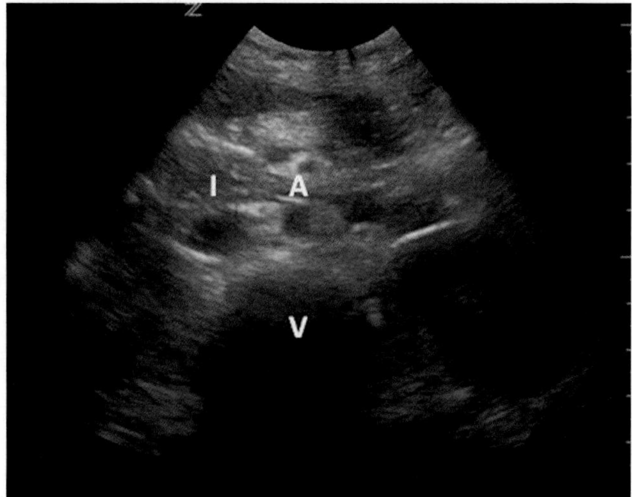

Figure 13.5
(*A*) Longitudinal and (*B*) transverse views of the inferior vena cava (I) just superior to the vertebral body shadow (V) and next to the aorta (A).

59% when compared to a reference standard of percent weight change. The World Health Organization dehydration scale had a sensitivity of 73% and a specificity of 43% when compared to this same standard [14].

Focused questions for pediatric ultrasound

The questions for pediatric abdominal ultrasound are as follows:

1. Is there a dilated (> 6 mm) appendix visualized and is it compressible?
2. Is there a large (> 5 cm) folded layer of bowel visualized?
3. Is there a dilated (> 4 mm) pylorus?

The questions for pediatric musculoskeletal ultrasound are as follows:

1. Is the long bone defect improved with reduction?
2. Is there a defect in the cortex of the long bone or the skull?
3. Is there a hip effusion > 5 mm, or a difference of > 2 mm between the symptomatic and the asymptomatic (contralateral) hip?

The questions for pediatric inferior vena cava ultrasound evaluation are as follows:

1. Does the longitudinal IVC collapse more than 50% with inspiration?
2. Is the transverse IVC/aorta ratio less than 1 : 1?

Anatomy

The gastrointestinal anatomy of the pediatric patient is essentially the same as the adult and is well described in Chapter 12. The only structure not mentioned previously is the pylorus, which is a thickened area of muscle between the gastric antrum and the duodenal cap. The pyloric muscle is hypoechoic and surrounds echogenic mucosa. A normal exam of the pylorus will document relaxation of the pyloric canal as fluid travels from the stomach to the duodenum.

Musculoskeletal anatomy of the pediatric patient is also essentially the same as the adult and is well described in Chapter 11. The only structure not mentioned in Chapter 11 is the hip. When the linear probe is held along the axis of the femoral neck, the bright shadow of the femoral head and neck are seen, with the intervening echolucent joint fluid. Just anterior to the fluid is the outer margin of the capsule, which is usually seen as an echogenic line mirroring the femoral neck and extending over the femoral head (Figure 13.6).

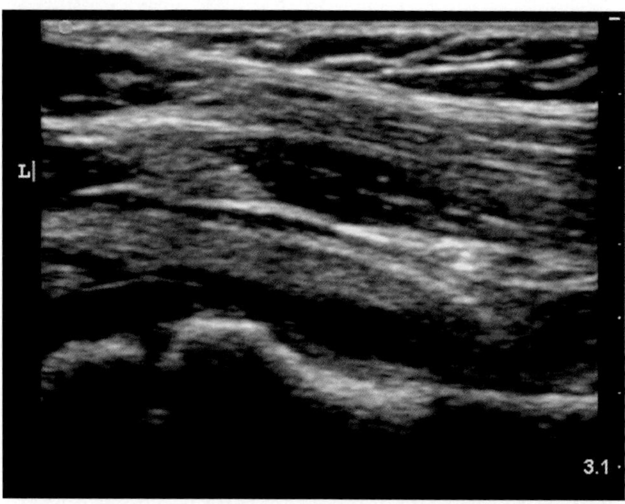

Figure 13.6
Normal hip. Note the echogenic line of the joint capsule.

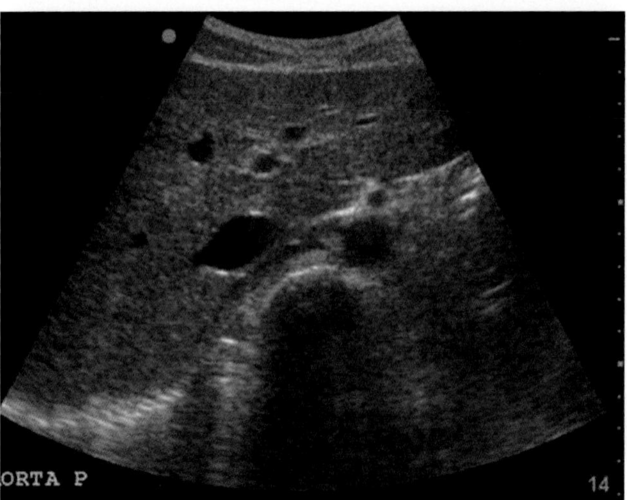

Figure 13.7
IVC/aorta ratio.

Aorta and IVC anatomy is also essentially the same as in the adult and is described in Chapters 4 and 14. Again, the most important landmark when evaluating these two vessels is to ensure that the vertebral shadow is well visualized and that the vessels are located just anterior to this shadow (Figure 13.7). Care must be taken when imaging the vena cava longitudinally that the probe does not slide over the aorta instead of the vena cava. Fanning side to side in the longitudinal plane can help to ensure that the probe is being held over the widest diameter and over the correct vessel.

Technique

Probe selection

Most pediatric applications use the high-frequency linear probe because most of the salient structures are at a relatively shallow depth. In pediatric gastrointestinal applications, unless there is a significant amount of soft tissue or abdominal fat, the linear probe will give images with the most detail. This is certainly also true for pediatric musculoskeletal applications, where the linear probe is used almost exclusively. When imaging the IVC, it depends on the size of the child. This is the one application where even small children may need to be imaged using the lower-frequency probe, since the structures of interest are often more than 5–6 cm deep.

Views

The scanning protocols for pediatric applications have all largely been discussed in previous chapters. In the acute or emergent setting, a good place to start is to ask the patient to point to the area of maximal pain and to begin the evaluation there – this is true for both gastrointestinal and musculoskeletal applications. Again, evaluating all structures in two planes is good practice, and better images can often be obtained when scanning the pediatric patient in the lap of a parent or caregiver.

Scanning tips

Trouble evaluating the abdomen?

- Remember that it is very difficult to visualize a normal appendix. Seeing no appendix means either the patient does not have appendicitis or your ultrasound is non-diagnostic.
- Making the decision to pursue alternative imaging depends on the clinical suspicion of disease. This holds true for all pediatric gastrointestinal applications, as ultrasound is best for *ruling in* disease but more challenging when *ruling out* disease.

Can't find a bony cortex defect?

- Look for secondary signs of bony injury. Cortex disruption should usually result in a hematoma overlying the fracture fragments. Identifying the hematoma first and then focusing on the underlying cortex can help to focus the exam.

Unsure of where to measure for a hip effusion?

- Remember that the best way to evaluate joints is to look at the asymptomatic contralateral side first. If there is a greater than 2 mm difference in the capsular-synovial thickness this is considered pathologic.

Not sure you are looking at the IVC?

- Always identify the vertebral shadow first and look for the fluid-filled structures just anterior to this shadow to find the aorta and vena cava. Color and pulsed-wave Doppler can help distinguish bowel loops or the gallbladder from vessels. Once the transverse IVC is identified, turn the probe longitudinally (usually in the mid-clavicular line) so that the probe marker is to the patient's head and slide up the IVC to see the atria junction and the confluence with the hepatic veins.

Normal images

Figures 13.8 and 13.9 demonstrate normal images.

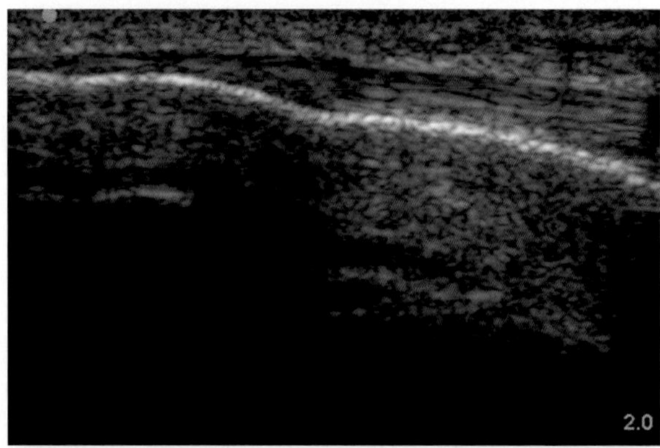

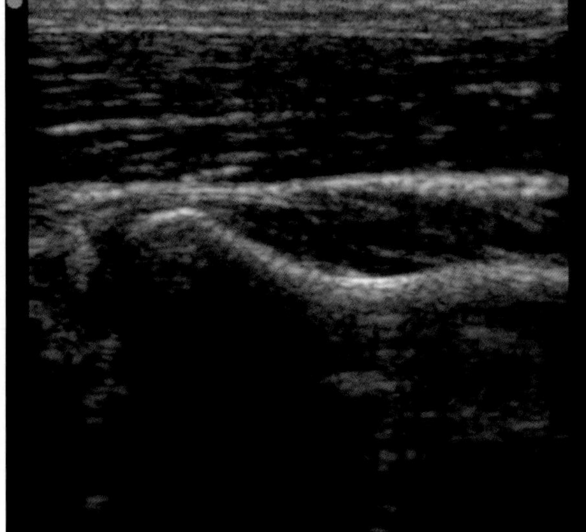

Figure 13.8
Normal smooth bony cortex.

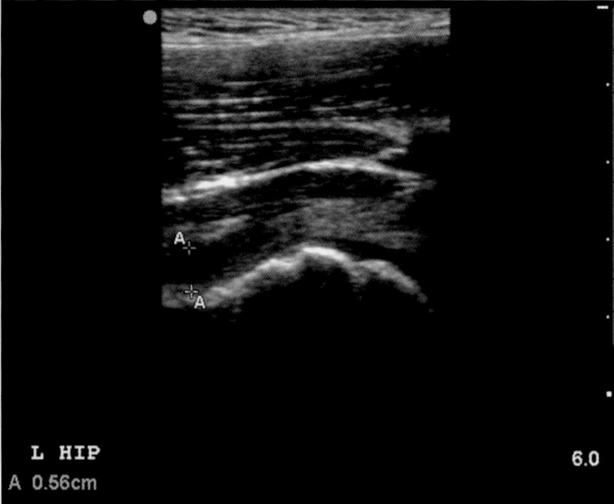

Figure 13.9
Normal hip.

Abnormal images

Figures 13.10–13.14 demonstrate abnormal images.

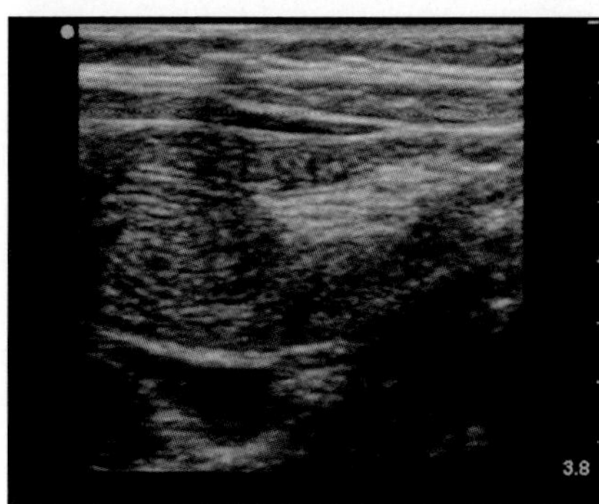

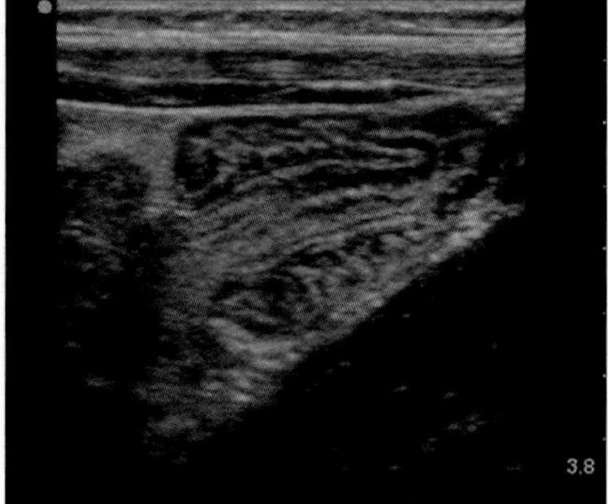

Figure 13.10
Intussusception. Note the "telescoping" appearance of the intussusceptum.

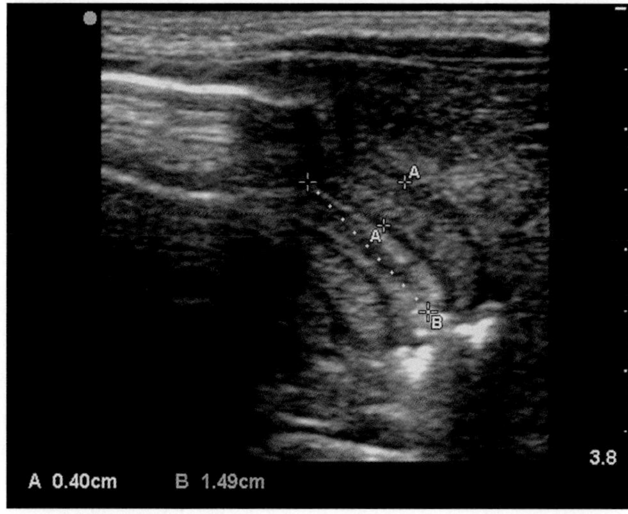

Figure 13.11
Pyloric stenosis.

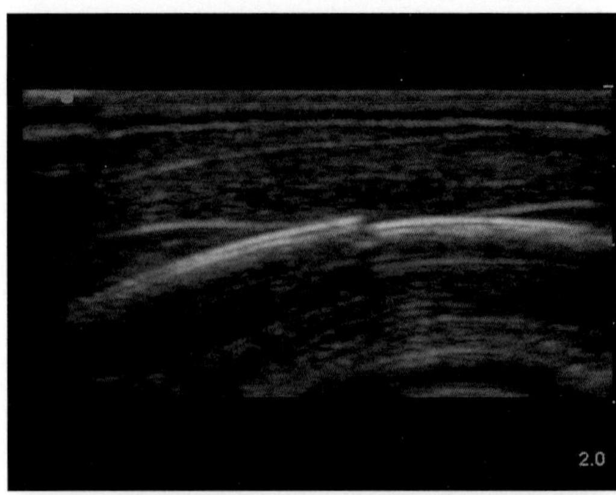

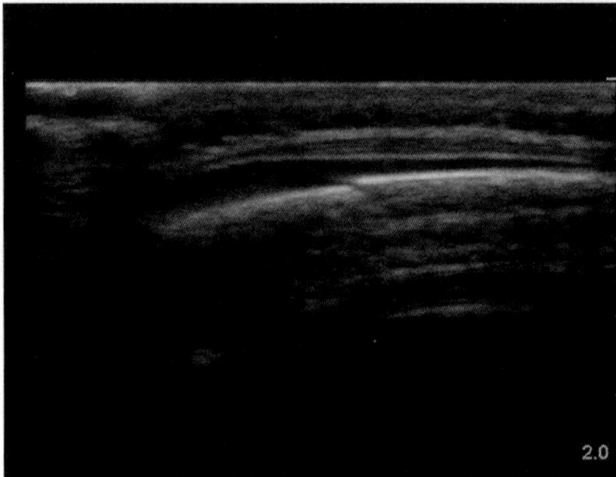

Figure 13.12

Skull fracture. It is important to distinguish between a suture line and a fracture. In both these images the fracture is identified by the angulation and the sharp edges. Suture lines have a brighter echogenic, smooth edge.

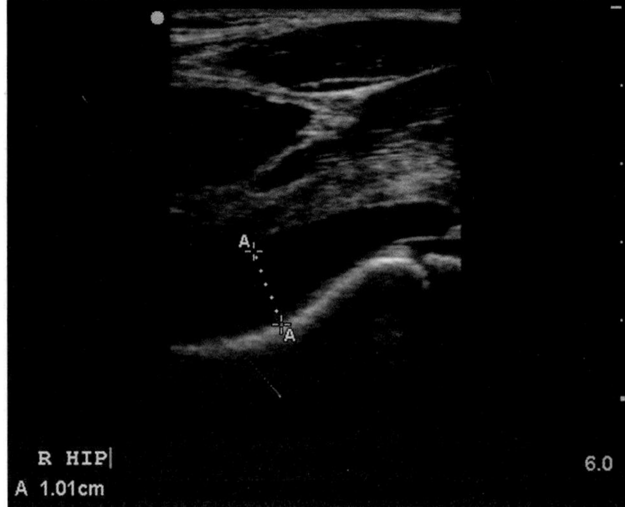

Figure 13.13

Hip effusion. Note that the joint diameter is greater than 5 mm.

Literature review

Reference	Methods	Results	Notes
Steiner *et al.* 1996 [9]	210 pediatric patients with head injury were evaluated with US. Positive findings were confirmed with further imaging.	All depressed skull fractures seen on US were confirmed by CT (6/6). 16/16 linear fractures were confirmed by x-ray. Negative US patients were not imaged further but "did well."	Study was performed in 1996 and is still waiting for prospective trial to confirm use of US as screening test where patients with negative US can be observed only.
Chen *et al.* 2007 [7]	Pediatric patients suspected of forearm fracture had both US and plain films performed.	46/48 pediatric patients had fracture location correctly identified by US (sensitivity 97%, specificity 100%). 24/26 had successful reduction using US only.	First study to show that point-of-care US could not only identify fractures but also help guide reduction.
Chen *et al.* 2007 [13]	Case–control study looking at IVC/aorta ratios in patients receiving fluids for dehydration and those who were clinically well.	36 pairs of subjects. IVC/aorta ratio lower in cases (mean 0.75) than in controls (1.01).	Easier to perform technique in children confirms ratio as a marker of dehydration.

New directions

One area of potential research that is pediatric-specific is the utility of ultrasound in looking at Salter–Harris I and II fractures. It is well documented that the lack of cortex mineralization in neonatal and pediatric patients makes these fractures difficult to identify with plain radiographs, and there is some evidence that ultrasound is better able to detect small breaks in the cortex or to identify the hyperintense fracture line seen with compression injuries [15]. In addition, outcome assessment trials are needed to evaluate the efficacy of pediatric head injury protocols that include ultrasound as a screening test.

References

1. Brenner D, Elliston C, Hall E, Berdon W. Estimated risks of radiation-induced fatal cancer from pediatric CT. *AJR Am J Roentgenol* 2001; **176**: 289–96.
2. Vasavada P. Ultrasound evaluation of acute abdominal emergencies in infants and children. *Radiol Clin North Am* 2004; **42**: 445–56.

3. Blumhagen JD, Maclin L, Krauter D, Rosenbaum DM, Weinberger E. Sonographic diagnosis of hypertrophic pyloric stenosis. *AJR Am J Roentgenol* 1988; **150**: 1367–70.
4. O'Keeffe FN, Stansberry SD, Swischuk LE, Hayden CK. Antropyloric muscle thickness at US in infants: what is normal? *Radiology* 1991; **178**: 827–30.
5. Hernanz-Schulman M, Sells LL, Ambrosino MM, *et al.* Hypertrophic pyloric stenosis in the infant without a palpable olive: accuracy of sonographic diagnosis. *Radiology* 1994; **193**: 771–6.
6. Hubner U, Schlicht W, Outzen S, Barthel M, Halsband H. Ultrasound in the diagnosis of fractures in children. *J Bone Joint Surg Br* 2000; **82**: 1170–3.
7. Chen L, Kim Y, Moore CL. Diagnosis and guided reduction of forearm fractures in children using bedside ultrasound. *Pediatr Emerg Care* 2007; **23**: 528–31.
8. Durston W, Swartzentruber R. Ultrasound guided reduction of pediatric forearm fractures in the ED. *Am J Emerg Med* 2000; **18**: 72–7.
9. Steiner S, Riebel T, Nazarenko O, *et al.* [Skull injury in childhood: comparison of ultrasonography with conventional xrays and computerized tomography] [German]. *Rofo* 1996; **165**: 353–8.
10. Trenchs V, Curcoy AI, Castillo M, *et al.* Minor head trauma and linear skull fracture in infants: cranial ultrasound or computed tomography? *Eur J Emerg Med* 2009; **16**: 150–2.
11. Chan YL, Cheng JC, Metreweli C. Sonographic evaluation of hip effusion in children. Improved visualization with the hip in extension and abduction. *Acta Radiol* 1997; **38**: 867–9.
12. Vieira RL, Levy JA. Bedside ultrasonography to identify hip effusions in pediatric patients. *Ann Emerg Med* 2010; **55**: 284–9.
13. Chen L, Kim Y, Santucci KA. Use of ultrasound measurement of the inferior vena cava diameter as an objective tool in the assessment of children with clinical dehydration. *Acad Emerg Med* 2007; **14**: 841–5.
14. Levine AC, Shah SP, Umulisa I, *et al.* Ultrasound assessment of severe dehydration in children with diarrhea and vomiting. *Acad Emerg Med* 2010; **17**: 1035–41.
15. Jones GP, Seguin J, Shiels WE. Salter-Harris II fracture of the proximal humerus in a preterm infant. *Am J Perinatol* 2003; **20**: 249–53.

14 Ultrasound in shock

Introduction

As we have seen throughout this book, individual organ assessment with ultrasound can be useful in answering focused questions such as the presence of gallstones or the diameter of the aorta. Many emergent conditions demonstrate pathology across multiple organ systems, however, and a more comprehensive approach can yield dramatic results.

The focused assessment with sonography in trauma (FAST) was the first multisystem approach to bedside sonography. Although early definitions of the examination included only an evaluation of the peritoneum, cardiac and thoracic assessments were added over the years to form a more comprehensive assessment for bleeding in the trauma patient. In the last decade several authors have applied similar diagnostic principles to the evaluation of the medical patient, to search for reversible causes of hypotension in the critical care setting.

The remainder of this chapter will describe an overall approach to hypotension evaluation using bedside sonography, as well as a review of the major approaches which have been described in the literature.

General approach to the patient in shock

The major focus of bedside ultrasound is to augment the diagnostic capacity of the clinician at the bedside. Thus, ultrasound will be employed to answer a series of focused questions in parallel with the physical examination and other available data (such as heart rate, blood pressure, and pulse oximetry).

This approach can be tailored to provide the highest-yield information for each given clinical scenario. An assessment of the aorta may not yield useful information in a septic pediatric patient, for example. And yet by surveying the heart, inferior vena cava (IVC), peritoneum, aorta, and thorax, a number of life-threatening and reversible processes may be diagnosed.

Cardiac ultrasound

As discussed in Chapter 3, cardiac ultrasound can be used to assess for cardiac contractility (including cardiac standstill), presence of right ventricular dilatation, pericardial effusion, or even tamponade. All of these states can create hypotension. Most of these assessments can be made using the subxiphoid four-chamber view or the parasternal long-axis view previously described.

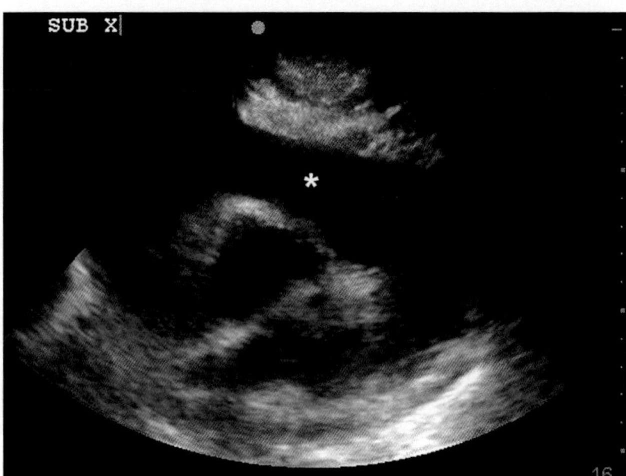

Figure 14.1
Cardiac tamponade. Note collapse of the right ventricular free wall due to fluid (asterix).

Cardiac tamponade

Assessment for pericardial effusion is part of the basic cardiac ultrasound assessment. It is important to note that tamponade physiology may develop in the setting of acute or chronic pericardial effusion. An increase in the amount of fluid surrounding the heart can acutely compromise ventricular function and cardiac output. In addition, decreasing preload (as can occur with hemodialysis, hemorrhage, sepsis, dehydration, diuresis, nitrates, etc.) can remove pressure necessary to offset the impact of the effusion. This can lead to tamponade without an acute change in the volume of pericardial effusion. Thus, tamponade should be suspected in any patient with pericardial effusion and hemodynamic compromise.

To review the findings discussed in Chapter 3, right atrial collapse during systole is the earliest sign of pericardial tamponade. As pressure increases, the right ventricular free wall will collapse during diastole (Figure 14.1). Pericardial effusion is best visualized by the subxiphoid four-chamber view; however, effusions may be visualized in any standard view. The four-chamber views are best for assessing right atrial and ventricular appearance throughout the cardiac cycle. Keep in mind that the parasternal views do not give the most accurate cross-section of the right heart and are less useful in assessing for tamponade. In the setting of tamponade, the IVC will demonstrate dilatation and diminished respiratory variation.

Right ventricular dilatation

A four-chamber cardiac view (subxiphoid or apical) is best for visualizing right ventricular size side-by-side with the left ventricle. A normal ratio

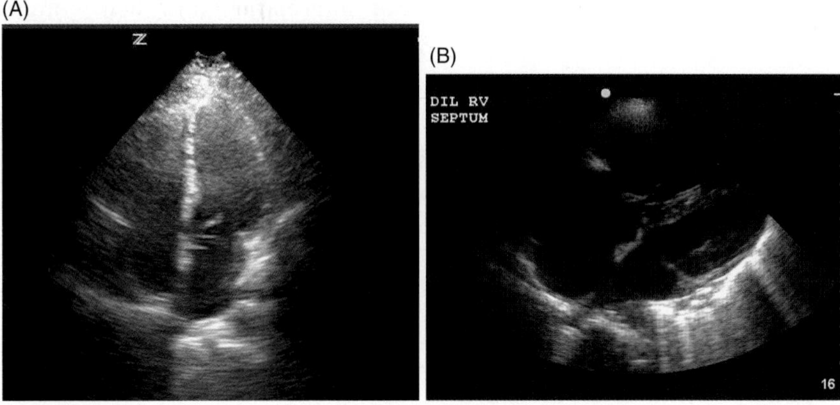

Figure 14.2
Dilatation of the right ventricle (RV) compared to the left ventricle (LV) in apical 4 chamber view (panel A) and subxiphoid view (panel B).

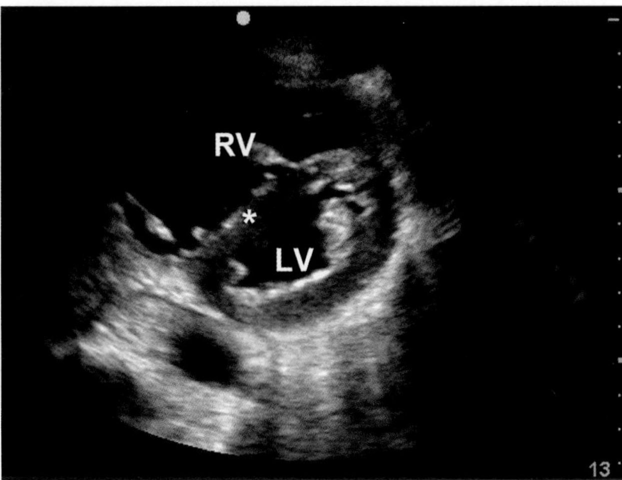

Figure 14.3
High right heart pressures flatten the interventricular septum (*) between the dilated right ventricle (RV) and left ventricle (LV).

of RV to LV size is 0.6 : 1. However, most authors consider RV dilatation definitive when the RV and LV appear equal in diameter at the level of the atrioventricular valves (Figure 14.2). Another finding consistent with increased right-side pressures is flattening of the ventricular septum or even bowing of the septum toward the LV (Figure 14.3). RV dilatation is found in pulmonary hypertension, pulmonary embolism, chronic obstructive pulmonary disease, and other chronic conditions. However, in the acutely decompensating patient the diagnosis of pulmonary embolism must be suspected. In this setting, an evaluation for DVT (described in Chapter 8) can provide additional information and help inform the diagnosis.

Hyperdynamic left ventricle

Increased contractility of the left ventricle, or near-complete obliteration of the LV cavity in systole, may be seen in a variety of conditions including hypertrophic cardiomyopathies, anemia, thyrotoxicosis, sepsis, and hypovolemia. In the acutely decompensating patient the latter two diagnoses are most likely, and distributive shock from blood loss, sepsis, or other acute cause must be considered.

Hypodynamic left ventricle

In contrast, global loss of contractility in the left ventricle can suggest a primary cardiac cause for the hypotension, as occurs with myocardial infarction or myocarditis but can also be seen with toxins, sepsis, or cardiac "stunning." It can also be found in congestive heart failure (CHF) and other chronic conditions. In either case, a diffusely hypokinetic left ventricle suggests that the patient will not respond well to fluid bolus, and inotropes or pressors may be of benefit.

Assessments of cardiac contractility are most useful when combined with an estimation of IVC size and respiratory variation. This helps rapidly inform the decision to use fluids or inotropes/pressors as the next management step in shock.

Inferior vena cava

Many authors have attempted to demonstrate a correlation between IVC appearance and central venous pressure (CVP), with varied success. Although measurement of the IVC diameter has been described from a transverse and longitudinal approach, many have described the longitudinal approach as more optimal in the adult patient, and the transverse approach more optimal in the pediatric patient. This view allows visualization of the IVC along with hepatic vein confluence and the IVC entry into the right atrium (Figure 14.4). Measurement of the IVC diameter is recommended at a point approximately 2 cm distal to the diaphragm.

During inspiration, negative intrapleural pressure causes negative intraluminal pressure and increases venous return to the heart, speeding blood through the extrathoracic IVC. Given that the extrathoracic IVC is such a compliant vessel, this causes the IVC diameter to decrease with normal inspiration (Figure 14.5). Therefore, in patients with low intravascular volume, the inspiration to expiration diameter ratios change much more than in patients with normal or increased intravascular volume. M-mode can be used to quantify the ratio of maximum and minimum diameters of the IVC during respiration.

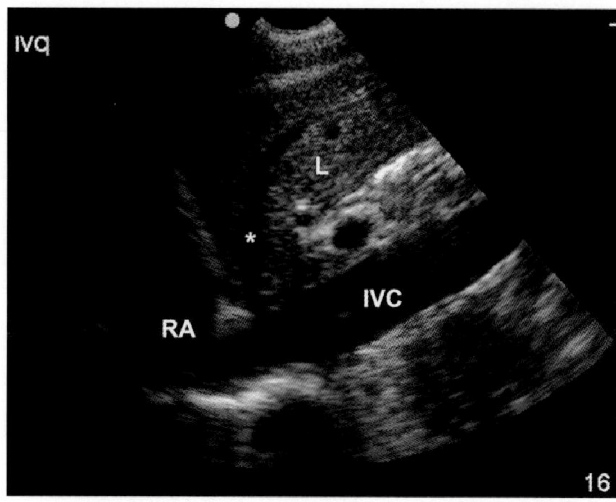

Figure 14.4

Inferior vena cava (IVC) draining into the right atrium (RA). The hepatic vein (*) drains through the liver (L) into the IVC.

(A)

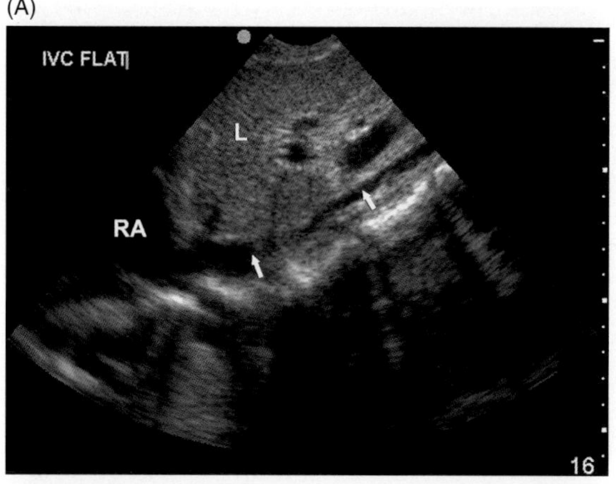

(B)

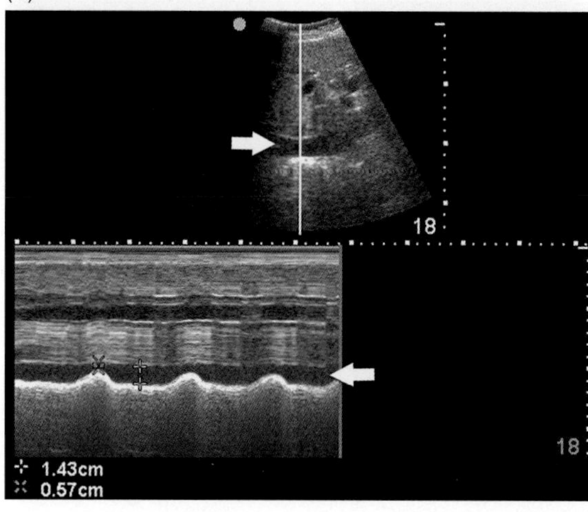

Figure 14.5

(*A*) Small-diameter IVC (arrows) behind liver (L) draining into right atrium (RA). (*B*) Variation in diameter during respiration measured using M-mode. This patient should be fluid-responsive.

Table 14.1 Inferior vena cava diameter, respiratory variation, and right atrial (RA) pressure

IVC (cm)	Respiratory change	RA pressure (cm H_2O)
< 1.5	Total collapse	0–5
1.5–2.5	> 50% collapse	5–10
1.5–2.5	< 50% collapse	11–15
> 2.5	< 50% collapse	16–20
> 2.5	No change	> 20
Reproduced with permission from Wong & Otto 2000 [1].		

(A)

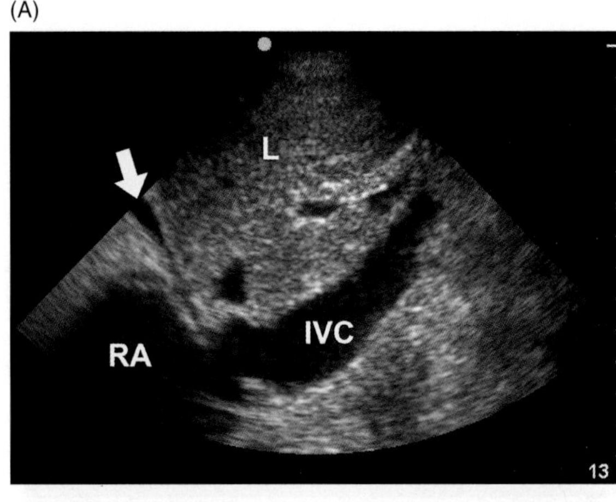

(B)

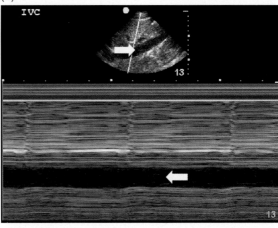

Figure 14.6

(*A*) Large-diameter IVC in a patient with fluid overload. A pericardial effusion (arrow) is also visible. In real time a lack of variation in IVC diameter would be noted by M-mode, as noted by the arrows in (*B*) another patient.

It may be more helpful to think of the extremes of IVC appearance on ultrasound and how that predicts fluid responsiveness in the hypotensive patient. Table 14.1 describes the range of IVC diameters and respiratory variation, and the expected correlation to CVP (right atrial pressure).

In spontaneously breathing patients, an IVC diameter of < 1.5 cm with complete inspiratory collapse is associated with a low CVP and fluid responsiveness [2–4]. Variation in IVC diameter with respiration is lower in patients with CHF than without CHF (5).

In contrast, patients with an IVC diameter of > 2.5 cm with no respiratory change are unlikely to respond to a fluid load and are likely to have a high CVP (> 20 cm H_2O) [2,4,6]. These patients may benefit more from inotropy or afterload reduction. Figure 14.6 demonstrates increased IVC diameter in a patient with fluid overload.

In mechanically ventilated patients, this phenomenon is reversed because inspiration now results in positive thoracic pressure. Therefore, IVC distensibility has been studied as a predictor of fluid responsiveness. Respiratory variation in IVC diameter of 13–18% was predictive of fluid responsiveness in two studies [7,8].

The FAST exam

Although the FAST exam was discussed in Chapter 2 as it relates to a trauma assessment, there are other disease states which can cause bleeding into the peritoneum or thoracic cavity. Ruptured ectopic pregnancy, bleeding from malignancies, postoperative complications, and other etiologies can cause hypotension from bleeding. In these settings the sonographic evaluation will be similar to the one performed as part of a trauma evaluation.

Note that the FAST exam is most sensitive for fluid when the patient is in the Trendelenberg position. Be cautious when performing and interpreting the examination when the patient is not in this position. For example, patients in an optimal position for mechanical ventilation (head of bed elevated 30 degrees) will not demonstrate fluid in Morison's pouch or the left upper quadrant until a significant amount of fluid is present. In those patients, the pelvic view (especially longitudinal) may be more helpful. For a variety of normal and abnormal FAST exam images, refer to Chapter 2.

Aorta

As discussed in Chapter 5, leaking abdominal aortic aneurysms can have profound hemodynamic consequences. Thus, a rapid assessment of the aorta caliber can be useful in the evaluation of the acutely hypotensive patient. Although an aorta diameter greater than 3 cm (and iliac vessel diameter greater than 1.5 cm) is considered aneurysmal, the actual diameter must be placed into the proper clinical context. Figure 14.7 demonstrates an aneurysmal aorta.

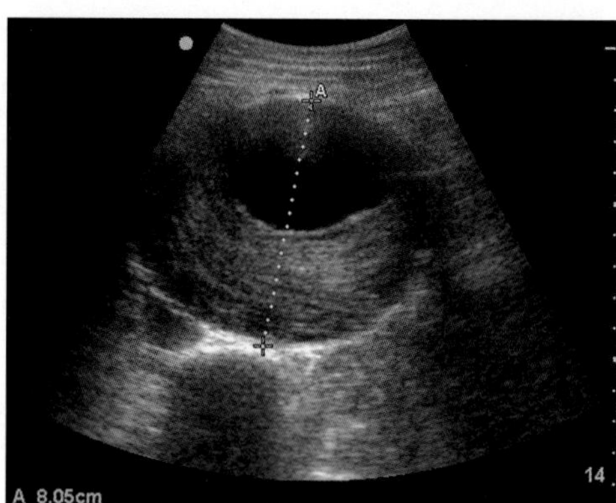

Figure 14.7
Aortic aneurysm, over 8 cm in diameter.

Pleura and lung

Pneumothorax is a common complication of trauma, medical illness such as chronic obstructive pulmonary disease (COPD) and asthma, and iatrogenic complications of mechanical ventilation, central line placement, and other critical care interventions. Thus, evaluation for pneumothorax (as detailed in Chapter 2) should be a standard part of the evaluation of the hypotensive patient. Some clinicians prefer to assess for pneumothorax using the same curvilinear, microconvex, or phased-array probe used for the rest of the hypotension evaluation. Others switch to a high-frequency linear probe for a more detailed examination of the pleural interface. The latter approach is likely to be more accurate. Figure 14.8 demonstrates the M-mode appearance of normal lung and pneumothorax.

In addition, using the appearance or disappearance of B-lines when evaluating the dyspneic or hypotensive patient can help assess cardiac function and can point to whether a patient is becoming fluid-overloaded or diuresing well. Because lung ultrasound is more dynamic than chest x-ray, patient monitoring with ultrasound can help guide clinical management more minutely. This is true not only with fluid overload but also with changes in the appearance of lung parenchyma with acute respiratory distress syndrome (ARDS), pneumonia, and other interstitial lung processes. Lung ultrasound is discussed in more detail in Chapter 9. Increasing clinician familiarity with lung imaging techniques has the potential to change how pulmonary function is monitored in critical patients.

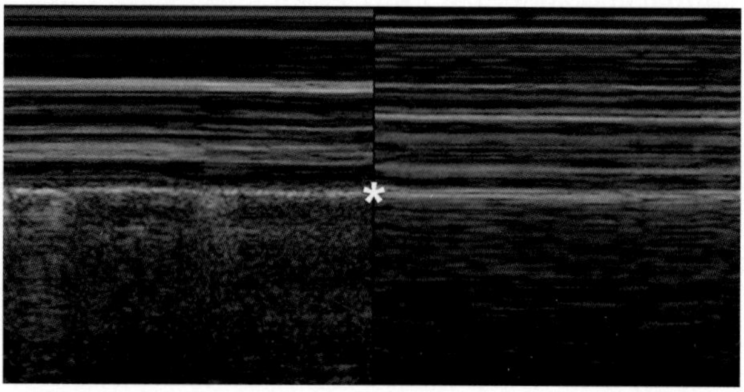

Figure 14.8
M-mode appearance of normal lung (*left*) and pneumothorax (*right*). Pleura (*) is visible in the middle of the screen.

Sample clinical protocol

Figure 14.9 demonstrates common probe positions for the evaluation of hypotension causes, using the rapid ultrasound in shock/hypotension (RUSH) protocol. Table 14.2 summarizes these views as well as common pathology and clinical actions to consider.

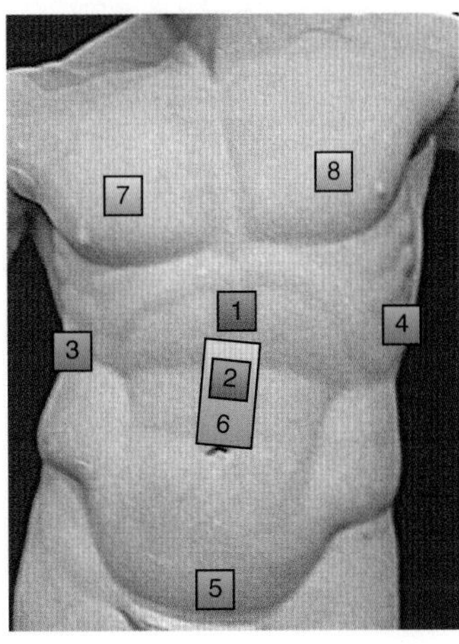

Figure 14.9

Probe positions for rapid ultrasound in shock/hypotension (RUSH): (1) heart, (2) IVC, (3, 4, 5) Morison's pouch and the FAST exam, (6) aorta, and (7, 8) pneumothorax.

Table 14.2 Multisystem assessment in hypotension

Assessment	Findings	Actions to consider
Heart	Cardiac standstill	Code termination
	Pericardial tamponade	Pericardiocentesis
	Right ventricular dilatation	Thrombolysis (if pulmonary embolism strongly suspected)
	Hyperdynamic left ventricle	Fluid bolus
	Hypodynamic left ventricle	Pressors, inotropes
IVC	Dilated ($>$ 2.5 cm), no respiratory variation	Diuresis or optimize cardiac management
	Small ($<$ 1.5 cm), collapse with inspiration	Fluid bolus
FAST exam	Peritoneal fluid	Search for cause of bleeding
	Thoracic fluid	Tube thoracostomy, search for cause of bleeding
Aorta	Aneurysm (diameter $>$ 3 cm)	Vascular surgery consultation, OR
Pleura	Pneumothorax	Tube thoracostomy
Deep veins	Deep vein thrombus	Thrombolysis or anticoagulation

Perhaps the most comprehensive sonographic assessment of the hypotensive patient was described by WINFOCUS (Figure 14.10).

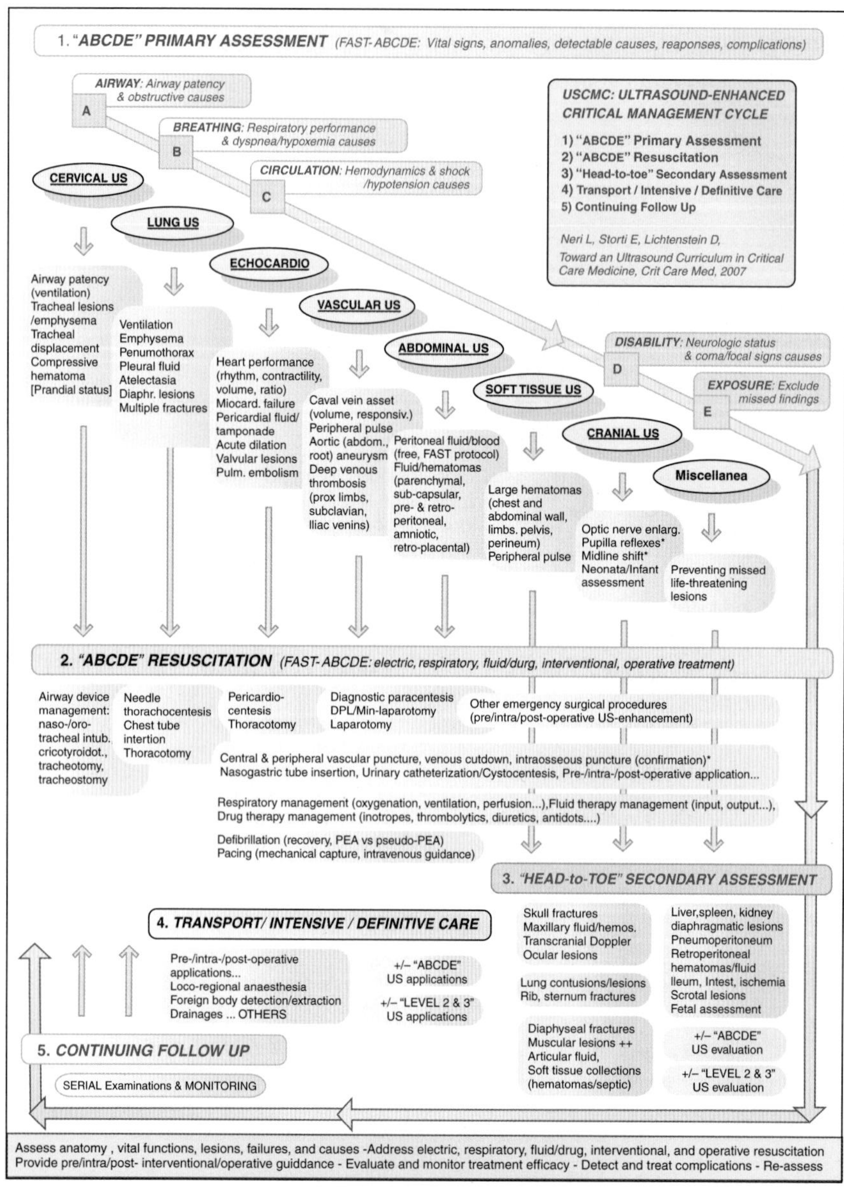

Figure 14.10

The WINFOCUS ultrasound life support algorithm. In step 1, a clinically driven ultrasound assessment is performed (ABCDE, *top row*). Next, step 2 describes possible interventions, which can be guided by the results of the sonography. Available at www.winfocus.org/uscme/uscmc/usls.

Literature review

Protocol and reference	Methods	Notes
UHP protocol Rose *et al.* 2001 [9]	Undifferentiated hypotensive patient: Morison's pouch, heart, aorta.	Case examples and protocol description.
Trinity protocol Bahner 2002 [10]	Cardiac, aorta, and FAST.	Case example and protocol description.
FATE Jensen *et al.* 2004 [11]	Focused assessed transthoracic echocardiography: heart, pleural effusion.	Protocol description, feasibility study and case series. Adequate images in 97% of 210 ICU patients.
RCT of US in hypotension Jones *et al.* 2004 [12]	FAST, heart, aorta, IVC: undifferentiated hypotension patients randomized to immediate vs. delayed (15 min) US assessment.	Early US yielded more focused differential diagnosis and more accurate physician impression of final diagnosis.
FEER Breitkreutz *et al.* 2007 [13]	Focused echocardiographic evaluation in resuscitation: heart.	Protocol description, including incorporation of US protocol into existing ACLS guidelines with minimal interruption of CPR.
CAUSE Hernandez *et al.* 2008 [14]	Cardiac arrest ultrasound exam: heart, pneumothorax.	Protocol description: search for tamponade, hypovolemia, massive PE, and pneumothorax as cause for cardiac arrest.
RUSH Weingart *et al.* 2009 [15]	Rapid ultrasound in shock and hypotension: HI-MAP: heart, IVC, Morison's/FAST, aorta, pneumothorax.	Protocol description.
ACES Atkinson *et al.* 2009 [16]	Abdominal and cardiac evaluation with sonography in shock: heart, IVC, aorta, FAST.	Protocol description and case examples.
RUSH Perera *et al.* 2010 [17]	Rapid ultrasound in shock: Pump: heart Tank: IVC, jugular veins, FAST, Pneumothorax assessment Pipes: aorta, DVT assessment	Protocol description.
WINFOCUS Neri *et al.* 2007 [18]	ABCDE for ultrasound: A – Airway (trachea, cricothyroid) B – Breathing (lung ultrasound – pneumothorax assessment and B-lines)	Protocol description

Protocol and reference	Methods	Notes
	C – Circulation (cardiac, IVC, FAST, aorta, DVT) D – Disability (optic nerve, cranial ultrasound) E – Exposure (extremities)	

References

1. Wong SP, Otto CM. Echocardiographic findings in acute and chronic pulmonary disease. In Otto CM (ed.), *Textbook of Clinical Echocardiography*, 2nd edn. Philadelphia, PA: Saunders; 2000: 747.
2. Adler C, Buttner W, Veh R. [Relations of the ultrasonic image of the inferior vena cava and central venous pressure] [German]. *Aktuelle Gerontol* 1983; **13**: 209–13.
3. Kircher BJ, Himelman RB, Schiller NB. Noninvasive estimation of right atrial pressure from the inspiratory collapse of the inferior vena cava. *Am J Cardiol* 1990; **66**: 493–6.
4. Simonson JS, Schiller NB. Sonospirometry: a new method for noninvasive estimation of mean right atrial pressure based on two-dimensional echographic measurements of the inferior vena cava during measured inspiration. *J Am Coll Cardiol* 1988; **11**: 557–64.
5. Blehar DJ, Dickman E, Gaspari R. Identification of congestive heart failure via respiratory variation of inferior vena cava diameter. *Am J Emerg Med* 2009; **27**: 71–5.
6. Minutiello L. [Noninvasive evaluation of central venous pressure derived from respiratory variations in the diameter of the inferior vena cava] [Italian]. *Minerva Cardioangiol* 1993; **41**: 433–7.
7. Barbier C, Loubieres Y, Schmit C, *et al.* Respiratory changes in inferior vena cava diameter are helpful in predicting fluid responsiveness in ventilated septic patients. *Intensive Care Med* 2004; **30**: 1740–6.
8. Feissel M, Michard F, Faller JP, Teboul JL. The respiratory variation in inferior vena cava diameter as a guide to fluid therapy. *Intensive Care Med* 2004; **30**: 1834–7.
9. Rose JS, Bair AE, Mandavia D, Kinser DJ. The UHP ultrasound protocol: a novel ultrasound approach to the empiric evaluation of the undifferentiated hypotensive patient. *Am J Emerg Med* 2001; **19**: 299–302.
10. Bahner D. Trinity: a hypotensive ultrasound protocol. *J Diagn Med Sonogr* 2002; **18**: 193–8.
11. Jensen MB, Sloth E, Larsen KM, Schmidt MB. Transthoracic echocardiography for cardiopulmonary monitoring in intensive care. *Eur J Anaesthesiol* 2004; **21**: 700–7.

12. Jones AE, Tayal VS, Sullivan DM, Kline JA. Randomized, controlled trial of immediate versus delayed goal-directed ultrasound to identify the cause of nontraumatic hypotension in emergency department patients. *Crit Care Med* 2004; **32**: 1703–8.
13. Breitkreutz R, Walcher F, Seeger FH. Focused echocardiographic evaluation in resuscitation management: concept of an advanced life support-conformed algorithm. *Crit Care Med* 2007; **35**: S150–61.
14. Hernandez C, Shuler K, Hannan H, *et al.* C.A.U.S.E.: Cardiac arrest ultrasound exam. A better approach to managing patients in primary non-arrhythmogenic cardiac arrest. *Resuscitation* 2008; **76**: 198–206.
15. Weingart SD, Duque D, Nelson BP. The RUSH exam: rapid ultrasound for shock/hypotension. text.emcrit.org/ultrasound/The%20RUSH%20Examfinal.htm.
16. Atkinson PR, McAuley DJ, Kendall RJ, *et al.* Abdominal and Cardiac Evaluation with Sonography in Shock (ACES): an approach by emergency physicians for the use of ultrasound in patients with undifferentiated hypotension. *Emerg Med J* 2009; **26**: 87–91.
17. Perera P, Mailhot T, Riley D, Mandavia D. The RUSH exam: Rapid Ultrasound in SHock in the evaluation of the critically ill. *Emerg Med Clin North Am* 2010; **28**: 29–56, vii.
18. Neri L, Storti E, Lichtenstein D. Toward an ultrasound curriculum for critical care medicine. *Crit Care Med* 2007; **35**: S290–304.

Section 2

Procedural ultrasound

Performing procedures on acutely ill patients can be one of the most rewarding and challenging aspects of emergency medicine and critical care practice. These patients present unique challenges to the clinician for a variety of reasons. Most notably, since they are acutely ill or decompensating, there is an urgency to perform procedures in suboptimal conditions. The patients themselves often pose unique challenges. Many patients have abnormal anatomy due to prior surgical procedures, scarring, trauma, or acute or chronic illness. In addition, obesity can obscure standard anatomic landmarks. Perhaps the clinician attempting to perform the procedure will not be the first operator or must navigate through a prior failed procedural attempt. Finally, because of the acuity of their illness, many patients do not have the functional capacity to remain in standard procedural positions (i.e., lying in the Trendelenburg position or sitting upright), and this often makes successful procedural outcomes more challenging. These conditions are found in many critical care settings – therefore, the benefits of ultrasound guidance for procedures are not limited to the emergency department.

Any advantage over standard surface anatomy or landmark-based techniques should be a welcome addition to the arsenal of all critical care physicians. As with the diagnostic applications of ultrasound, ultrasound for procedure guidance is meant as an adjunct to the physical examination. When the sternocleidomastoid muscle cannot be seen or felt, ultrasound can help visualize the internal jugular vein and obviate the need for such landmarks. When clinical acumen alone cannot distinguish a subcutaneous abscess from an area of induration, ultrasound can help make the distinction.

The chapters that follow describe techniques whereby ultrasound can aid in the performance of common and often lifesaving procedures. As with all ultrasound use, the skills described here are operator-dependent. But then so is the interpretation of electrocardiograms or laceration repair. This should not be an excuse, but a call to practice and to build comfort with the techniques described. In addition, the same tenet of a simple, algorithmic approach toward procedural ultrasound should apply. In the case of procedure guidance, the questions may be "How deep is the effusion?", "Is there an abscess at this site?", or "Where exactly is my needle with respect to the vein?".

There is an ever-increasing body of literature to support the use of ultrasound for procedures, and patient safety is becoming a leading priority for both federal and private healthcare agencies. As ultrasound use becomes more widespread, and as its impact on patient satisfaction, safety, and operator preference becomes more pronounced, we may see the end of the era of procedures performed without the use of radiographic guidance.

15 Vascular access

Introduction

Vascular access is one of the most basic skills required of the critical care physician. Many factors, including body habitus, volume depletion, shock, history of intravenous drug abuse, prior cannulation, scarring, thromboses, congenital deformity, and cardiac arrest, can make vascular access difficult or even dangerous. Traditionally, surface anatomy and anatomic landmarks have served as the only guides for locating central veins. The incorporation of ultrasound into the procedure allows for more precise assessment of vein and artery location, vessel patency, and real-time visualization of needle placement.

The paradigm for radiology is to perform invasive procedures such as vascular access under real-time direct visualization so as to reduce complications. Although patients may have complicating medical problems, those scheduled for procedures in radiology are usually hemodynamically stable. Why, then, would critical care physicians perform invasive procedures on more unstable patients without the same tools and techniques to increase safety?

Real-time bedside ultrasonography facilitates rapid and successful vascular access [1–6]. Indeed, there is increasing institutional and literature support for performing cannulation under direct visualization as the technology spreads throughout the hospital. This is not limited to the emergency department but is applicable to any critical care unit or patient care area in the hospital.

Focused questions for vascular access

The questions for vascular access are as follows:

1. Where is the target vein?
2. Is it patent?

This chapter will cover techniques to make this assessment seem second nature.

Anatomy

The most common venous cannulations assisted by ultrasound guidance are internal jugular, femoral vein, and peripheral venous cannulations. Ultrasound-guided subclavian vein cannulation has been described but is technically more challenging because the clavicle serves to obstruct ultrasound waves and imaging can be difficult.

Anatomic landmarks for internal jugular and femoral vein cannulation are well described. However, a brief review of relevant anatomy as it applies to sonographic evaluation is warranted.

Internal jugular anatomy

Figure 15.1 shows variations in the anatomy encountered when the ultrasound probe is placed at the apex of the sternocleidomastoid muscle triangle (where the sternal and clavicular heads of the muscle meet near the level of the larynx). This is not predictable using landmarks to guide cannulation, but is readily apparent using ultrasound. The internal jugular in most patients will be strikingly obvious, and with compression it will be easy to identify whether the vessel is patent and thus amenable to cannulation. Variations in the internal jugular–carotid relationship occur with neck position as well; this can be assessed in real time under ultrasound.

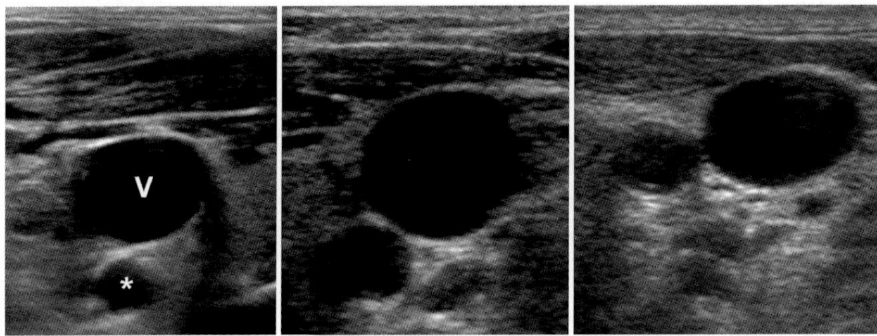

Figure 15.1

Variations in the relationship between the internal jugular vein (V) and carotid artery (*) visualized using ultrasound. Note that the relative position of the vessels differs between patients and with neck position.

Femoral triangle anatomy

Just distal to the inguinal ligament is the femoral triangle. From lateral to medial, this space contains the femoral nerve, artery, and vein, then empty space and lymphatics. This arrangement is sometimes recalled using the mnemonic "NAVEL." Typically, one would palpate for a pulse in this area and then direct a needle medially to find venous blood. Figure 15.2 shows the image obtained when the ultrasound probe is placed just distal to the inguinal ligament over the common femoral vein.

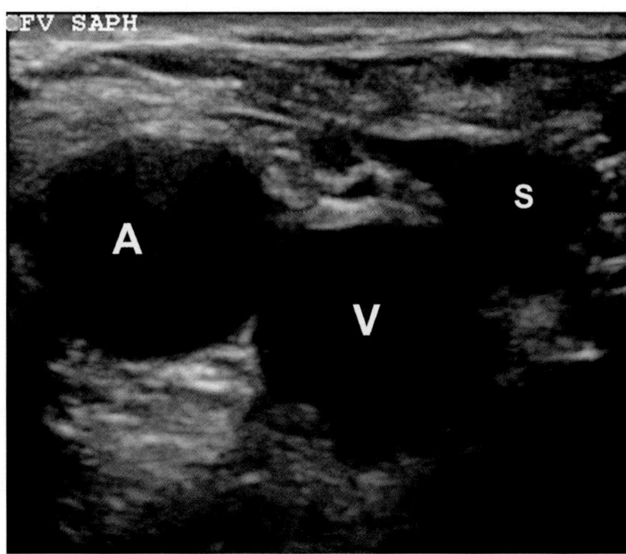

Figure 15.2
Common femoral artery (A) and vein (V). The greater saphenous vein (S) is visible at this level as well.

If the same ultrasound probe were then guided more distally along the vein, an image like that in Figure 15.3 would be obtained. Here, the superficial femoral vein is demonstrated. At this level, the common femoral artery has bifurcated to superficial and deep femoral arteries. The common femoral vein has also bifurcated into superficial and deep, and usually the superficial is the only vessel seen at this level. It is also quite common at this level to find the artery quite close to the vein, or even overlying it. The femoral vein is most reliably medial to the artery at a point just distal to the inguinal ligament; ultrasound evaluation of the vessels distal to this site will reveal how variable the anatomy can be as one travels caudally. As described in Chapter 8, patent veins will completely compress to a thin line with probe pressure. If they do not, a clot is present, and cannulation should be attempted on another vessel.

Although it is helpful to have color flow to show patency and spectral Doppler to distinguish flow patterns, it is not necessary. In fact, it can sometimes be misleading because partial vein occlusion will still demonstrate flow, and transmitted pulsations can affect spectral wave forms. The most important distinguishing characteristic is that veins have thinner walls, and are therefore easily and completely compressible. If the vein is not completely compressible, a clot or thrombosis should be suspected and another vessel selected (see Chapter 8). Moreover, it is instructive to observe a vessel throughout the respiratory cycle before attempting cannulation, because the level of respiratory variation and change in caliber or diameter that is observed is quite surprising. This is even more marked in dehydrated or septic patients and thus, if observed, may require more reverse Trendelenburg positioning.

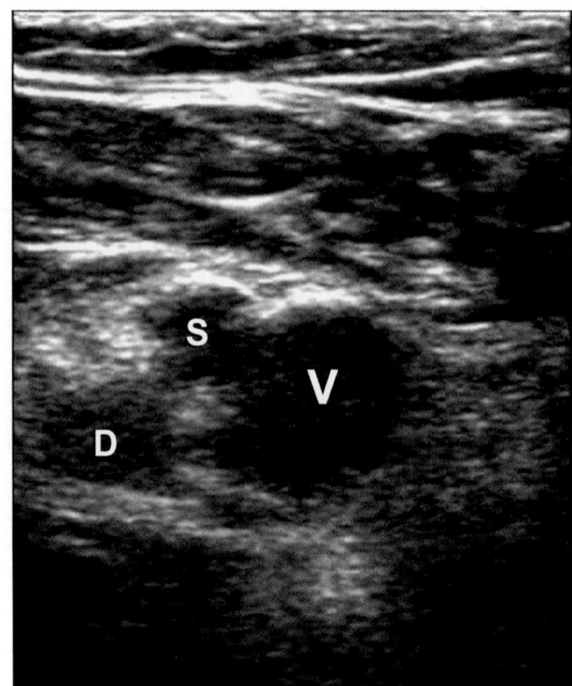

Figure 15.3

Superficial femoral vein (V), superficial (S) and deep (D) femoral arteries.

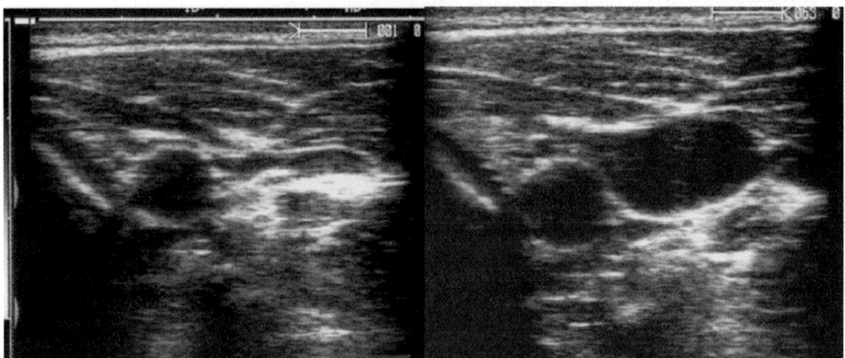

Figure 15.4

Internal jugular vein and carotid artery. When the patient is not lying flat (*left*), the carotid is seen as a round anechoic structure but the jugular vein is collapsed. When the Valsalva maneuver and Trendelenburg position are applied (*right*), the highly distensible internal jugular vein fills with blood and is easily seen to the right of the carotid.

Figure 15.4 shows the same patient with and without Valsalva and increased Trendelenburg positioning. These techniques make the internal jugular vein much easier to visualize, and the increased caliber will improve cannulation success.

Technique

Probe selection

Generally, a high-frequency (5–10 MHz) linear probe is used for vascular access (Figure 15.5). The higher frequency generates higher-resolution pictures, and the linear image display makes needle guidance and identification somewhat more intuitive.

Special equipment

A sterile probe cover (Figure 15.6), typically packaged with sterile conducting gel, should be used when performing the venous access with maximal sterile barrier technique. Sterile gloves can be used as a substitute probe cover if these packages are not available.

Approaches

Two general approaches are used during vascular access: *static* and *dynamic*. Ultrasound is used to verify the vessel location prior to using a standard external landmark-based approach (static technique), or it is used for real-time imaging of the venipuncture (dynamic technique). The dynamic technique may use a short-axis approach (also known as out-of-plane or transverse, where cross-sectional anatomy of the vessel is visualized) or a long-axis approach (also known as in-plane or longitudinal, using the longitudinal view of the vessel and needle). Each technique has benefits and

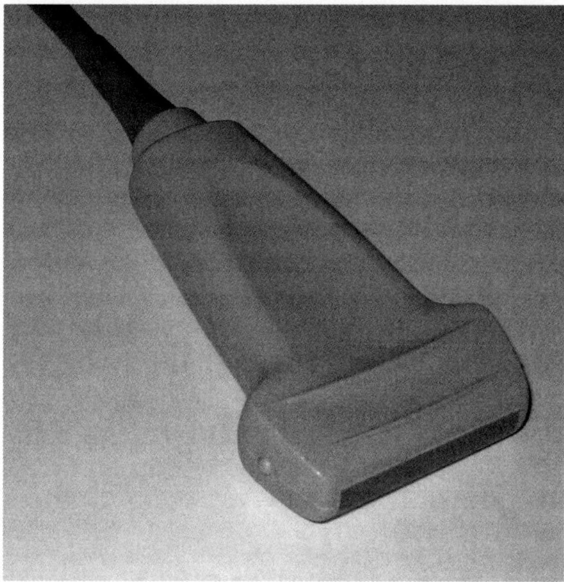

Figure 15.5
A high-frequency linear probe.

Table 15.1 Static versus dynamic techniques

Approach	Benefits	Drawbacks
Static	Transducer is not needed during the sterile portion of the procedure	No real-time guidance for trajectory, dynamic changes in anatomy
Dynamic long axis	Clear view of needle depth and trajectory throughout procedure	Technically difficult, no guidance laterally for left–right trajectory changes
Dynamic short axis	Provides view of structures surrounding vessel, allows for lateral trajectory correction	More difficult to visualize the needle tip

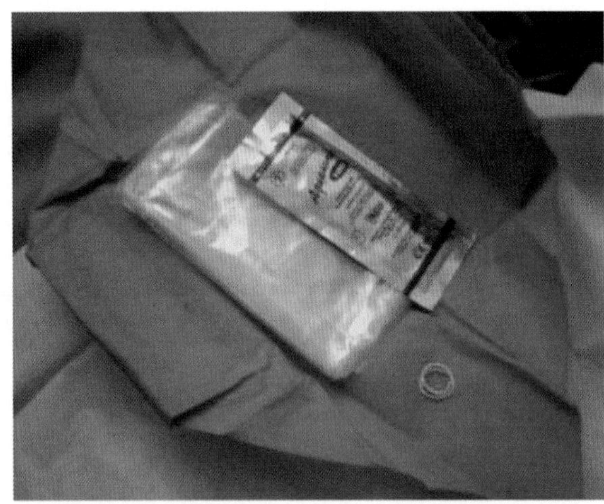

Figure 15.6
A typical sterile probe cover kit, consisting of a clear plastic probe cover and sterile ultrasound gel (in the silver packet). The rubber bands can be applied to help keep the probe cover from sliding out of place on the transducer.

drawbacks, some of which are highlighted in Table 15.1. When first learning the technique, it is preferable to use the dynamic short-axis view. This is because the relative location of the artery and vein is easier to appreciate, and the risk of veering off course from the vein to the artery is reduced. When a level of comfort is reached with ultrasound guidance for cannulation, some operators favor the long axis and some the short. There is some controversy over which is the better method, and often patient positioning and operator preference dictate the optimal approach in any individual case.

The procedure can be performed by a single operator or by two people, with one person holding the ultrasound probe and one performing the procedure. When a two-operator approach is used, the more experienced ultrasound operator should be the one holding the ultrasound probe, while the more novice operator performs the cannulation. For either technique, the preparation and probe orientation are the same.

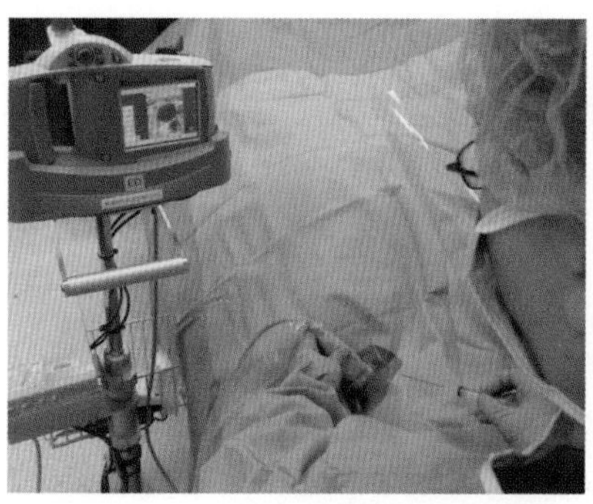

Figure 15.7

Patient positioning for central venous access. Note that the probe marker should face the operator's left, so that the left of the screen and the left of the probe are aligned.

Setup

This book assumes familiarity with the standard techniques for the procedures described. Thus, Chapters 15 and 16 highlight only the techniques related to ultrasound use.

Patient positioning

Position the patient as you would normally (Figure 15.7). The ultrasound machine should be placed immediately next to the patient so you can visualize the relevant patient anatomy and the ultrasound image at the same time. The operator will therefore be facing both the patient and the ultrasound machine.

If a *static approach* is employed, the vessel should be visualized at this point, and patency should be checked (using compressibility as described in Chapter 8). Center the target vessel on the screen – this places the transducer over the center of the vessel. A mark should be placed on the skin at the midpoint of the transducer to mark vessel location. To assess vessel trajectory, repeat this process once more at a point on the vessel 1–2 cm away. Thus, the two points marked on the skin will define a line and act as a better guide for needle direction than a single point.

For *dynamic approaches*, the patient should be draped and prepped in the usual sterile fashion. Next, the transducer should be prepped in a sterile fashion.

Transducer preparation

The sterile probe cover kit (or a sterile glove if kits are unavailable) should be placed on the sterile field. A non-sterile assistant should hold the probe upright and apply standard (non-sterile) conducting gel to the transducer. The probe is then inserted into the sterile sheath and placed on the sterile field. Sterile gel (from silver lubricant packages) can then be placed on the sterile glove on top of the probe (Figure 15.8).

Probe orientation

Note the location of the probe marker. The probe marker and the screen marker (see Chapter 1) should be pointing in the same direction. That is, the

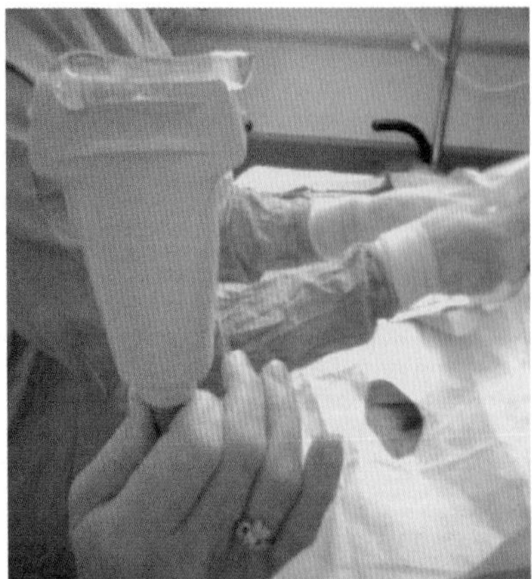

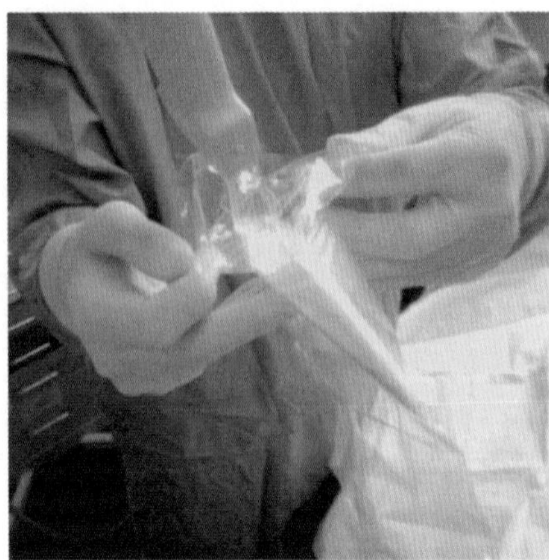

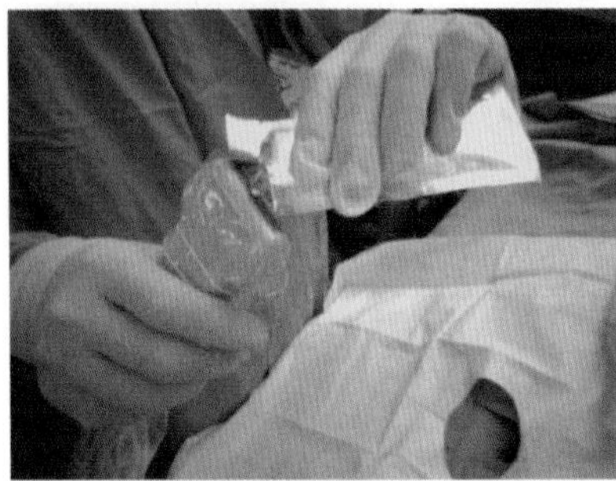

Figure 15.8
Probe preparation.

probe marker should correspond to the left side of the operator (not necessarily the left side of the patient) and the left side of the ultrasound image on the screen. This way, if the needle moves to the left of the probe, it will also move to the left on the screen. For an in-plane (long-axis) approach, most operators hold the probe marker toward themselves so that the needle will be visualized coming in from the left side of the screen.

Holding the probe

Proper hand position was described in Chapter 1. A comfortable and stable hand position is even more important when the probe is used to guide the placement of a needle. As shown in Figure 15.9, the first three fingers should hold the probe, leaving the remaining fingers and heel of the hand free for stabilization. Hand position is a compromise between stability, comfort, and safety: be sure to keep your fingers away from the needle!

Vessel identification

Place the transducer at the site of anticipated needle placement. Search for the vessel using local ultrasound landmarks as a guide (sternocleidomastoid

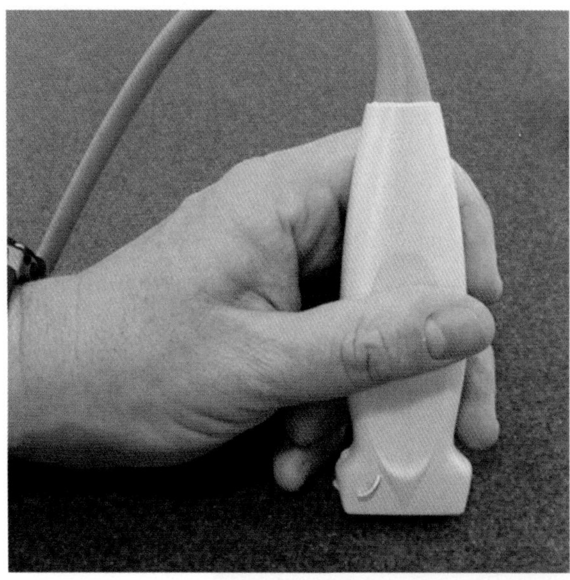

Figure 15.9
Holding the ultrasound probe in the non-dominant hand.

muscle, carotid artery for the internal jugular approach; femoral artery for the femoral vein approach). Check compressibility of the vein. This serves to distinguish artery from vein and reduces the risk of attempting catheter placement at the site of a deep vein thrombus. At this point, the center of the vessel should be held in the center of the screen. This means that the vessel is beneath the center of the probe.

For a short-axis approach

Center the cross-section of the vein on the screen. One simple way to assess the proper distance from the transducer is to use the geometry of a 45°–45°–90° triangle, or the Pythagorean theorem. As shown in Figure 15.10, measure the depth from the surface to the vessel (D_2). This is equal to the distance from the transducer to where the skin puncture should be made (D_1), as long as the needle enters the skin at a 45-degree angle. When a more shallow angle is desired, the distance from the transducer (for a given vessel depth) must be increased. For a 45-degree approach the hypotenuse (H) is roughly equal to $1.4 \times D_2$. Thus, if the vessel is centered 1 cm beneath the skin, puncture the skin 1 cm toward the operator from the transducer and the vein will be punctured by 1.4 cm of needle depth. If the vein is 2 cm deep, puncture 2 cm from the transducer and hit the vessel when the needle has traveled 2.8 cm. It is useful to make this calculation before attempting cannulation, to avoid complications. If the needle is at distance H and the vessel has not been cannulated, then the trajectory is not correct and the needle should be repositioned before injuring deeper structures such as the carotid or femoral artery. Puncturing the skin at a point too close to the transducer position will yield a steep trajectory and will make cannulation more difficult.

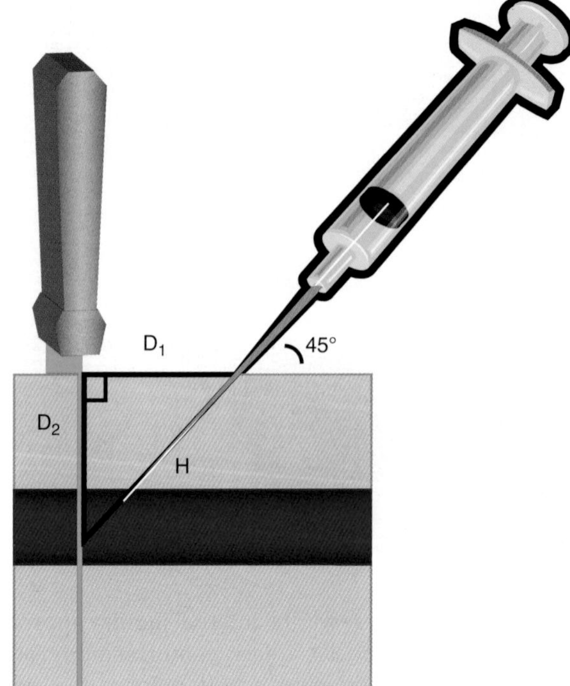

Figure 15.10
Pythagorean theorem: needle orientation in a simplified 45–45–90 degree triangle where $D_1 = D_2$. The hypotenuse (H) is roughly equal to $1.4 \times D_2$.

In the short-axis approach, the needle is only visible at the point where it crosses the ultrasound plane perpendicular to it. The needle will be seen as a dot, often with either a faint shadow (black) or reverberation artifact (white) deep to the needle. However, often the needle itself will not be visualized. This is because the needle width is quite small, and during the initial portion of the path, the needle has not yet crossed the plane of the ultrasound beam. It is possible to angle the probe toward the needle to ensure that it is traveling along the correct trajectory. Signs of the needle pushing through tissue will be seen (muscle displacement, tenting in of the vein when the needle is attempting to pierce the wall) even if the needle itself is not well visualized.

Note that the appearance of the needle tip and needle shaft will be identical on ultrasound. The cross-section of a line (the needle) is a dot, no matter which part of the line is cut by a plane (the ultrasound beam). Figure 15.11 demonstrates an approach to ensuring it is the tip, and not the shaft, of the needle that is visualized in the short-axis approach. The tip of the needle is the area at which the dot is just barely visible – moving the probe slightly should cause the dot to disappear if you are at the tip (because the beam will slide past the needle). If you are visualizing the shaft, the dot will be visible in either direction. Since one great weakness of the short-axis approach is visualizing the tip of the needle, it is important that operators become

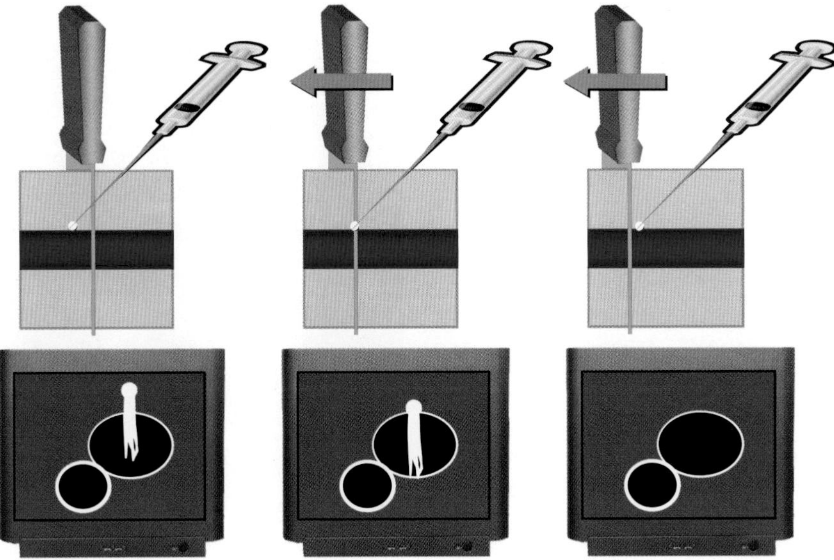

Figure 15.11

Moving the probe (sliding or tilting) from the shaft of the needle (*left*) toward the tip (*center*) and beyond (*right*). When the needle is about to disappear from view, the tip is being visualized.

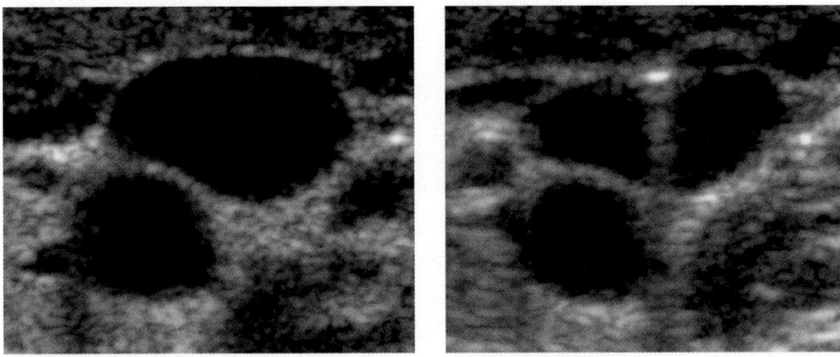

Figure 15.12

The needle tenting the internal jugular vein (*right*) as it is about to puncture the vessel. Note that the vessel is pushed inward as compared to the image prior to cannulation (*left*).

comfortable with the concept of ensuring that they can see the tip of the needle by moving the ultrasound plane appropriately.

As the needle approaches the vessel, the walls of the vessel will tent downward and then pop back when the wall is punctured. In Figure 15.12, the needle cross-section is visualized as a bright point with some reverberation artifact. Tenting of the internal jugular vein is also seen in Figure 15.13.

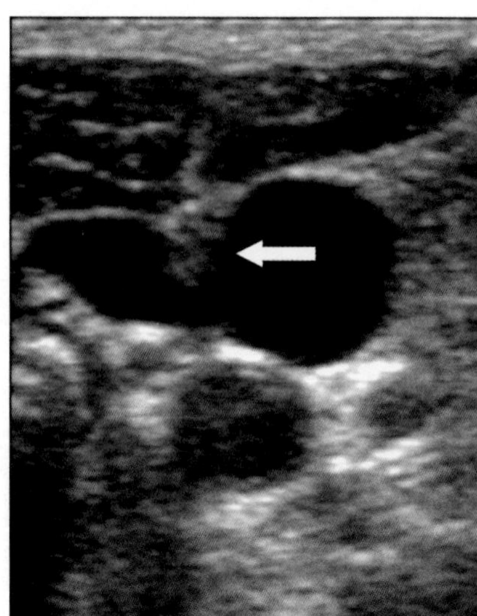

Figure 15.13
Another view of a needle tenting the anterior wall of the vein (arrow).

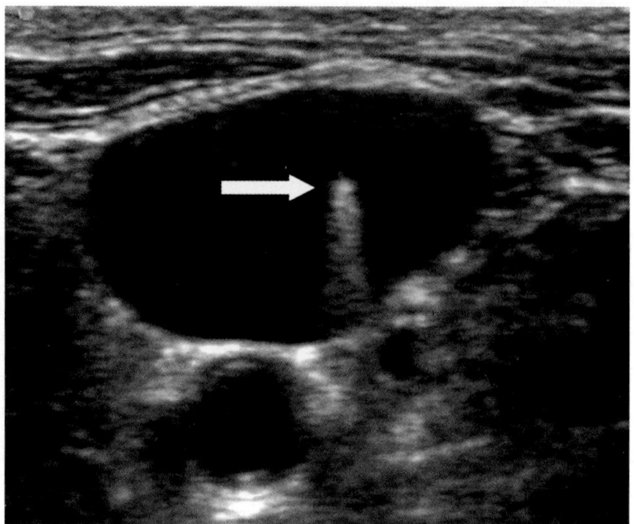

Figure 15.14
Needle tip (arrow) visible within vein lumen.

After the vein is punctured, a flash should be seen in the syringe, and the tip of the needle should be visible within the vessel (Figure 15.14). Proceed with normal cannulation techniques (guidewire, introducer) from this point onward.

Many authors advocate the use of ultrasound to confirm venous (and not arterial) cannulation after the flash is obtained. The guidewire can be visualized within the vein (Figure 15.15) and the catheter can often be seen as well (Figure 15.16). Doppler can be used to demonstrate flow near the catheter tip

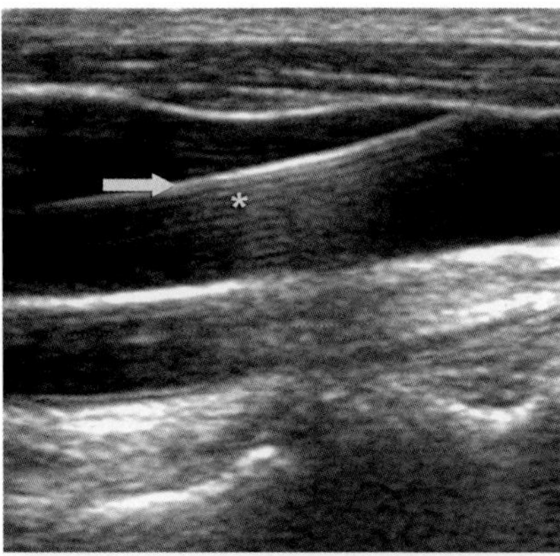

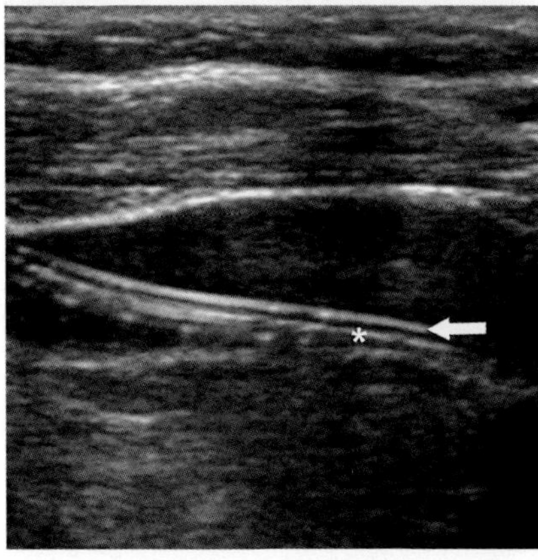

Figure 15.15
Guidewire (arrow) visualized within vein. Note reverberations (*) distal to the wire.

as a small flush of saline is infused. Saline flow can also be seen as microbubbles in the right heart when pushed through a subclavian or internal jugular central line (Figure 15.17).

For a long-axis approach

Again, it is recommended that the short-axis approach be mastered before attempting the dynamic long-axis approach, because the technique is similar. Center the long axis of the vein on the screen. To ensure that you are in the center, focus on the largest diameter of the vessel. Hold the needle in line with the trajectory of the vessel, which should be in the same plane as the ultrasound beam (Figure 15.18).

With this technique, it is important to keep the transducer steady over the center of the vessel. If the needle is misdirected out of the plane (seen as losing the image of the needle), the needle should be withdrawn toward the skin and redirected. *Do not* redirect the ultrasound beam to find the needle, instead redirect the *needle* toward the *beam*.

(A)

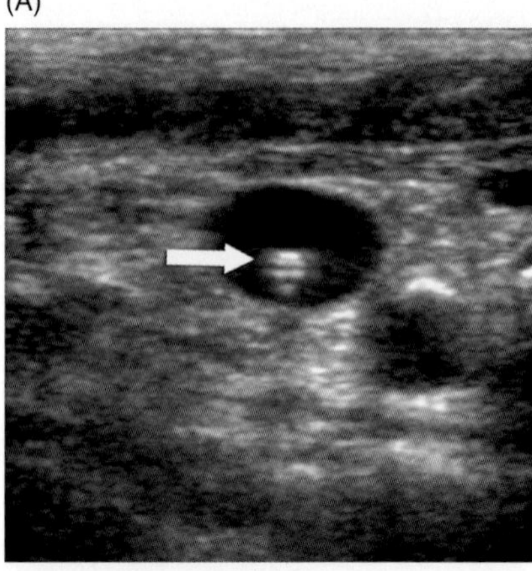

(B)

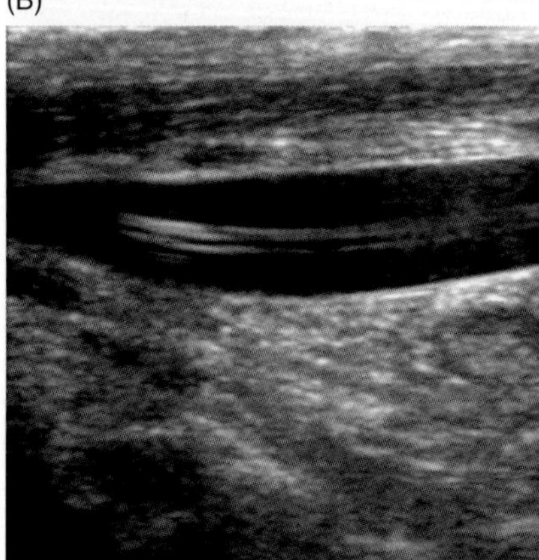

Figure 15.16

Catheter (arrow) visualized within the vein in (*A*) transverse and (*B*) longitudinal views.

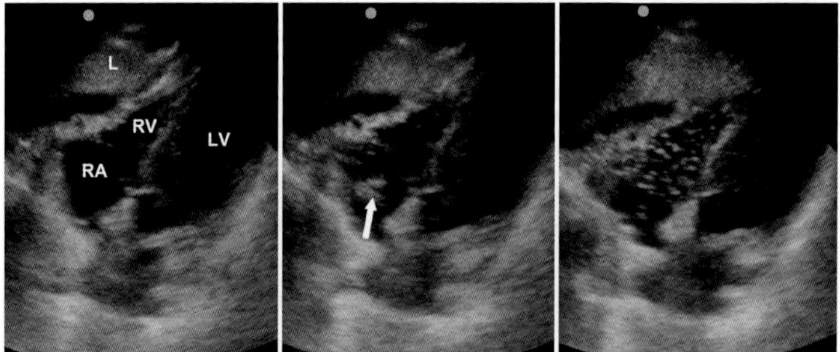

Figure 15.17

Subxiphoid view of the heart with right atrium (RA), right ventricle (RV), left ventricle (LV), and liver (L) visible. Several mL normal saline is pushed into the central line and a blush of agitated saline (microbubbles) is visible as it enters the right atrium (arrow, *center*). The microbubbles then spread throughout the right side of the heart (*right*). This effect occurs almost instantly and lasts just a few seconds.

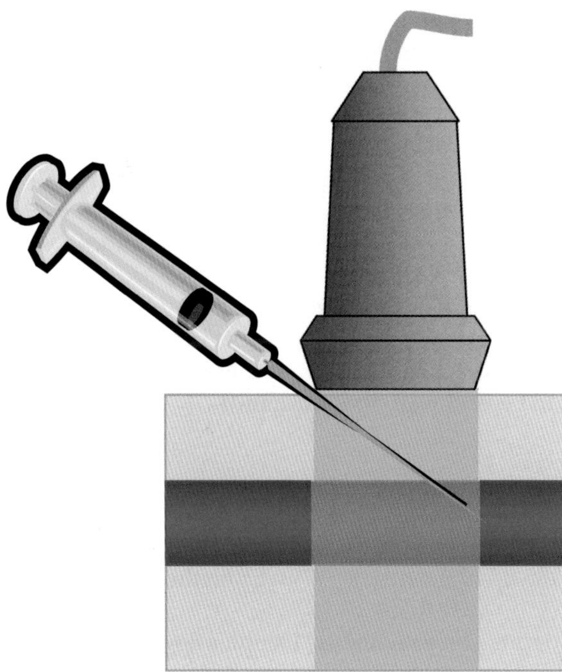

Figure 15.18
Long-axis positioning. Note that the needle and the vessel are both in the plane of the ultrasound beam.

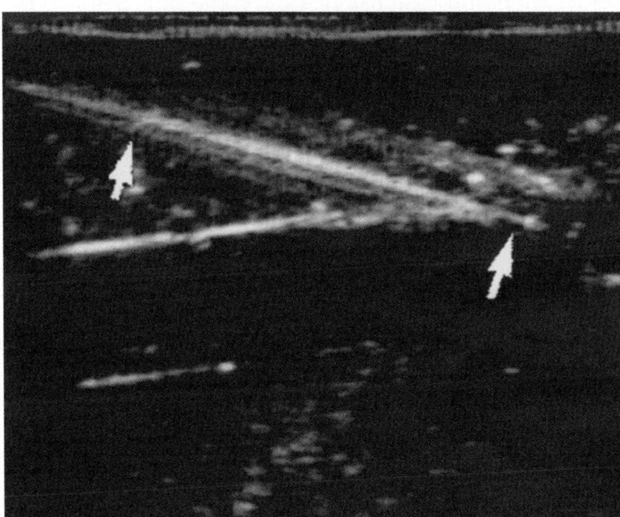

Figure 15.19
Long-axis visualization of the needle puncturing the vessel. The arrows point out the highly conductive metal needle with reverberation artifact emanating parallel to it.

When visualizing the long axis of the needle and vessel, the entire length of the needle (including the all-important tip) can be visualized (Figure 15.19).

For the novice user, it can be challenging to correlate movements of the needle with changes in appearance of the image on the screen. However, it is important to stress that the ultimate goal of ultrasound use is vessel cannulation. Thus, one cannot lose sight of the syringe and needle during the procedure. It is easy to focus on the screen and miss a flash of blood, or to focus on the syringe and miss the needle veering dangerously off course on the screen. With practice, it becomes easier to simultaneously focus on the screen and the syringe, just as one focuses on both the road ahead and the rearview mirror when driving a car. It is also quite useful to apply negative pressure on the syringe as soon as the tip of the needle punctures the skin. Creating a slight vacuum using only one hand on the syringe is a useful skill to develop for many procedures involving a needle. As soon as a vessel is punctured, the negative pressure will facilitate the flash. With a bit of practice this sudden pressure change can be felt by the operator, providing an additional sensory clue to successful cannulation (in addition to seeing a flash and visualizing tenting of the vessel wall on ultrasound).

Scanning tips

- Tilt probe toward needle tip when using a short-axis approach.
- Remember to image the tip of the needle. Visualizing the needle shaft is not useful.
- Be sure to check for depth, compressibility, Doppler flow, and location of nearby arteries.
- Note how subtle changes in patient positioning, Trendelenburg, and so on impact vessel location and distension. Take some time prior to the procedure to maximize the positioning, using ultrasound as a guide.
- When using a two-person technique, the more experienced sonographer should hold the probe, and the less experienced one should direct the needle.

Pitfalls

- Keep the vein centered on the screen in the short-axis view. Remember that the needle will be inserted at the center point of the transducer. If the transducer is not centered over the vein, the needle will be directed to the wrong location.
- After the flash of blood, the procedure is no longer facilitated by ultrasound. At this point, put the probe down and continue the procedure as you normally would.
- Be sure to angle or slide the transducer (in the short-axis technique) to visualize the tip of the needle. If the transducer remains in a static position, it cannot be relied on to demonstrate the needle trajectory accurately. In the short-axis approach, the plane follows the needle tip.
- In the long-axis approach, the opposite is true. Keep the probe (and plane of the ultrasound beam) steady in the optimal position. If the needle deviates from the plane, the needle (and not the probe) should be redirected. In the long-axis approach, the needle follows the plane.

Cannulation of the subclavian vein

The use of ultrasound with the infraclavicular approach to subclavian vein cannulation is limited by the large acoustic shadow created by the clavicle. However, the take-off of the subclavian vein from the internal jugular vein can often be visualized by placing the probe in a supraclavicular position. Using the same basic principles outlined previously, identify the proximal subclavian vein and the internal jugular vein.

Cannulation of the external jugular vein

Because the external jugular vein is superficial, it is often readily identified by visualization and palpation. However, some cases are limited by a patient's range of motion or adiposity. In such instances, ultrasound guidance may prove useful. Figure 15.20 demonstrates the sonographic appearance of the external jugular vein, along with the internal jugular vein. The technique of vessel cannulation is identical to that of the internal jugular vein as described previously. Of note, the superficial external jugular vein is easily collapsed with even slight pressure of the transducer on the skin.

Peripheral venous cannulation

Peripheral venous cannulation can sometimes be unsuccessful after multiple attempts – even with attempts at the relatively larger antecubital veins. In this case, one might consider attempting cannulation of the brachial or cephalic veins. These veins lie deeper in the structures of the upper arm and are not readily palpable. Consequently, these veins are not generally used for

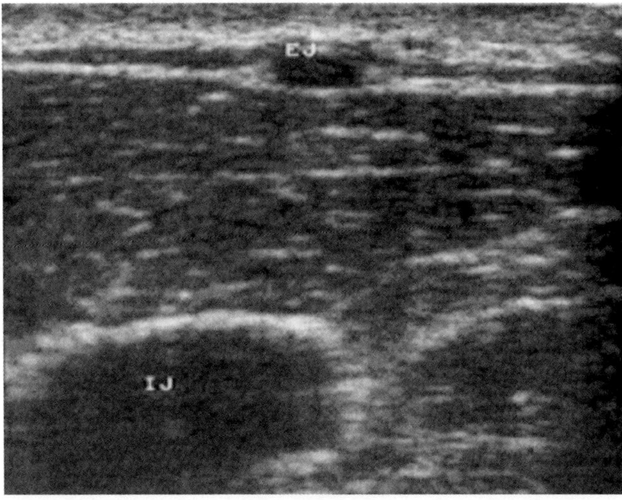

Figure 15.20
Transverse view of external jugular (EJ) and internal jugular (IJ) veins.

intravenous catheter placement in the absence of ultrasound guidance. In most patients, the depth of these vessels requires that a longer intravenous catheter (1.75–2.0 in [4.4–5.0 cm]) be used. Caution should be exercised with the more proximal brachial vein because it lies immediately adjacent to the ulnar and median nerves. More distal peripheral veins (such as in the antecubital fossa or forearm) may be cannulated as well using the techniques described here.

Focused question

1. Where is the target vein?

Anatomy

The axillary vein divides into the cephalic vein, which runs superficially toward the lateral (dorsal) aspect of the upper arm; the basilic vein, which courses superficially along the inferior and medial (ventral) aspect of the arm; and the brachial vein, which runs deeply inferior to the biceps muscle (Figure 15.21).

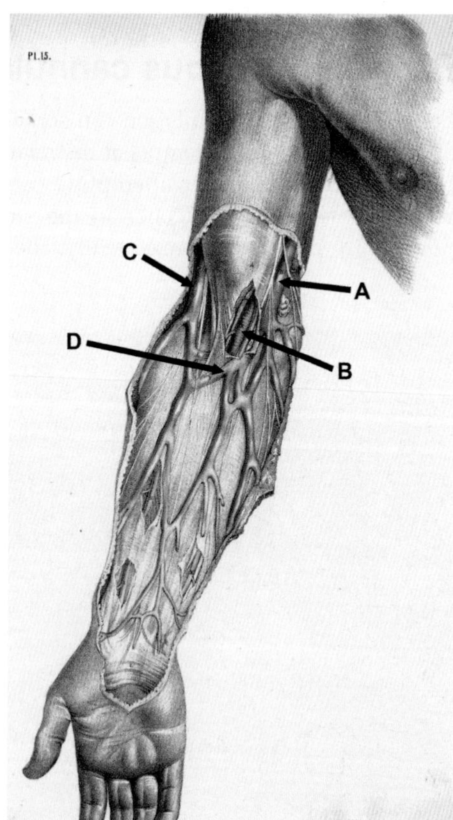

Figure 15.21

Upper arm vasculature. The basilic vein (A), brachial artery (B), cephalic vein (C), and median antecubital vein (D) are visualized. The superficial and deep brachial veins are not visible here, but flank the brachial artery. Image reproduced from *Maclise's Surgical Anatomy*, Plate 15. Philadelphia, PA: Blanchard and Lea, 1859 (image out of copyright).

The basilic and cephalic veins rejoin in the antecubital fossa, and the brachial vein runs deep in this location. Frequently, the brachial vein will be found as paired superficial and deep brachial veins.

Technique

Probe selection

Generally, a high-frequency linear transducer is used.

Special equipment

For deep vein cannulation, a longer catheter is required (at least 2 in [5 cm]). Sterile probe covers can be used for sterile peripheral access.

Setup

As usual, the ultrasound machine should be placed in a position where the target anatomy on the patient and the ultrasound screen are both readily visible (Figure 15.22). Thus, the operator will generally be facing both. The patient should be placed in the standard position for the procedure.

A single-operator approach can be used, as described previously. Alternatively, one operator can demonstrate the vessel using ultrasound while another cannulates the vein. This approach can be incredibly useful when ultrasound is used to demonstrate vessel location and depth so that an experienced nurse can place the intravenous line.

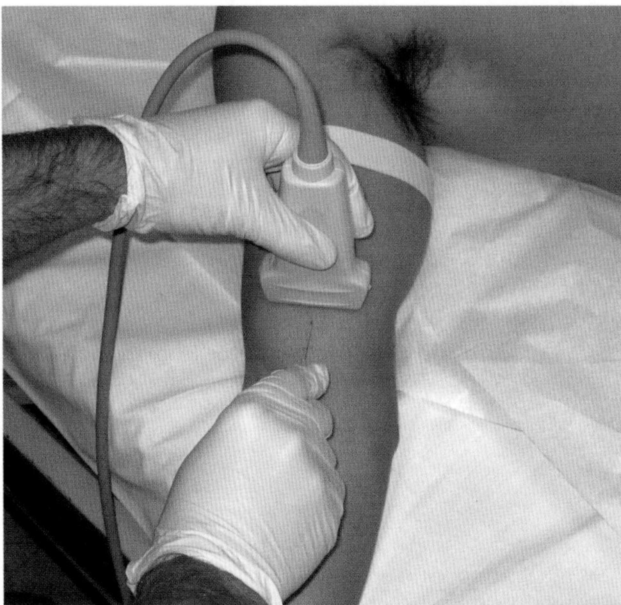

Figure 15.22 Positioning for ultrasound-guided peripheral vein cannulation.

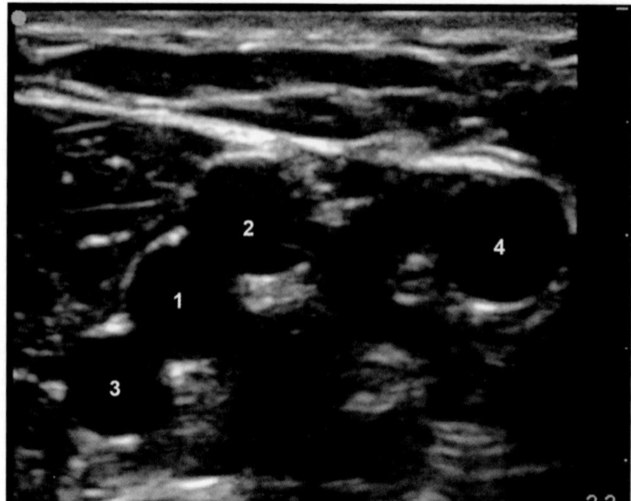

Figure 15.23
The brachial artery (1) and adjacent superficial (2) and deep (3) brachial veins are visualized. The basilic vein (4) is seen to the right.

Procedure

As described for central venous cannulation, survey the vessels of interest using the transducer in the transverse plane. Either the static or the dynamic technique can be employed. In Figure 15.23, the brachial artery is seen adjacent to the superficial brachial and deep brachial veins. The basilic vein is visualized as well.

It is important to check compressibility and vessel patency. Smaller veins and arteries often do not have sufficient flow to generate a brisk Doppler signal, but differences in compressibility often highlight the veins from the arteries. The brachial and basilic veins readily compress, but the brachial artery remains patent (Figure 15.24). In real time, even small arteries can be seen to pulsate when pressure is placed on them. Once the target vein is identified, the process of intravenous catheter placement is largely unchanged (except for the use of a longer catheter).

Tips

Peripheral veins are more superficial, inconstant, and fragile than central veins. All the care and finesse one usually employs in cannulating a difficult peripheral vein should still be used with ultrasound.

Use the least amount of pressure possible with the transducer when imaging the veins. Often, no veins are visible because they have all been collapsed by too much pressure.

Pitfalls

Difficult veins are difficult veins. Ultrasound can help find veins that would otherwise be invisible, but it cannot prevent veins from rolling or collapsing, and nor does it melt away valves.

(A)

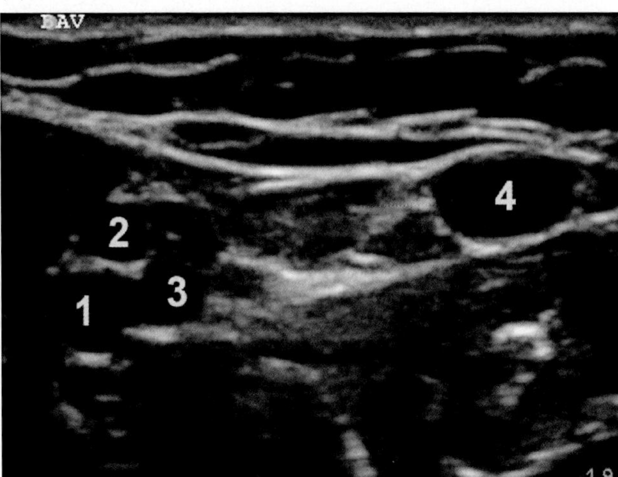

(B)

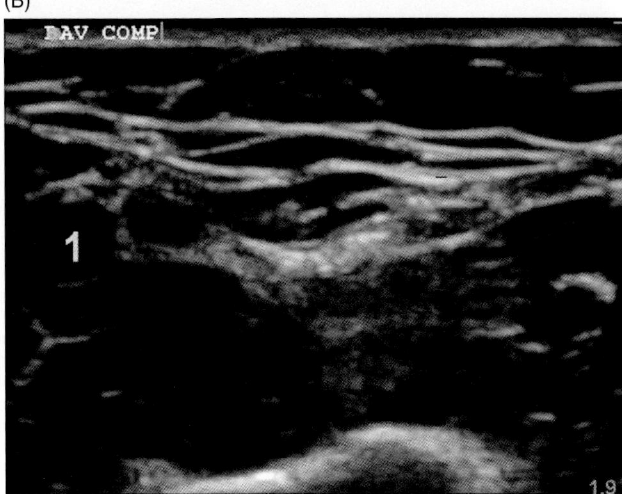

Figure 15.24

(*A*) The brachial artery (1) and adjacent superficial (2) and deep (3) brachial veins are visualized. The basilic vein (4) is seen to the right. (*B*) With slight compression, the veins collapse entirely and only the brachial artery remains patent. In real time, the artery would visibly pulsate with compression.

Do not approach peripheral veins with a catheter at an acute angle. Remember that getting *to* the vessel is only the first step – you must thread the catheter *into* the vessel. If you would normally place an IV at a 15- to 30-degree angle to the skin, ultrasound cannot make a 60-degree angle of approach feasible. A commonly used guide to catheter length is that two-thirds of the length of the catheter should reside within the vessel for it to

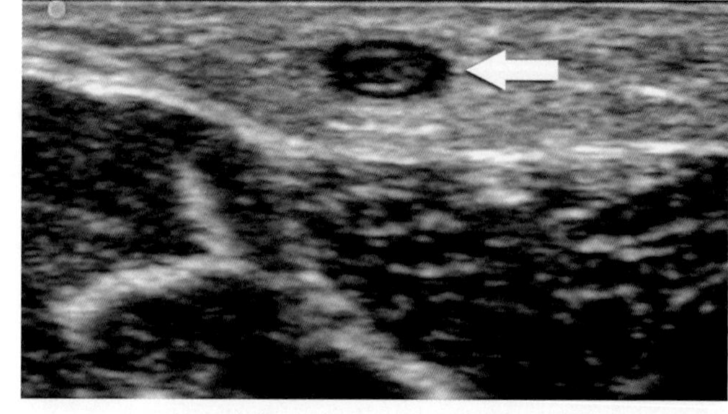

Figure 15.25 Superficial thrombophlebitis (arrow). Note echogenic material within the vein, which does not compress.

remain stable in its position. Catheters typically used for peripheral venous access are designed for vessels just beneath the skin surface; it is better to overestimate the length needed rather than underestimate when approaching a deeper vessel.

Occasionally, thrombophlebitis of the peripheral veins is encountered (Figure 15.25). As with DVT of the central veins, it is not recommended that cannulation is attempted in thrombosed vessels.

Literature review

Ultrasound use in central venous access was first described in the early 1990s. Since then, dozens of studies have sought to assess the efficacy of the technique. In 2005, Milling *et al.* randomized patients to landmark-based, static ultrasound, or dynamic ultrasound guidance for central venous cannulation [1]. The study found that ultrasound guidance was associated with a higher success rate. In 1997, Hilty *et al.* found a reduction in the number of attempts and complication rates when using ultrasound [2]. Notably, the authors determined that the femoral pulsation felt during cardiopulmonary resuscitation (CPR) was frequently venous and not arterial. This finding should call into question common assumptions about venous anatomy during chest compressions, and the technique of directing the needle medial to the pulse felt during CPR.

Several meta-analyses have examined pooled data from studies of patients in a variety of settings (intensive care unit, transplant unit). Hind *et al.* found that use of ultrasound reduced the risk of failed catheter placement (relative risk reduction of 0.14) [3]. A similar analysis by Randolph *et al.* found that ultrasound guidance in seven patients would prevent one complication [4]. A review article by McGee and Gould noted the high complication rates of central venous access (Table 15.2) and recommended ultrasound be used for line placement when available [5].

The US Department of Health and Human Services published recommendations in 2001 regarding techniques to reduce medical errors. Among

Table 15.2 Summary of complication rates for central venous access approaches

	Frequency (%)		
Complication	**Internal jugular**	**Subclavian**	**Femoral**
Arterial puncture	6.3–9.4	3.1–4.9	9–15
Hematoma	< 0.1–2.2	1.2–2.1	3.8–4.4
Hemothorax	NA	0.4–0.6	NA
Pneumothorax	< 0.1–0.2	1.5–3.1	NA
Total	**6.3–11.8**	**6.2–10.7**	**12.8–19.4**

Reproduced with permission from McGee DC, Gould MK. Preventing complications of central venous catheterization. *N Engl J Med* 2003; **348**: 1123–33 [5].

the recommendations (which included handwashing guidelines and pre-anesthesia checklists) was the recommendation that ultrasound should be used to guide the placement of central venous catheters [6].

Several studies have examined the use of ultrasound in gaining peripheral intravenous access. Studies in the emergency [7–9] and anesthesia [10] literature have demonstrated higher success rates using ultrasound in patients deemed to be difficult venous access cases or in whom prior (non-ultrasound-guided) approaches had failed. Ultrasound can identify peripheral vein characteristics associated with higher cannulation success rates as well [9].

References

1. Milling TJ, Rose J, Briggs WM, *et al.* Randomized, controlled clinical trial of point-of-care limited ultrasonography assistance of central venous cannulation: the Third Sonography Outcomes Assessment Program (SOAP-3) Trial. *Crit Care Med* 2005; **33**: 1764–9.
2. Hilty WM, Hudson PA, Levitt MA, Hall JB. Real-time ultrasound-guided femoral vein catheterization during cardiopulmonary resuscitation. *Ann Emerg Med* 1997; **29**: 331–6.
3. Hind D, Calvert N, McWilliams R, *et al.* Ultrasonic locating devices for central venous cannulation: meta-analysis. *BMJ* 2003; **327**: 361.
4. Randolph AG, Cook DJ, Gonzales CA, Pribble CG. Ultrasound guidance for placement of central venous catheters: a meta-analysis of the literature. *Crit Care Med* 1996; **24**: 2053–8.
5. McGee DC, Gould MK. Preventing complications of central venous catheterization. *N Engl J Med* 2003; **348**: 1123–33.
6. Rothschild JM. Ultrasound guidance of central vein catheterization. In Shojania KG, Duncan BW, McDonald KM, *et al.*, eds. *Making Health Care Safer: a Critical Analysis of Patient Safety Practices.* Evidence

Report/Technology Assessment No. 43. AHRQ Publication No. 01-E058, Rockville, MD: Agency for Healthcare Research and Quality; 2001. www.ncbi.nlm.nih.gov/bookshelf/br.fcgi?book=erta43 .

7. Costantino TG, Parikh AK, Satz WA, Fojtik JP. Ultrasonography-guided peripheral intravenous access versus traditional approaches in patients with difficult intravenous access. *Ann Emerg Med* 2005; **46**: 456–61.
8. Keyes LE, Frazee BW, Snoey ER, Simon BC, Christy D. Ultrasound-guided brachial and basilic vein cannulation in emergency department patients with difficult intravenous access. *Ann Emerg Med* 1999; **34**: 711–14.
9. Panebianco NL, Fredette JM, Szyld D, *et al*. What you see (sonographically) is what you get: vein and patient characteristics associated with successful ultrasound-guided peripheral intravenous placement in patients with difficult access. *Acad Emerg Med* 2009; **16**: 1298–303.
10. Sandhu NP, Sidhu DS. Mid-arm approach to basilic and cephalic vein cannulation using ultrasound guidance. *Br J Anaesth* 2004; **93**: 292–4.

16 Ultrasound for procedure guidance

Introduction

Using techniques similar to those described in Chapter 15, ultrasound can be used to guide an ever-growing number of common bedside procedures. Many clinicians find that using ultrasound guidance for one set of procedures (venous access, for example), translates well to other areas.

Pleural effusion and thoracentesis

Pleural effusions typically appear as an echo-free or hypoechoic space on ultrasound. Internal echoes, however, may be present in the fluid, and the echogenicity of the pleural effusion can assist the clinician in determining the cause of the effusion (Table 16.1) [1]. Still, definitive diagnosis requires aspiration for culture and cell counts.

The positive identification of pleural fluid requires the demonstration of dynamic signs such as a change in shape of the echo-free space during the respiratory cycle, atelectatic or compressed lung, and swirling motion in the echo-free space.

Focused questions

1. Is there pleural fluid?
2. Where is the optimal site for needle placement?

Table 16.1 Pleural effusions: appearances and etiologies

Characteristic	Appearance	Common etiologies
Anechoic	Totally echo-free fluid	Transudate, some exudates
Complex non-septated	Echogenic material inside anechoic effusion	Exudate
Complex septated	Floating fibrin strands or septae present	Exudate
Homogeneously echoic	Homogeneous echodensity, not anechoic	Exudate, hemorrhage, empyema

Anatomy

Fluid accumulates between the visceral and parietal layers of the pleura. It collects in the most dependent portions of the pleura (the costophrenic angles) and rises from that level as more volume accumulates. One of the first signs of pleural fluid is the loss of the normal mirror image artifact caudal to the diaphragm and liver or spleen. In Figure 16.1 the liver, kidney, diaphragm, pleural fluid, and lung are all visible.

Technique

Probe selection

Ultrasound of the pleural space may be performed with a 2.5–5.0 MHz transducer.

Special equipment

A marking pen is useful for many procedures where ultrasound mapping and static guidance is used (Figure 16.2).

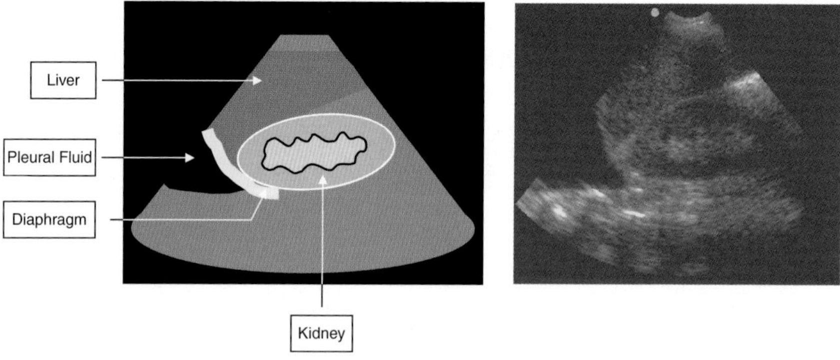

Figure 16.1
Black pleural fluid is demonstrated superior to the diaphragm and liver. The kidney is also well visualized in this view.

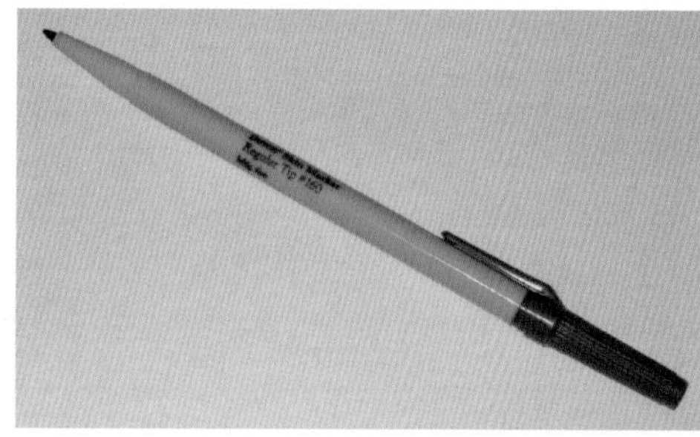

Figure 16.2
Marking pen.

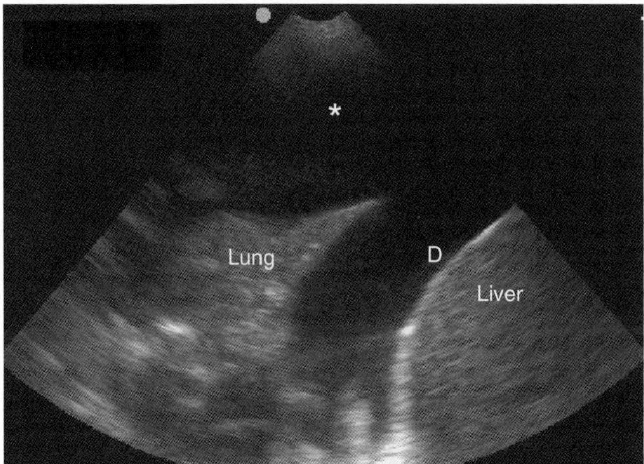

Figure 16.3
Pleural fluid (*) is noted above the diaphragm (D) and liver. Lung tissue is normally not well visualized because of the large amount of air. In this case the pleural fluid provides a good acoustic window, and the normally aerated lung tissue has been compressed somewhat and made more dense by the additional fluid pressure in the thorax.

Setup

The patient is positioned in a seated-upright position when possible. Scanning is performed from the anterior axillary line to the paravertebral space and from the superior and inferior aspects of the fluid collection. The feasibility of thoracentesis requires the demonstration of a sonographic window to the fluid *persisting* throughout the respiratory cycle. There is no formal lower limit of effusion size beneath which thoracentesis is contraindicated. However, many operators recommend that a visceral to parietal pleural distance of at least 10 mm is preferable to minimize the risk of an adverse outcome. Moreover, incursions of lung or diaphragm during the respiratory cycle into the sonographic window are considered absolute contraindications to thoracentesis at that site. Positive identification of the diaphragm plus liver or spleen is required to avoid puncture of these organs. If no safe sonographic window is identified, seriously consider aborting the procedure.

After identifying a suitable sonographic window, note the angle of the transducer. In addition, measure the depth required to achieve penetration into the pleural space containing fluid (Figure 16.3). Last, mark the skin at the site of planned needle entry.

Procedure

Immediately following ultrasound examination, prepare the site in a sterile fashion and perform thoracentesis in the usual fashion (Figure 16.4), taking care not to alter the patient's position.

Duplicate the angle of the transducer with the thoracentesis needle or catheter during the procedure. Direct visualization of needle entry is not necessary if the prior steps are followed.

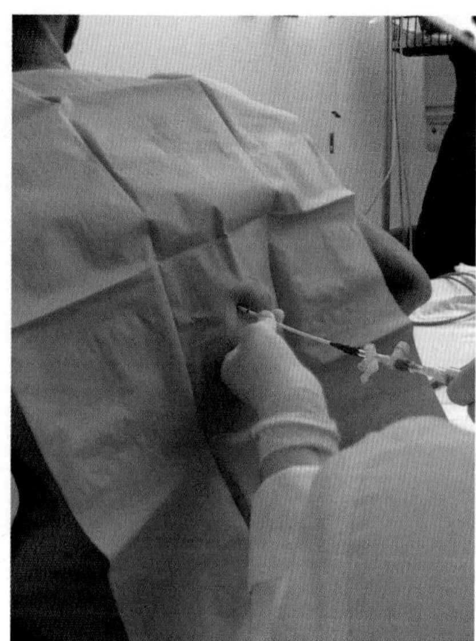

Figure 16.4
Thoracentesis setup. Note that needle placement and patient position are the same as for a standard landmark-based technique.

Tips

Measuring the depth from the skin to the parietal pleura allows for needle entry to a depth that should yield fluid while lowering the risk of puncturing the visceral pleura.

Pitfalls

Observe the proposed puncture site during the entire respiratory cycle. Significant changes in diaphragm position occur during respirations.

Literature review

Ultrasound was first used as a rescue method for failed or difficult thoracentesis. One early study demonstrated ultrasound-guided thoracentesis was successful in 88% of previously failed landmark-based attempts. The authors noted that scanning over the initial attempt sites found it to be above or below the effusion in 69% of the cases, and that the initial attempt was directly over the spleen, liver, or kidney in 58% of the cases [2]. Ultrasound guidance has a high success rate, even in cases where no fluid is visible on chest x-rays [3]. More recently, a study by interventional radiologists demonstrated a low complication rate (2.5% pneumothorax) when using ultrasound guidance, compared to historic pneumothorax rates of 4–30%. Interestingly, this study also noted that complications were not correlated to the amount of fluid removed during the procedure [4]. A retrospective study of ultrasound guidance versus landmark-based techniques demonstrated a significantly lower pneumothorax rate in the ultrasound guidance group (4.9% vs. 10.3%) [5].

Ascites and paracentesis

Detection of ascites by ultrasound is useful in the patient presenting with abdominal distension. Many patients without a known history of ascites present with abnormal transaminase levels and distension, and the presence of ascites is often incorrectly assumed. Beyond the diagnostic utility in confirming the diagnosis, ultrasound is helpful in choosing the optimal site for paracentesis.

Focused questions

1. Is there free fluid (ascites) in the abdomen?
2. Where is the optimal location for paracentesis?

Anatomy

Ascites accumulates in a gravity-dependent fashion within the peritoneum, similar to blood in trauma, as discussed in Chapter 2. Unless prior surgery, infections, or scarring alter the anatomy, the fluid tends to be free flowing. If loculations are present, the location of fluid pockets will be highly variable, and bowel may not "float" in the ascites as it normally would.

Technique

Probe selection

Ultrasound of the abdomen may be performed with a 2.5–5.0 MHz transducer.

Special equipment

A marking pen may be used.

Setup

Place the patient in the normal preferred position for paracentesis. Some authors prefer a decubitus position, while others have the patient sitting upright. The ultrasound technique employed is similar to that used in the FAST examination. In addition to the left and right upper quadrant exam, check the lower quadrants for fluid collections, and note the position of bowel, mesentery, and bladder. Note the echogenicity of any detected intraperitoneal fluid. On ultrasound, ascitic fluid appears anechoic with occasional echogenic strands (Figures 16.5 and 16.6).

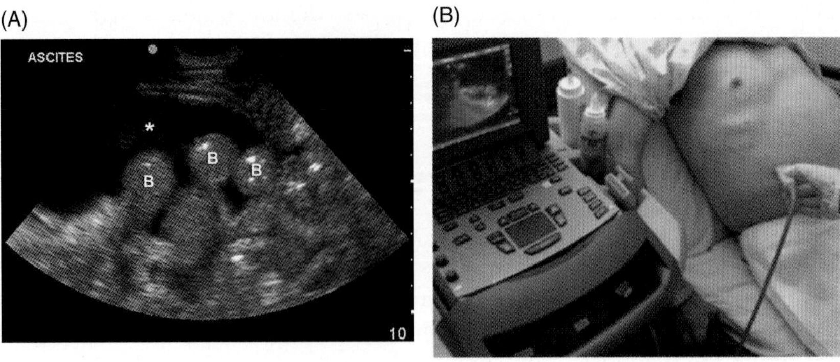

Figure 16.5
(*A*) Right lower quadrant view showing ascites (*) and bowel loops (B). (*B*) Patient positioning for ultrasound assessment of ascites.

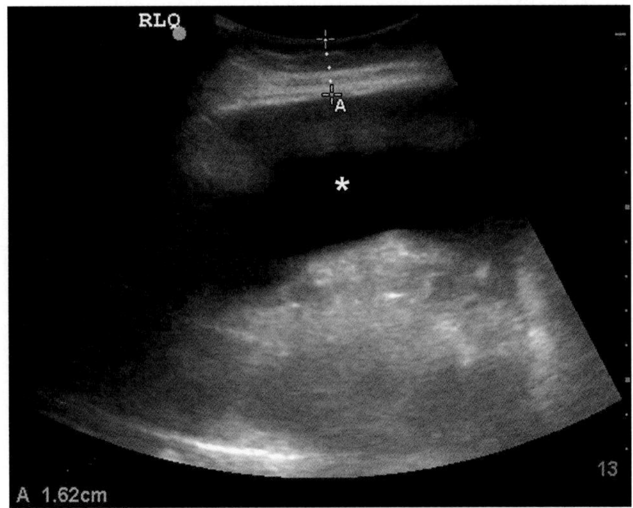

Figure 16.6
Left lower quadrant showing ascites (*) and bowel loops. The distance from skin to peritoneum is measured with calipers.

Recall that this fluid may be transudate, exudate, malignant, or blood. The depth from the surface of the skin to the ascites should be measured using the caliper function on the ultrasound machine or the depth gauge on the side of the screen. The inferior epigastric vessels may be visualized in the anterior lateral abdomen (Figure 16.7) and should be avoided.

Procedure

After a puncture site is identified and marked, the patient should remain in the same position for the paracentesis. Alternatively, real-time scanning can be used to guide the trajectory of the needle, similar to the dynamic approach in central venous cannulation. Ultrasound can also be used after a large-volume paracentesis to assess the adequacy of drainage.

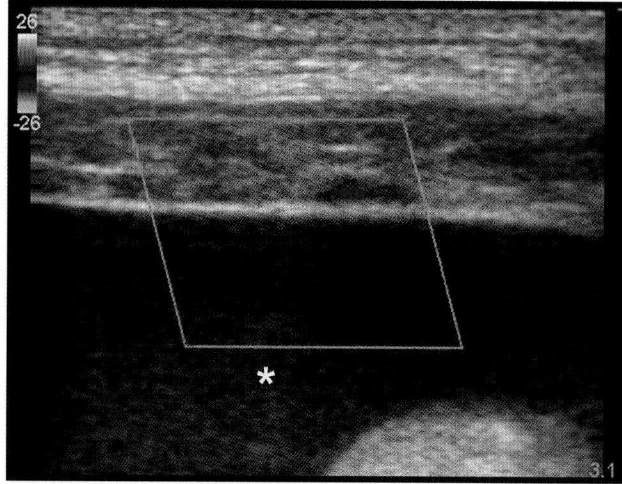

Figure 16.7
The inferior epigastric vessels are visualized using color Doppler, superficial to the peritoneum.

Tips

Although the left lower quadrant approach is most commonly cited as best when using a landmark-guided technique, ultrasound allows for more latitude in site selection. Any site where ascites is present without nearby bowel, bladder, or vascular structures would be appropriate, including a midline approach. This approach, through the linea alba, would be inappropriate if the exact location of the bladder or potential adhesions were not known.

Pitfalls

Be sure that the patient's position does not change from the time of scanning to the time of the procedure.

Bowel can sometimes move quite dynamically. Be sure the site of proposed paracentesis remains free of bowel for a minute or so before attempting needle puncture.

Literature review

When performed in a conventional blind manner, paracentesis is safe [6]. In a prospective study of 229 paracenteses performed on 125 patients, only two major complications (transfusion-requiring abdominal wall hematomas) and two minor complications (non-transfusion-requiring hematomas) occurred, yielding complication rates of 0.9% each. None of the procedures resulted in spontaneous bacterial peritonitis or death.

Some studies, however, suggest that the safety and efficacy of paracentesis may be improved through the use of ultrasound guidance. Bard *et al.* studied 27 consecutive patients with ascites detected by ultrasound [7]. In six of the eight patients with fluid in the flank region, air-filled loops of bowel were interposed between the abdominal wall and the fluid collection. It was suggested that a blind approach could have injured the bowel. Overall, the investigators concluded that ultrasound is helpful for selecting the puncture site so as to avoid intraperitoneal structures during the paracentesis.

A more recent study randomized patients to ultrasound-guided versus standard paracentesis. In patients where fluid was visualized, there was a 95% success rate in paracentesis, compared to 65% success without the use of ultrasound. Of the failed paracenteses in the landmark-based group, ultrasound guidance found no fluid in two cases and was able to guide successful aspiration in all others [8].

Joint effusions and arthrocentesis

Ultrasound is more accurate and reproducible than clinical evaluation for effusions [9,10]. There are multiple clinical situations where it is not obvious that there is an effusion. Ultrasound can not only assist in making this diagnosis but can also guide aspiration to ensure success.

Focused questions

1. Is there a joint effusion?
2. Where is the optimal location for arthrocentesis?

Anatomy

In visualizing joints on ultrasound, recall that fluid appears anechoic, and bone will be a bright reflector with distal shadowing. Thus, in normal joint sonography, the intersection of two bones will appear as a V-shaped gap, sometimes referred to as the "seagull sign" (Figure 16.8).

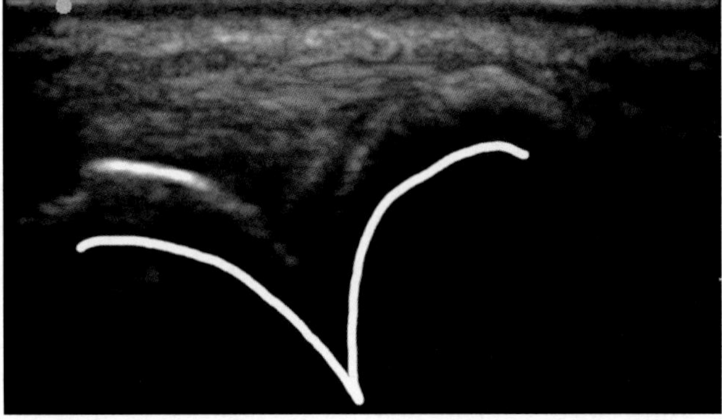

Figure 16.8
Joint anatomy. Note the bright, crisp white lines delineating bone, and the V-shaped space (superimposed white lines) between adjacent bones creating the joint space.

Technique

Probe selection

Ultrasound of the joints should be performed with a high-frequency (5–10 MHz) linear probe.

Special equipment

A marking pen may be used.

Setup

Place the patient in a comfortable position (based on which joint is involved) for the procedure. Scan over the area in question to search for signs of effusion in the joint space. Using the bony landmarks discussed previously (the "seagull sign") can be helpful if the superficial anatomy is obscured by edema or effusion. When an area demonstrating adequate fluid is located, mark the spot with a pen, and prep and drape the area in the usual sterile fashion.

Procedure

The rest of the procedure should be carried out using standard technique, being careful to maintain the same position used when mapping the fluid collection. In some cases it is useful to directly visualize the path of the needle from skin to joint. This is performed using an in-plane (long-axis) dynamic guidance approach as detailed in Chapter 15.

Hip

Visualization of the hip is useful in suspected sepsis of the joint, as well as in the evaluation of synovitis. Figures 16.9 and 16.10 demonstrate normal hip

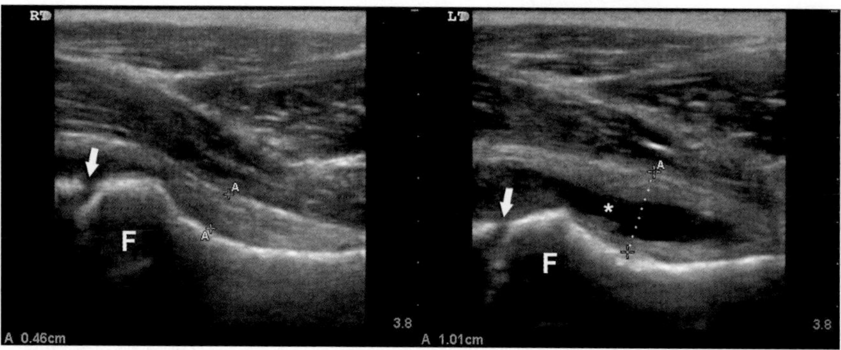

Figure 16.9

Normal hip (*left*) and synovitis (*right*). Note the anechoic fluid (*) within synovium lateral to the femur (F). The growth plate (arrow) is visible as well in this pediatric case.

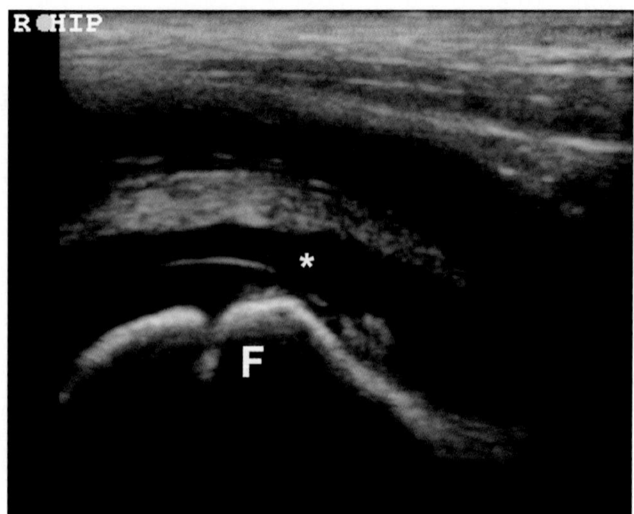

Figure 16.10
Hip effusion (*) is demonstrated lateral to femur (F) in another pediatric patient with hip pain and limp.

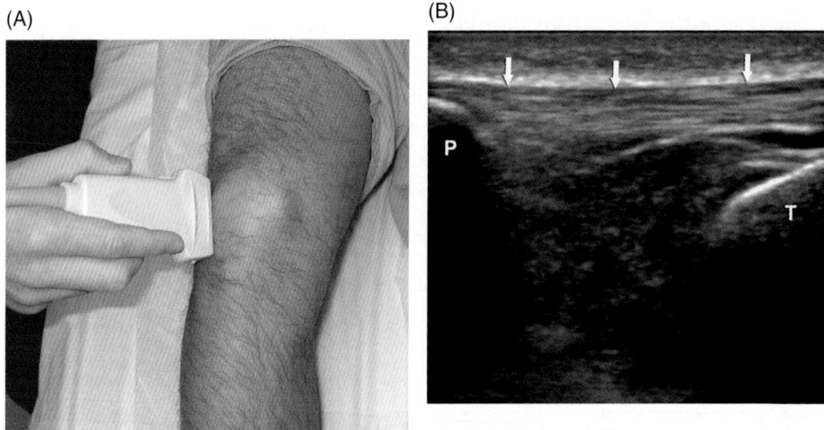

Figure 16.11
(*A*) Lateral placement of probe for knee arthrocentesis. (*B*) Image seen on screen, demonstrating patella (P), tibia (T), and patellar tendon (arrows).

anatomy as well as effusions. The diagnosis of hip effusions is discussed in more detail in Chapter 13.

Knee

The knee joint may be well visualized from a medial or lateral approach. In Figure 16.11, a standard probe position and normal joint appearance is demonstrated. In Figure 16.12, abnormal fluid is visualized in the joint.

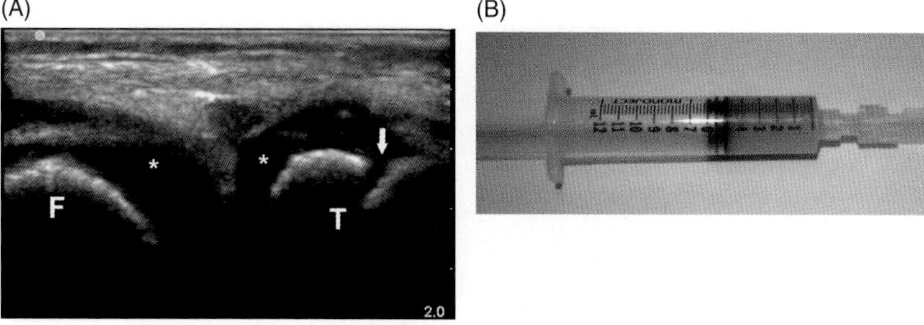

Figure 16.12
(*A*) Black fluid collection (*) within knee joint in child. Note the femur (F), tibia (T), and growth plate (arrow). (*B*) Pus aspirated from knee joint in the same patient.

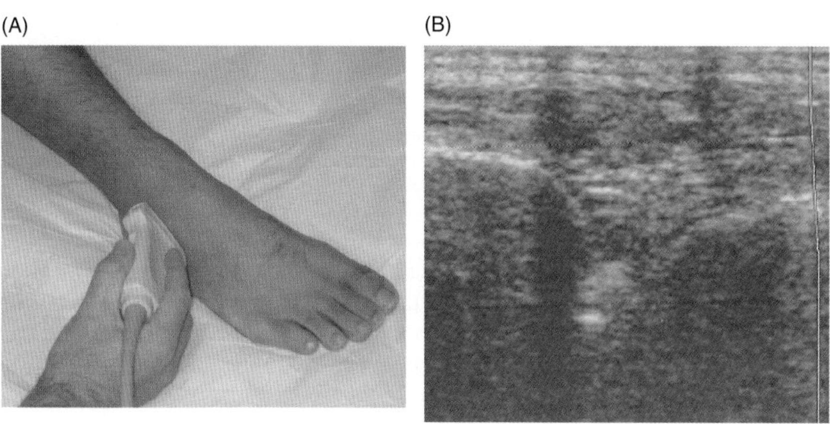

Figure 16.13
(*A*) Ankle probe position. (*B*) Ultrasound image obtained at this site.

Ankle

Figure 16.13 demonstrates placement of the probe longitudinally across the joint. Again, note the "seagull sign," which directs the search for black fluid in the "V." Fluid in this location, often accompanied by displacement of the bright echogenic joint capsule, represents an effusion.

Shoulder

Look for biceps tendon in bicipital groove (Figure 16.14). Here fluid is observed in the subdeltoid bursa. It is extra-articular, because it does not displace the biceps tendon.

Tips

When only a small amount of fluid is seen on ultrasound, it is sometimes useful to place some pressure on the joint at a different location to bring more

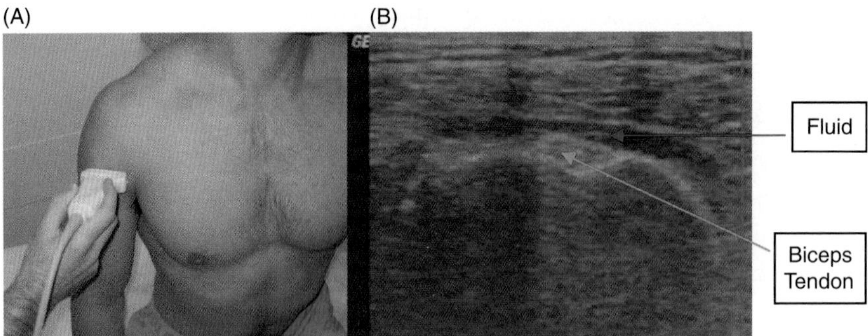

Figure 16.14
(*A*) Shoulder probe position. (*B*) Ultrasound image obtained at this site.

fluid to the puncture site. For example, suprapatellar pressure can increase the size of the synovial space inferior, medial, and lateral to the patella, and make aspiration of the joint at these sites simpler.

Pitfalls

Even slight movements of the joints will have a major impact on the location and depth of fluid collections. Be sure the patient is in his or her final position for the procedure when beginning ultrasound. Alternatively, ultrasound can be used to assess the optimal joint position in real time, and the patient can hold that position for the procedure.

Literature review

Although well described in the orthopedic and rheumatology literature, few studies describe ultrasound-guided arthrocentesis by emergency physicians. Some authors have reported success when using the modality in ankle arthrocentesis [9] and hip arthrocentesis [10]. Recently a randomized controlled trial of ultrasound versus landmark-guided knee arthocentesis in the emergency department found similar success rates with both techniques [11]. However, less pain and shorter procedure time was reported in the ultrasound group.

Foreign body identification/localization

Ultrasound can also be used to identify foreign bodies – either by direct visualization (metal) or by shadowing (wood, stones) or edema (inflammation and secondary tissue effects from wood or organic material). Physical exam can be extremely challenging in these situations, and a patient's own foreign-body sensation can often be misleading. Many common foreign bodies (e.g., wood) are not well visualized by x-ray, and triangulating the exact location of a small foreign body can be difficult and time-consuming using standard radiographic techniques.

Focused questions

1. Is there a foreign body?
2. Are there vascular structures near the foreign body?

Anatomy

The appearance of normal superficial tissues is shown in Figure 16.15. Note that the subcutaneous fat has a speckled appearance, which is slightly hypoechoic when compared to the appearance of organs such as the liver or spleen. Muscle appears "marbled" because hypoechoic muscle tissue is divided by hyperechoic fascial planes. Vascular structures will appear anechoic and will be compressible. Bone will act as a strong reflector, creating a bright boundary beyond which only shadowing will be visible.

Technique

Probe selection

Ultrasound of the superficial soft tissue should be performed with a high-frequency (5–10 MHz) linear probe.

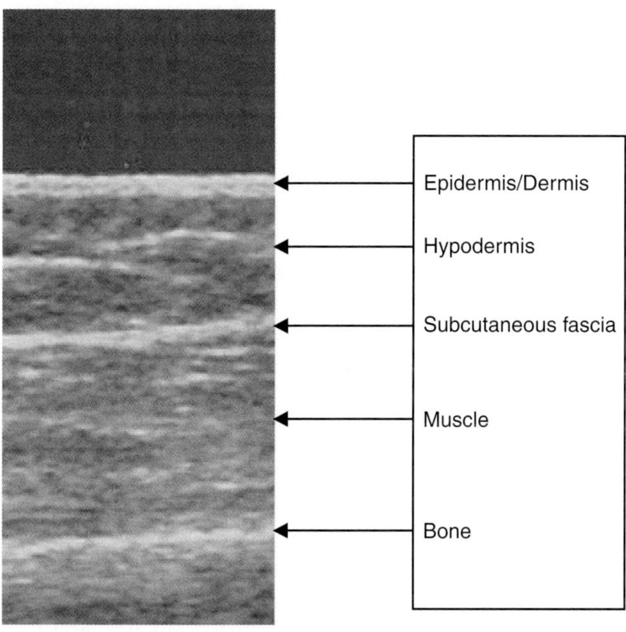

Figure 16.15 Normal dermal tissue, with component layers.

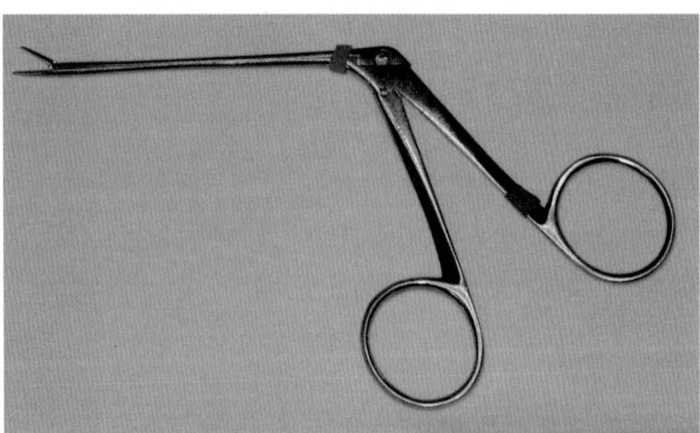

Figure 16.16
Alligator forceps.

Special equipment

The following special equipment is required:

- Lidocaine or other local anesthetic
- Water bath or standoff pad for superficial structures

Note: Be sure to check the manufacturer's instructions regarding the safety of water-bath use with your particular transducer. Any transducer with a cracked housing should *not* be used, because the gel may conduct electrical signals to the operator or the patient. Thus, a cracked housing would be *extremely dangerous* when used with a water bath.

- Alligator forceps (Figure 16.16) or other small grasping implement
- Sterile wire (e.g., Kopans wire) or needle if this will be used to guide a dissection

Setup

The patient should be placed in a comfortable position. As with other ultrasound-guided procedures, the ultrasound will be performed in the same position as the procedure itself.

Scan over the area of suspected foreign body and note the appearance of bright reflectors and/or shadowing in the area. Familiarize yourself with the appearance of normal bony anatomy (bright reflector with shadowing, described previously) as well as soft tissue, tendons, and vascular structures. Common foreign bodies such as wood or metal have a characteristic appearance on ultrasound (Figures 16.17–16.19). Glass is sometimes visualized on ultrasound, but small pieces may frequently be missed using this technique.

Procedure

Once the foreign body is localized, several techniques can be employed to remove it. One simple method is to guide a needle or wire to the foreign body

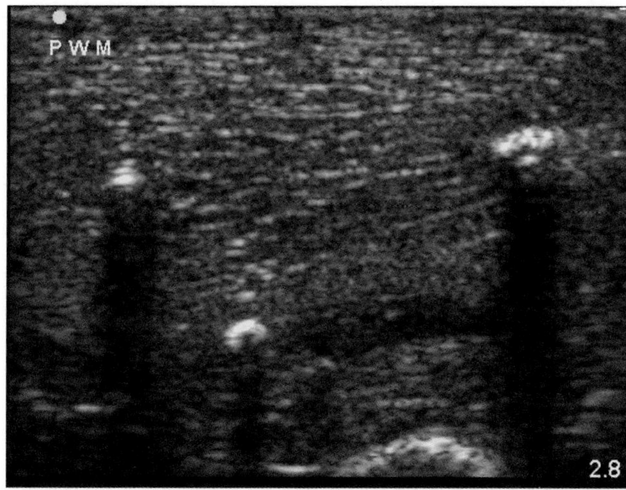

Figure 16.17
Transverse images of plastic, wood, and metal foreign bodies (left to right) are demonstrated. Note the shadows deep to each structure.

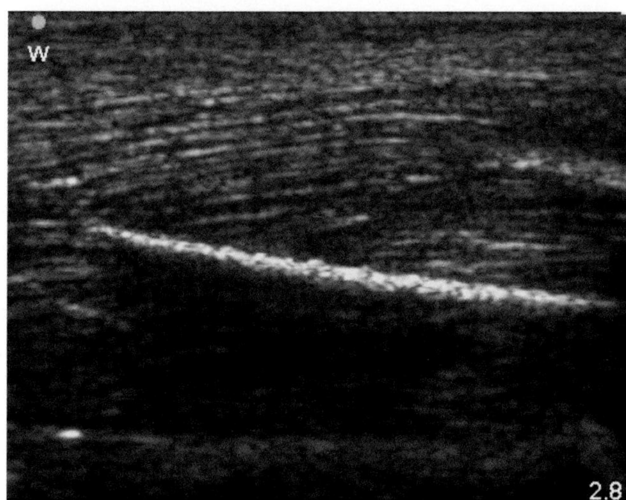

Figure 16.18
A wooden foreign body is demonstrated in the long axis.

using ultrasound, and then dissect to the foreign body using the metal guide. Kopans wires, often used for radiographic localization of breast masses prior to dissection, have been used by some operators. This technique can be useful when guiding the dissection for a consultant who will then use standard techniques.

Alternatively, many foreign bodies can be directly removed using ultrasound to guide the entire procedure. First, localize the long axis of the foreign body (splinters, toothpicks, and many metal foreign bodies are quite linear). Keeping the long axis of the foreign body centered on the screen, guide a needle with anesthetic solution to the foreign body using the same long-axis

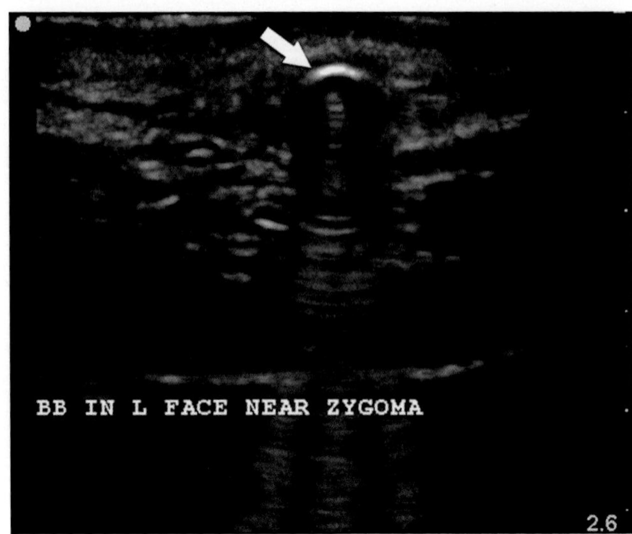

Figure 16.19
Metal foreign body (arrow) in soft tissue over zygoma.

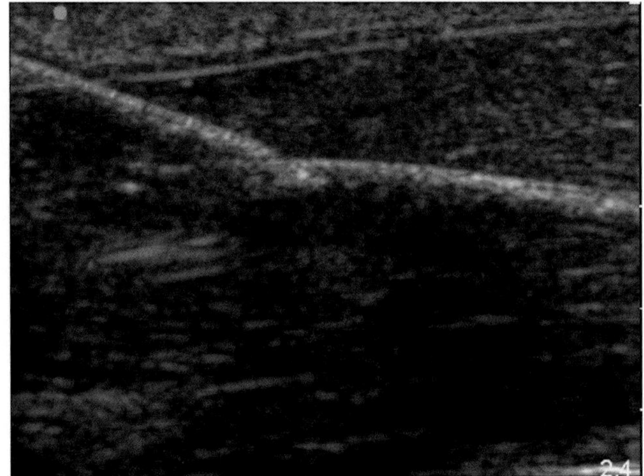

Figure 16.20
The needle (left side of screen) approaches the wooden foreign body.

approach described in Chapter 15. It is often easiest to enter the needle into the skin at the puncture point for the foreign body. Once contact with the foreign body is felt at the end of the needle (sometimes a tap can be heard as well), inject a generous amount of anesthetic at the site of contact (Figure 16.20).

In most cases, the solution will track around the entire foreign body, with three consequences. First, the foreign body will be better visualized as it is now surrounded by a rim of anechoic fluid. Second, the area will be well

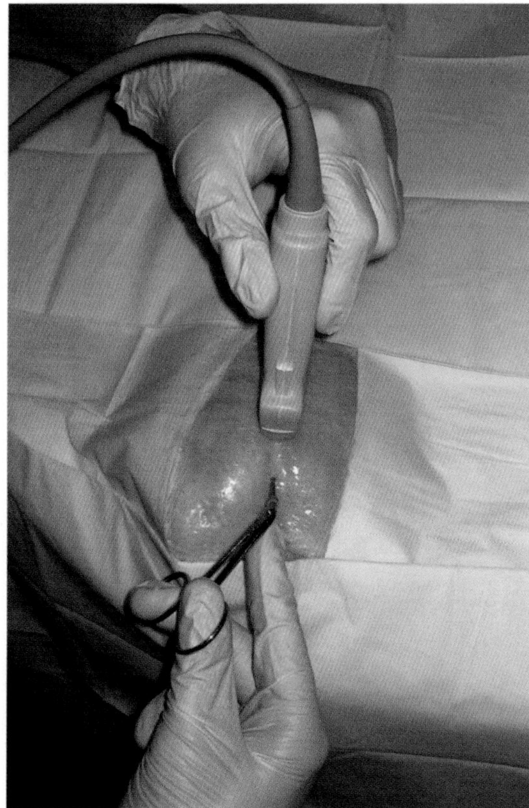

Figure 16.21
Probe positioning during procedure.

anesthetized without the need for multiple injections. Third, the foreign body will often be "loosened" a bit by the extra fluid.

Now that a track of anesthetic has been deployed from the surface of the skin down to the foreign body, the object can be removed under direct visualization. Make a small nick in the skin (or use the entry point for the foreign body) at the site of desired entry. Using the same long-axis technique, use an alligator forceps to follow the same path the anesthetic needle just took. Be sure to keep the forceps in the plane of the ultrasound beam. If the forceps veers off course, then back up toward the skin surface and redirect into the plane. Once contact with the foreign body is felt at the end of the forceps (sometimes a tap can be heard as well), open the jaws slightly to grasp the end of the object. The object can then be withdrawn along the previously anesthetized track.

Proper hand positioning is demonstrated in Figure 16.21. The non-dominant hand holds the probe along the long axis of the foreign body. The dominant hand then guides the forceps in the same plane.

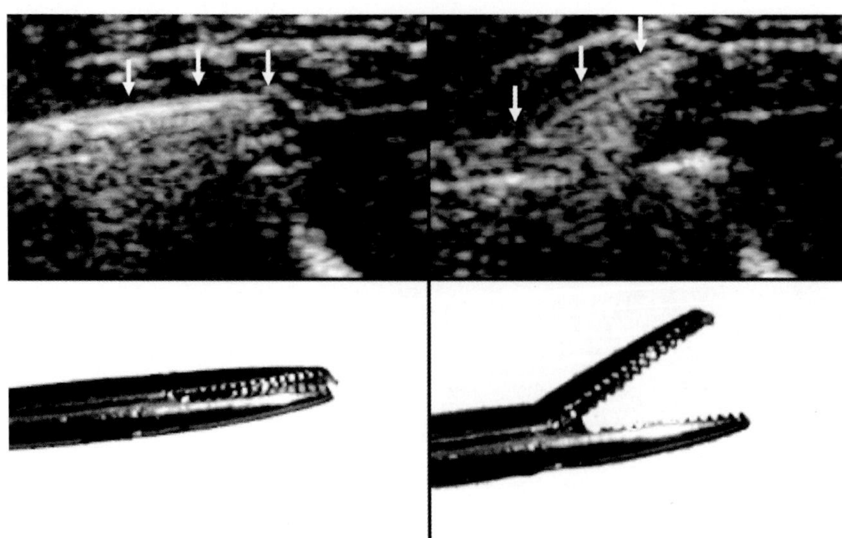

Figure 16.22
Sonographic appearance of the forceps while closed (*left*) and open (*right*).

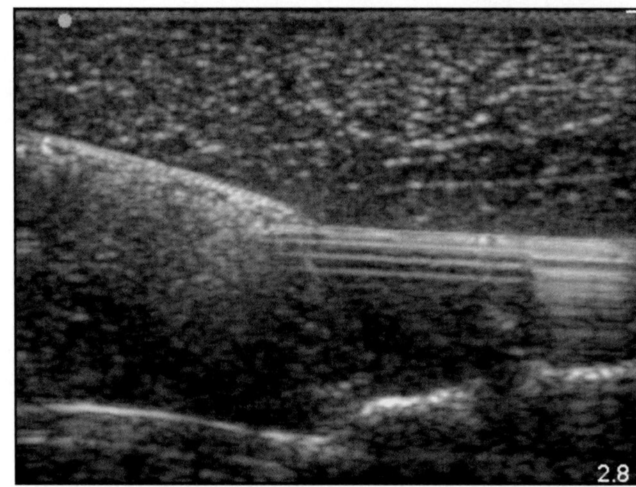

Figure 16.23
Grasping a foreign body. The forceps is visualized coming in from the left of the screen, and a metallic foreign body (with reverberation artifact) is seen on the right.

Figure 16.22 depicts the closed and open positions of the forceps and their appearance on ultrasound. The superficial aspect of the forceps will be visualized, but beam scatter will obscure the deeper portion.

Figure 16.23 shows the forceps approaching from the left, nearing a metallic foreign body. Note the reverberation artifact commonly seen with metallic objects on ultrasound.

Tips

The long-axis approach is better than a short-axis method for this technique due to the small size of most foreign bodies, and it is the method preferred by most interventional radiologists.

Generous use of local anesthetic increases patient comfort and also mechanically facilitates the procedure.

Pitfalls

The long-axis approach is technically more challenging and requires more practice. Familiarize yourself with the mechanics of the procedure using a model such as a chicken breast with embedded toothpicks.

Be sure to pull out long foreign bodies in line with their long axis. When grasped from an oblique or perpendicular angle, the object will act as a barb and remain fixed.

Literature review

Many studies of ultrasound detection of foreign bodies have determined the accuracy of the technique in cadaveric or simulated models. One study demonstrated a sensitivity of 93% for detection of wooden objects and 73% for plastic in human cadaver legs [12]. Another study demonstrated similar accuracy in the detection of wooden foreign bodies by a radiologist (83%), ultrasound technicians (85%), and emergency physicians (80%) in a chicken thigh model [13]. A study of foreign-body detection in a porcine model showed sensitivities of 97% by emergency physicians and 86% by trainees [14]. Other authors have described the use of ultrasound in localizing radiolucent foreign bodies in live human subjects, especially in the extremities [15].

Abscess drainage

Differentiation of cellulitis and abscess is discussed in Chapter 11. Once an abscess is confirmed, ultrasound can help identify any nearby neurovascular structures, assess the size and depth, and can be used to guide a needle for drainage. Of course, an open incision and drainage may be performed after the abscess is confirmed and characterized as well.

Focused questions

1. Is there an abscess?
2. Are there vascular structures near the abscess?

Anatomy

Abscesses will appear hypoechoic or dark (Figure 16.24), often with gray heterogeneous swirling material inside. They often demonstrate posterior enhancement, because they do not attenuate sound waves as much as the surrounding tissue (as described in Chapter 1). Assessment of nearby vascular structures should be undertaken once abscess is confirmed (Figures 16.25 and 16.26).

Technique

Probe selection

Ultrasound of the superficial soft tissues should be performed with a high-frequency (5–10 MHz) linear probe.

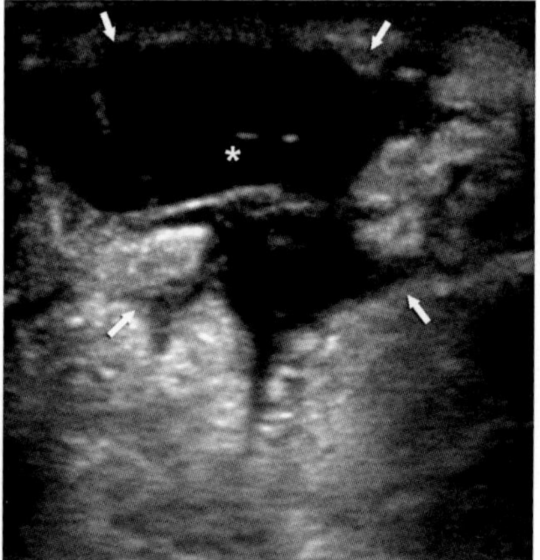

Figure 16.24

Ultrasound-visualized soft-tissue abscess (arrows) and heterogeneous material (*).

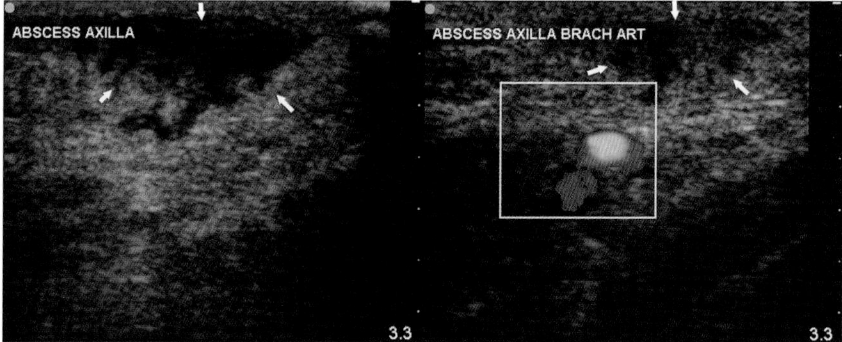

Figure 16.25

Axilla abscess (arrows) with axillary vessels seen in far field (*right*).

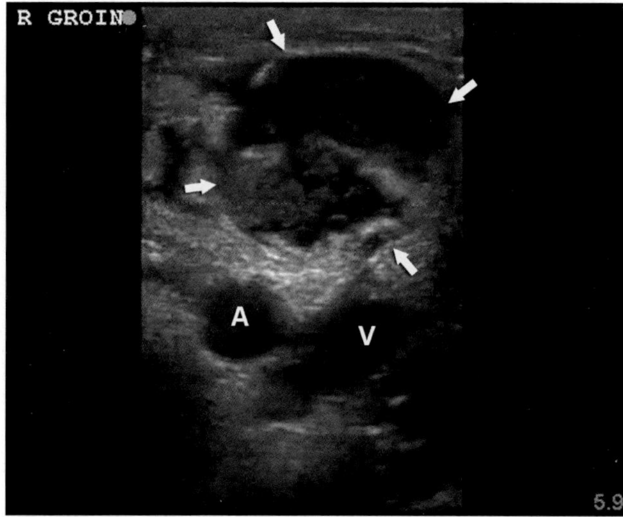

Figure 16.26
Groin abscess (arrows) with femoral artery (A) and vein (V) deep to this.

Special equipment

A marking pen may be used.

Setup

Position the patient as you normally would for the procedure. Scan over the area of greatest fluctuance or over any suspicious area. Note the presence or absence of any abscess cavity, as well as any nearby vascular structures that would preclude safe incision and drainage. Also note any deeper or lateral extension of the fluid collection. Ultrasound can sometimes highlight that the superficial inflammation was only the "tip of the iceberg" and drive the operator to obtain further imaging or consultation before embarking on a deep dissection. Using the caliper function, measure the depth from the surface of the skin to the cavity. A marking pen may be used to note the location of the cavity.

Procedure

The remainder of the procedure can commence without further use of ultrasound. Alternatively, ultrasound can be used to guide needle placement for aspiration in real time using the same long-axis technique described in Chapter 15.

Peritonsillar abscesses

The technique for peritonsillar abscess is the same as for other abscess ultrasounds. The only difference is that the high-frequency intracavitary probe is the most conducive to identifying these abscesses because its shape allows

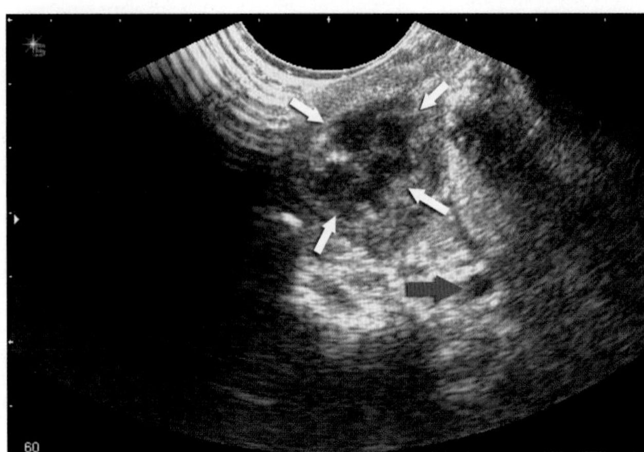

Figure 16.27
A peritonsillar abscess is seen in the near field (small white arrows), and the carotid artery is visualized in the far field (large red arrow).

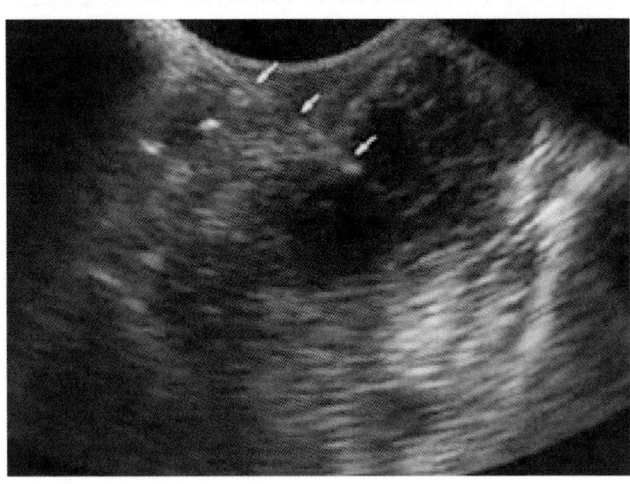

Figure 16.28
Peritonsillar abscess drainage via needle aspiration (arrows). Image courtesy of Dr. Michael Blaivas, Professor of Emergency Medicine, Northside Hospital Forsyth, Atlanta, GA.

placement in the posterior pharyngeal space, and its high frequency makes the image generated easy to interpret. Gel is applied to the end of the probe, and a sterile cover shields the patient from the probe. Again, an abscess is identified as a hypoechoic space over the area of maximal swelling. The use of ultrasound in this setting has several potential benefits. First, it may be possible to avoid the discomfort of a "dry tap" where there is induration but no abscess. Second, color Doppler may be used to identify the depth and location of the carotid artery so it can be avoided during the incision and drainage procedure (Figure 16.27).

In Figure 16.28, the needle is visualized as the abscess cavity is drained. As with vessel cannulation, static localization or dynamic cavity aspiration is possible and may depend on the patient's ability to tolerate continuous ultrasound imaging.

Literature review

Ultrasound is more accurate than physical exam alone in detecting abscess (positive predictive value 93% vs. 81%; negative predictive value 97% vs. 77%) [16]. Thus, the number of non-therapeutic incision and drainage procedures could be reduced using ultrasound guidance. Another study of soft-tissue infections in the emergency department demonstrated that ultrasound changed the management of nearly 50% of patients. Management changes included recognition of occult abscess where only cellulitis was expected, deferring incision and drainage where no abscess was found, and obtaining further diagnostic studies or consultation [17].

In the setting of possible peritonsillar abscess, ultrasound has demonstrated promise in preliminary studies. One study demonstrated negative aspirates in three patients without abscess identified on ultrasound, and positive aspirates in three patients with sonographic findings of abscess [18].

Lumbar puncture

One of the classic landmark-guided procedures, lumbar puncture, can be quite challenging in patients without classic landmarks. In many emergency department patients, spinous processes are not readily palpable, and it is not uncommon for the iliac crests to be obscured by certain body proportions as well. Ultrasound can be used to locate the orientation and depth of the spinous processes, which can be a huge advantage for a critical diagnostic procedure.

Focused questions

1. Where is the interspinous space?
2. How deep is the interspinous ligament?

Anatomy

The goal of lumbar puncture (using a midline approach) is to place the needle through the skin and subcutaneous tissues, into the interspinous ligament, through the ligamentum flavum, and into the subarachnoid space. Ultrasound can demonstrate much of the target anatomy. In some patients, the ligamentum flavum can be visualized, but more commonly, at least the spinous processes are well visualized on ultrasound.

Technique

Probe selection

Ultrasound can be performed with a high-frequency (5–10 MHz) linear probe or a lower-frequency (2–5 MHz) curvilinear probe.

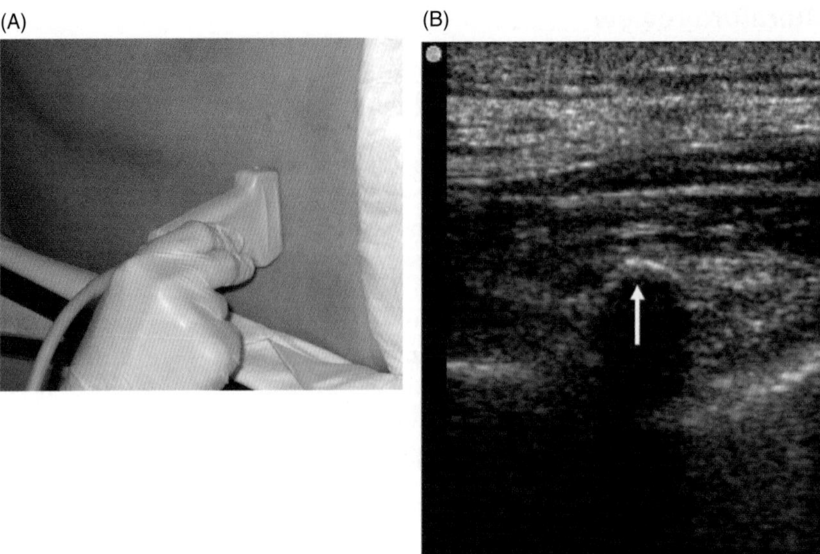

Figure 16.29

(*A*) Transverse probe positioning and (*B*) the image obtained at this level. Note the crisp white line and posterior shadowing which delineates the spinous process.

Special equipment

A marking pen is used.

Setup

Place the patient in the desired position for lumbar puncture (lateral decubitus or sitting upright). Using the linear transducer, locate the midline at the desired lumbar spine level in a transverse and longitudinal orientation. Note the appearance of the spinous processes on ultrasound. They will appear as bright echogenic crescents with shadowing posteriorly. When using a transverse approach, note the location of the spinous processes above and below the desired puncture site (Figure 16.29). Using a curvilinear probe is advocated by some authors in the setting of larger patient body habitus, or to visualize more lateral and deep anatomy (Figure 16.30).

It is often easier to use a longitudinal approach, where two spinous processes are visualized simultaneously (Figure 16.31). When the ultrasound image is obtained, the probe is oriented in the midline of the spinous processes (sagittal hash marks on the patient in Figure 16.32), and the interspinous space is centered in the middle of the probe (transverse hash marks on the patient). The initial needle puncture can then be made at the center of the "cross-hairs," which should line up with the interspinous space.

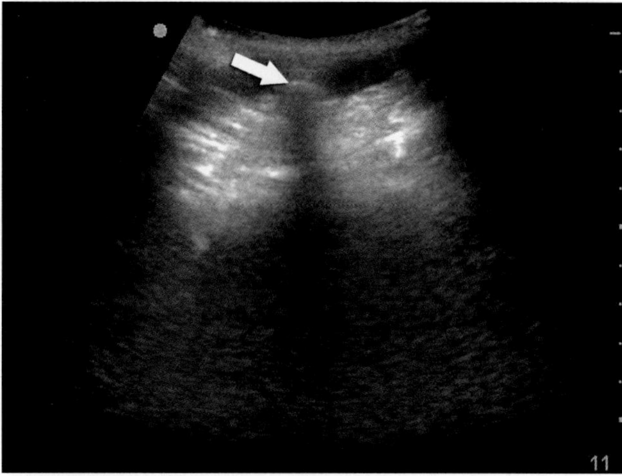

Figure 16.30

Transverse image of lumbar spine obtained using curvilinear probe. Spinous process (arrow) visible with distal shadowing.

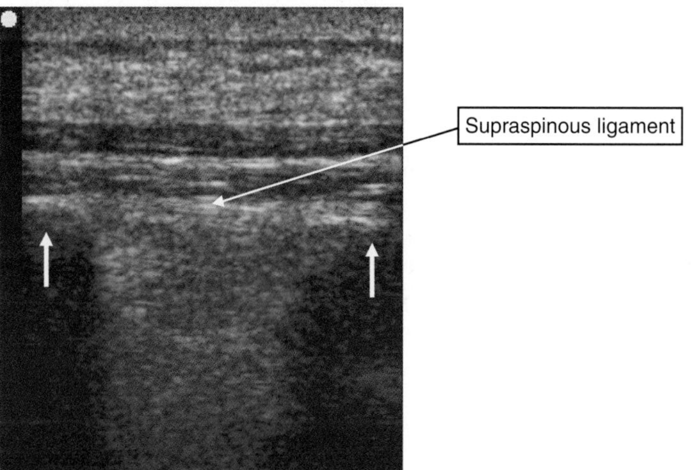

Figure 16.31

Ultrasound image of interspinous space. Bold arrows mark vertebral shadows.

Procedure

Once the optimal entry point is found and the distance from the skin to the interspinous space is measured, the patient can be prepped and draped in the standard fashion for the procedure. No real-time guidance is used for this technique.

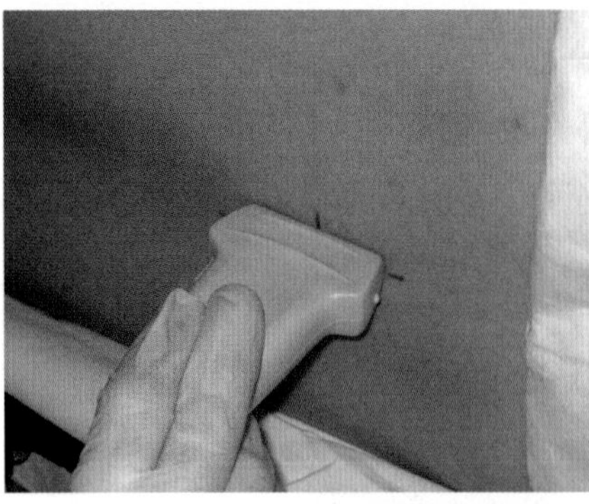

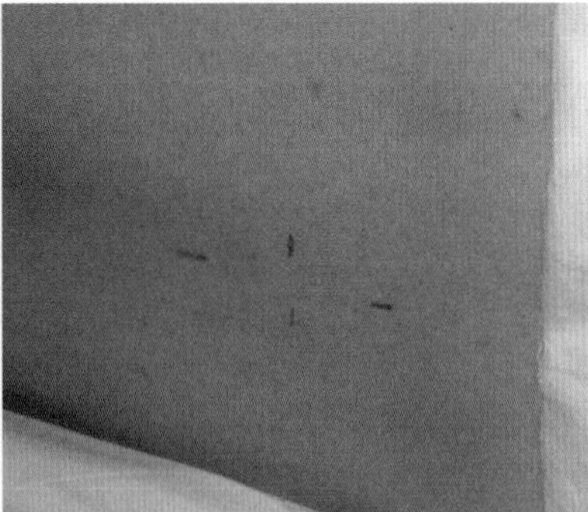

Figure 16.32
Marking interspinous space.

Tips

Take the time to note the optimal location for needle entry. The remainder of the procedure is not guided by ultrasound, so thorough setup is key.

Measuring the depth to the interspinous space is crucial. In larger patients, longer needles must often be used, and it is better to know this in advance.

Pitfalls

Be sure to direct the needle along the same trajectory as the ultrasound beam. Knowing the right vertical and horizontal coordinates for puncture is not useful if an incorrect trajectory is taken from the skin to the deeper tissues.

As with other procedures, the patient should not be moved after ultrasound localization. The relationship between the skin surface and deeper landmarks can change considerably with motion, and this is more pronounced in larger patients.

Literature review

Ultrasound has been used to guide the placement of epidural catheters in laboring women without palpable landmarks [19]. Although there was no difference in success rates (100%) using ultrasound or standard techniques, pain scales and number of attempts were reduced in the group where ultrasound guidance was used. A case series of successful use of ultrasound in challenging cases has been described in the emergency medicine literature as well [20]. Ultrasound was used to demonstrate optimal positioning for lumbar puncture in pediatric [21] and adult [22] populations, though these two studies did not assess success rates or randomize patients to landmark- versus ultrasound-guided techniques.

Pericardiocentesis

Pericardiocentesis is the aspiration of fluid from the pericardial sac. Typically, it is performed in a blind fashion by directing the needle from the subxiphoid region toward the left nipple until blood is aspirated. This method necessitates needle placement through the liver. Cardiac ultrasound has been shown to help guide pericardiocentesis in a subxiphoid, parasternal, or apical approach [23–25]. When ultrasound is used to guide the procedure, a parasternal approach may be used, which involves a more direct anatomic approach to the heart than the subxiphoid approach. Note that some operators prefer the parasternal approach for its shorter course, and others avoid this approach due to concern over the risk of coronary artery laceration. Thus, the optimal approach may depend on operator preference and patient factors.

Visualization of the needle entering the pericardial space or visualization of agitated sterile saline injections in the pericardial space helps confirm correct placement of the cardiac needle. Also, the depth markers on the ultrasound display screen can aid in determining how deep the cardiac needle must be advanced to be in the pericardial space. Use of cardiac ultrasound in this manner may help prevent cardiac lacerations, pneumothorax, pneumopericardium, and liver laceration [23–25].

Detection of pacing capture

In transcutaneous and transvenous pacing, visualization of ventricular contraction by cardiac ultrasound subsequent to the pacing spikes indicates that capture has been obtained. In addition, proper placement of transvenous pacing wires can be confirmed using bedside cardiac ultrasound. Transvenous wires will appear bright or hyperechoic and can be seen within the right ventricle (Figure 16.33). Ultrasound can ensure that the wire is against the right ventricular wall and in good position (and also that perforation and hemopericardium have not occurred!). [26,27].

Bladder aspiration

Ultrasound can be used to ensure adequate volume exists within the bladder prior to catheterization. This has been shown to reduce the rates of "dry tap," which can save time and reduce frustration and unneccesary discomfort. In cases where catheterization is unsuccessful, infeasible, or contraindicated and a suprapubic aspiration is indicated, ultrasound can be used to guide needle placement.

Focused question

1. What is the volume of the bladder?

(A)

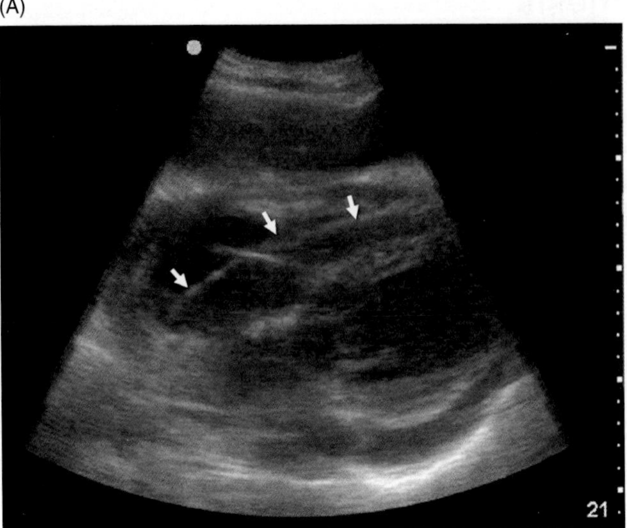

(B)

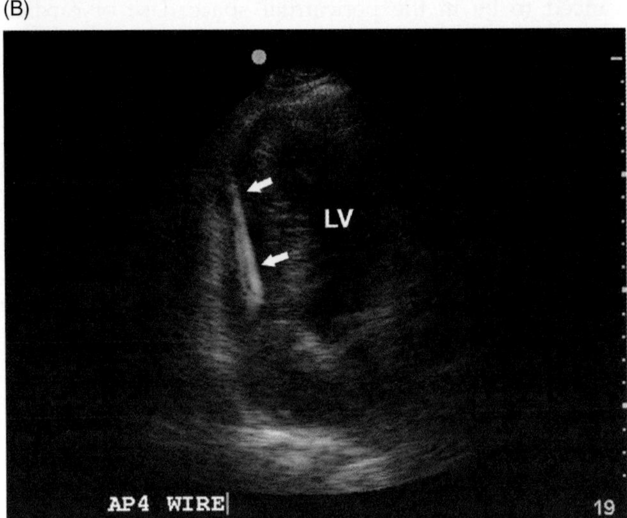

Figure 16.33

Ultrasound appearance of pacing wire in the right ventricle in (*A*) a subxiphoid view and (*B*) an apical view. Note the linear, bright echogenic appearance of the wire, in contrast to the anechoic black of the ventricle. LV, left ventricle.

Anatomy

Pelvic anatomy including the bladder has been described in Chapters 2 and 6. The bladder lies inferior and deep to the pubic symphisis, and expands cephalad into the abdomen as it distends with urine.

Technique

Probe selection

As described in Chapters 2 and 6, bladder ultrasound should be performed with a curvilinear or phased-array probe.

Special equipment

A sterile probe cover should be used if real-time needle guidance is to be attempted. Otherwise no special equipment is necessary.

Setup

Position the patient as you normally would for suprapubic bladder aspiration or transurethral bladder catheterization. If you are assessing bladder volume prior to catheterization of an infant, it is important to have the catheterization setup ready, as occasionally the suprapubic pressure of sonography (or even just the genital exposure to cool air!) will elicit spontaneous urination.

Procedure

The rest of the procedure should be carried out using standard technique, being careful to maintain the same position used when mapping the fluid collection. In some cases it is useful to directly visualize the path of the needle from skin to bladder. This is performed using an in-plane (long-axis) dynamic guidance approach as detailed in Chapter 15.

Suprapubic bladder aspiration

Locate the bladder in transverse and longitudinal planes with the probe placed just above the pubic symphysis, as described in Chapter 6. Calipers or depth markers on the side of the screen can be used to determine depth from skin to bladder (as was done with other aspiration procedures). Ensure that the bladder is large enough to allow for successful aspiration; a very empty bladder deep behind the pubic symphysis may not yield success. Note the location and angle of the ultrasound probe when placed directly over the bladder. Remove the ultrasound probe, sterilize the skin, and continue the procedure as usual, guiding the needle at the same angle and location as the probe was held. Alternatively, the entire procedure can be performed under sterile conditions, using a sterile sheath over the ultrasound probe. With this technique the needle can be observed from skin to bladder.

Urethral bladder catheterization

Prepare the patient (and any assistants to stabilize the patient) as well as any catheterization equipment and urine collection containers. Prep the patient's

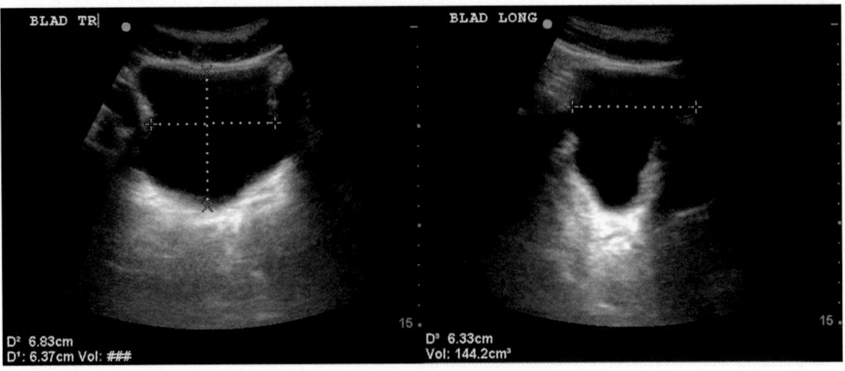

Figure 16.34

Calculation of bladder volume can be performed by measuring the diameter of the bladder in three planes: sagittal, transverse, and coronal.

urethra for the catheterization as usual. Once you are in position where you could catheterize as the next step, use the ultrasound probe to ensure adequate volume exists in the bladder. Bladder volume can be calculated using the equation [0.75 × length × width × height] or presets on your ultrasound machine (Figure 16.34). However, an easy rule of thumb is that a transverse diameter of 2 cm should yield sufficient urine (> 2.5 mL) for samples to be sent successfully [28]. If sufficient urine is present, put the probe away and perform sterile catheterization as usual. If the bladder is contracted, the procedure can be deferred.

Tips

As described with other procedures, ultrasound should be performed just prior to to the procedure. Urination in infants is unpredictable at best, and presence of urine in the bladder at time zero does not predict presence of urine in the bladder five minutes later. Providers should also be prepared for spontaneous urination.

If sufficient urine was noted within the bladder but suprabubic aspiration is unsuccessful, recheck the bladder volume (in case urination occurred unnoticed) and consider real-time (dynamic) guidance.

Pitfalls

For suprapubic bladder aspiration, be sure to use a needle long enough to reach the bladder.

It is also important to recreate the exact position and angle of the ultrasound probe with your needle. It is very common for providers to use a different angle and miss the target.

Literature review

Ultrasound guidance for evaluating placement of suprapubic cystostomy tubes has been described in the emergency department setting. Real-time sonographic guidance was used in a series of 17 patients with 100% success after ultrasound confirmation of urinary retention [29].

Pediatric emergency physicians used a portable ultrasound device to assess bladder volume and performed catheterizations only after confirmation of adequate urine volume. This process carried a 96% success rate, compared to 72% for patients where bladder volume was not assessed [30]. A randomized controlled trial of emergency department nurses trained in bladder volume assessment had higher catheterization success rates as well (92% with ultrasound vs. 67% without) though a longer mean time to catheterization was noted in the ultrasound group (28 versus 12 minutes) [28].

Regional nerve blocks

Nerve blocks can be incredibly useful in providing analgesia for procedures or for pain control. Sucessful nerve blocks can obviate the need for procedural sedation, decrease analgesia requirements, and reduce or eliminate the need for local anesthetic infiltration.

Focused questions

1. Where is the nerve?
2. Are there any vascular structures in the path of a potential nerve block?

Anatomy

Relevant anatomy specific to each nerve block is described below. In general, nerves appear hyperechoic on ultrasound. The fascicles are hypoechoic and are surrounded by hyperechoic perineural connective tissue (Figure 16.35). Often they are difficult to visualize because of anisotropy. Anisotropy refers to the difference in echogenicity seen in tendons and nerves based on the angle of the ultrasound beam (Figure 16.36). Thus, be sure to angle the probe back and forth if difficulty is encountered visualizing nerves in their expected locations.

Technique

Probe selection

Peripheral nerve blocks are generally performed with a high-frequency (5–10 MHz) linear probe.

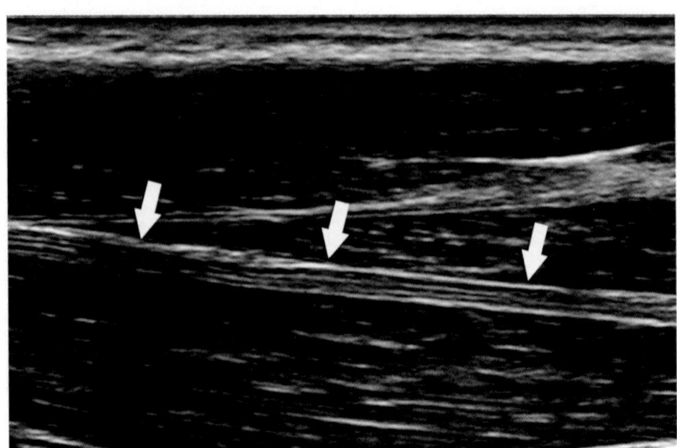

Figure 16.35
Longitudinal appearance of the ulnar nerve (arrows). Note the dark, continuous fascicles and bright perineurium.

(A)

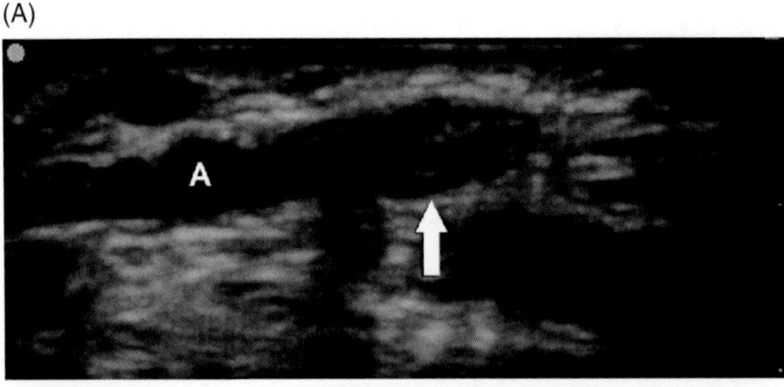

(B)

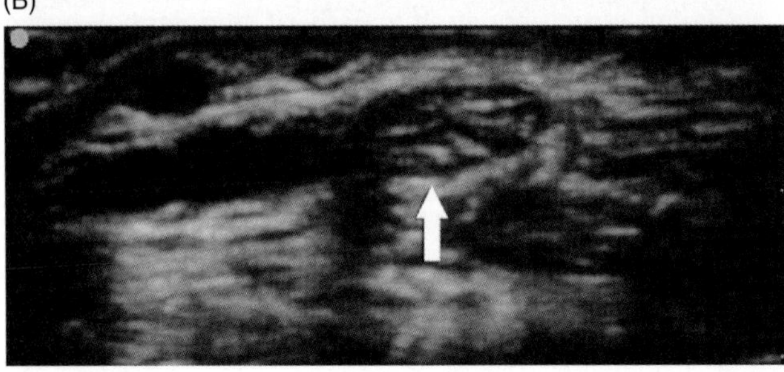

Figure 16.36
(*A*) The radial nerve (arrow) appears dark when the ultrasound beam is held at a shallow angle. The radial artery (A) is visible, with veins on either side. (*B*) When the probe is held at 90 degrees to the nerve, it appears much more echogenic and is more easily visualized.

Special equipment

A marking pen may be used to highlight surface anatomy. Often a stopcock and flexible tubing is attached from the needle to the anesthetic-filled syringe. This allows a second provider to administer anesthetic while the primary operator guides and stabilizes the needle in the optimal location. It is also less cumbersome when large volumes (> 10 mL) of anesthetic are to be infiltrated. Blunt (non-cutting) needles are generally recommended for nerve blocks, to minimize tissue injury, and some authors advocate the use of ultrasound-optimized needles. These needles appear more echogenic (and often more so at the tip) and are easier to visualize, but are also more expensive.

Setup

Position the patient as usual for any nerve block procedure. Ensure that you can visualize the ultrasound screen easily while you are in your typical position. As with vascular access, you should be able to see the patient's anatomy and the ultrasound image equally well and without putting yourself in an awkward position.

Procedure

Nerve blocks are performed using real-time dynamic guidance, typically in the long-axis (in-plane) view.

Femoral nerve block

The femoral nerve lies lateral to the femoral artery, superficial to the iliopsoas muscle. With the affected leg in neutral position, identify the inguinal crease. Scan the groin to reveal the femoral nerve, artery, and vein. The nerve is generally visible as an echogenic, roughly triangular structure in the short axis (Figure 16.37). Occasionally the nerve itself is not well visualized, and the needle will instead be directed lateral to the artery toward the nerve's

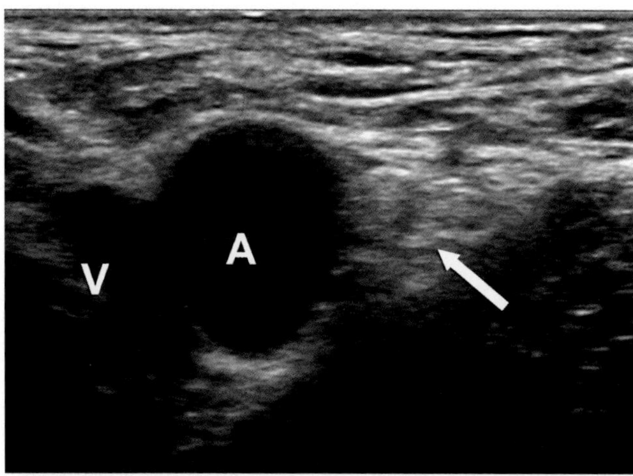

Figure 16.37
Femoral vein (V), artery (A), and nerve (arrow) from medial to lateral in the left inguinal crease.

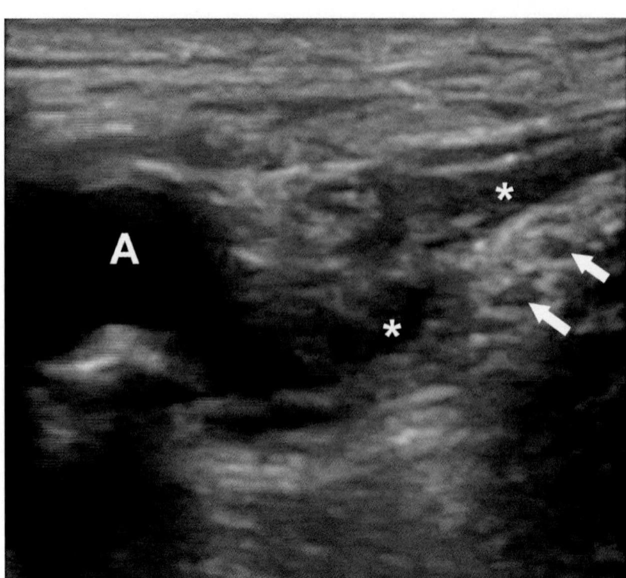

Figure 16.38
Local anesthetic (*) infiltrated near femoral nerve (arrows). The femoral artery (A) is visible medially.

expected location. The appearance of local anesthetic infiltrated around the femoral nerve is demonstrated in Figure 16.38.

Distal upper extremity nerve blocks

There are two methods for locating the radial, median, and ulnar nerves. It may be simplest to begin at the wrist [31]. The radial and ulnar nerves can be located next to their corresponding arteries at the wrist, and the median nerve can be located in the center of the wrist near the flexor digitorum muscle. Once located, the nerves can be traced proximally to the mid forearm. Alternately, the nerves can be located more proximally and traced distal toward the mid forearm. The radial nerve can be found above the elbow near the deep brachial artery, deep to the triceps muscle. The median nerve lies medial to the brachial artery near the elbow, superficial to the brachialis muscle. The ulnar nerve lies near the medial epicondyle at the elbow. Figures 16.39–16.41 demonstrate the radial, median, and ulnar nerves at the forearm, and Figure 16.42 shows local anesthetic infiltrated around the ulnar nerve.

Interscalene nerve block

The brachial plexus nerve roots can be found in the interscalene groove near the C6 level (Figure 16.43). Imaging in a transverse plane, begin medially and visualize the carotid artery and internal jugular vein with the sternocleido-mastoid muscle. This anatomy should be familiar, as it is demonstrated in internal jugular venous cannulation. Sliding the probe laterally, the anterior

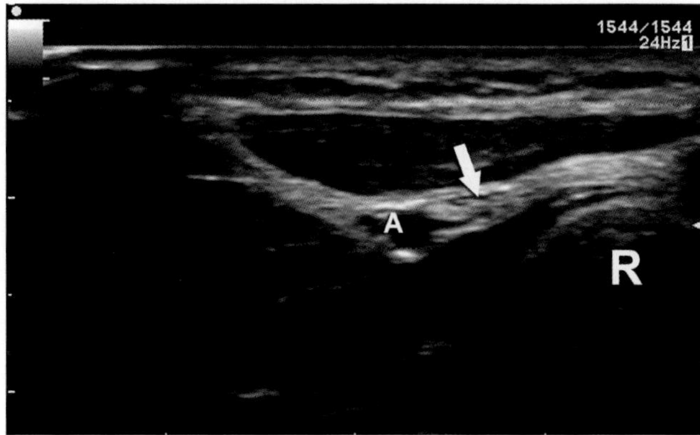

Figure 16.39
Radial nerve (arrow) near radial artery (A) and radius (R).

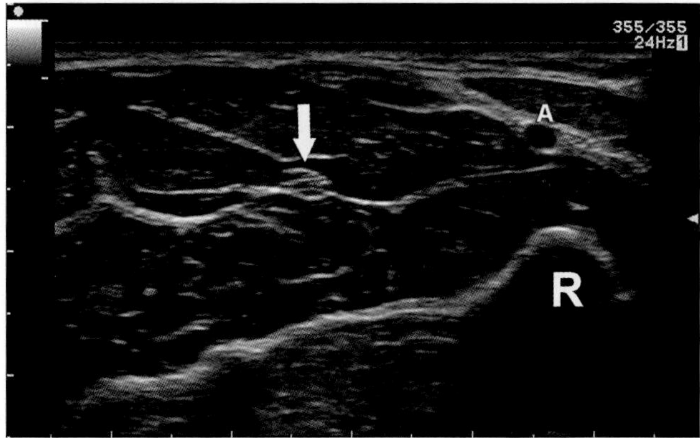

Figure 16.40
Median nerve (arrow), radial artery (A) and radius (R).

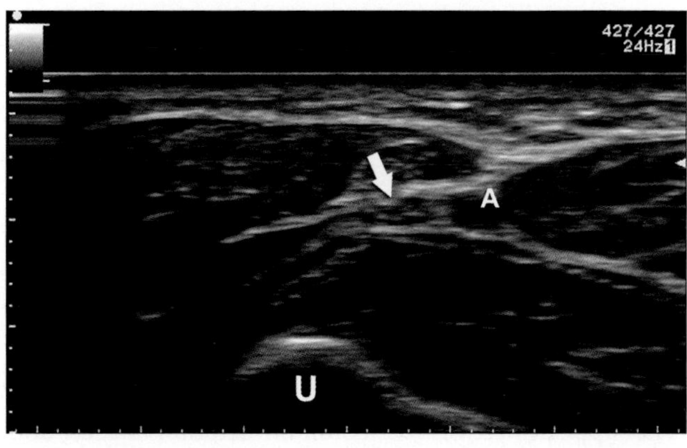

Figure 16.41
Ulnar nerve (arrow), ulnar artery (A) and ulna (U).

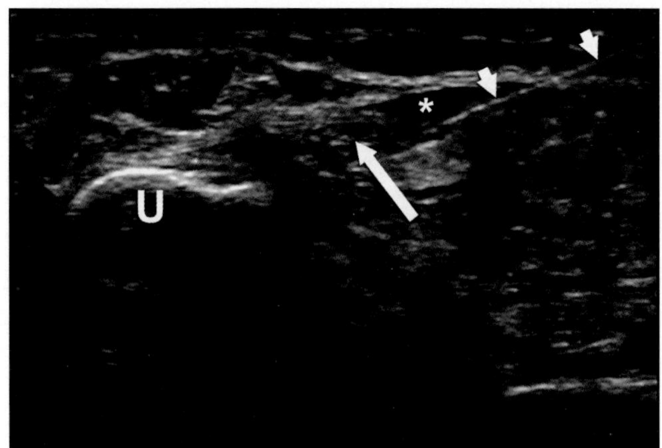

Figure 16.42
Local anesthetic (*) infiltrated around ulnar nerve (long arrow). The ulna (U) is visible, and the needle (small arrows) is visualized in the longitudinal plane.

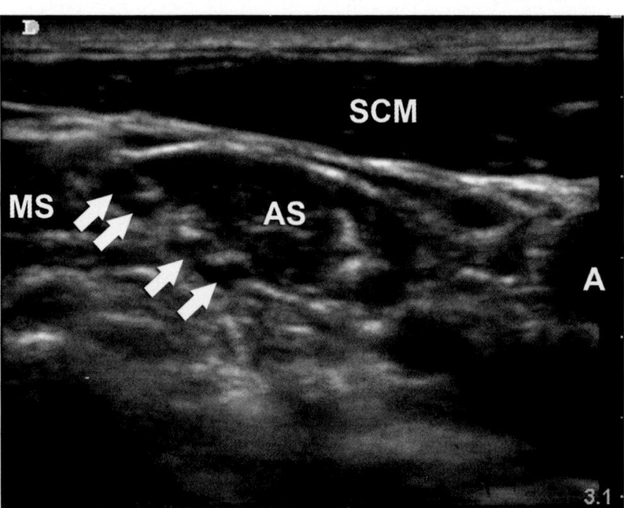

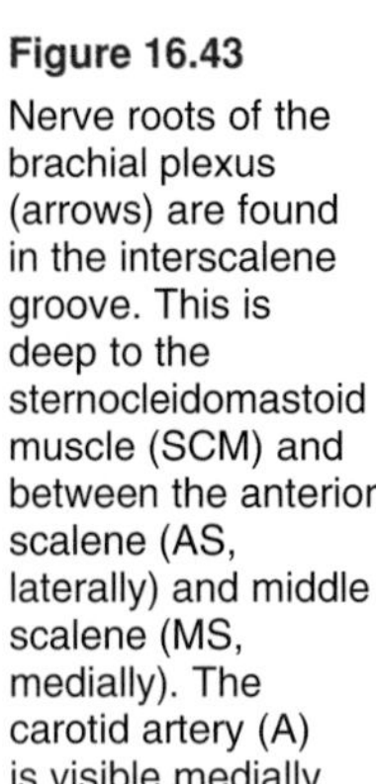

Figure 16.43
Nerve roots of the brachial plexus (arrows) are found in the interscalene groove. This is deep to the sternocleidomastoid muscle (SCM) and between the anterior scalene (AS, laterally) and middle scalene (MS, medially). The carotid artery (A) is visible medially.

scalene muscle will be encountered deep to the sternocleidomastoid. The brachial plexus should be visualized just lateral to that.

Note that the phrenic nerve is located quite close to this region, in between the sternocleidomastoid and anterior scalene muscles. The phrenic nerve is commonly affected by interscalene blocks, and this can lead to diaphragmatic paralysis. Operators should be prepared for this occurrence, and obviously should only select patients with good respiratory reserve for this block.

Tips

For femoral nerve blockade it is helpful to remain quite proximal, near the inguinal ligament. The appearance of the common femoral artery and vein, and the proximal branch point of the greater saphenous vein, should help confirm the proper location for anesthetic administration. Some authors advocate the use of an out-of-plane (transverse) approach toward needle guidance for the femoral nerve block. As with other procedures, patient anatomy and operator comfort should determine the optimal approach

It may be easier to visualize the interscalene nerve roots closer to the clavicle; once seen, trace them caudal for the block.

Pitfalls

With any peripheral nerve block, it is mandatory that anesthetic not be injected within the nerve. No pressure is required for these blocks, and they should not be painful. Pain and increased resistance to injection may be warning signs of intraneural injection.

As with venous access (Chapter 15), nerve blocks require significant hand–eye coordination. Position the patient, ultrasound machine, and operator in a comfortable position. The operator should be able to view the ultrasound image easily, and his or her hands should be in a position of comfort and stability.

Aspiration prior to injection is wise with any procedure; this is even more important given the larger volumes of anesthetic employed for regional blocks (up to 20 or more mL for large nerves).

Most importantly, motor blockade is common with regional nerve blocks; be sure to pad sensitive areas (such as the hip) to avoid injury or ulcer formation in the setting of a numb and immobilized extremity.

Literature review

A recent Cochrane review of 18 randomized controlled trials concluded that ultrasound-guided peripheral nerve blocks had success rates similar to those of other methods of nerve localization. However, ultrasound was shown to reduce complication rates and improve onset time. In addition, ultrasound may improve block quality [32].

Peripheral nerve blocks have been described in the anesthesia literature, and a feasibility study of 22 forearm blocks performed by emergency physicians (EPs) demonstrated the efficacy of the technique [31]. The feasibility of EP-performed femoral nerve blocks was demonstrated in elderly patients with hip fracture. Reduced pain scores were noted in patients receiving the block [33]. Stone *et al.* compared supraclavicular brachial plexus blocks to procedural sedation in 12 patients with upper extremity injury [34]. The authors found decreased length of stay in the nerve block group, and no significant complications in either group.

References

1. Yang PC, Luh KT, Chang DB, *et al.* Value of sonography in determining the nature of pleural effusion: analysis of 320 cases. *AJR Am J Roentgenol* 1992; **159**: 29–33.
2. Weingardt JP, Guico RR, Nemcek AA, Li YP, Chiu ST. Ultrasound findings following failed, clinically directed thoracenteses. *J Clin Ultrasound* 1994; **22**: 419–26.
3. Lichtenstein D, Hulot JS, Rabiller A, Tostivint I, Meziere G. Feasibility and safety of ultrasound-aided thoracentesis in mechanically ventilated patients. *Intensive Care Med* 1999; **25**: 955–8.
4. Jones PW, Moyers JP, Rogers JT, *et al.* Ultrasound-guided thoracentesis: is it a safer method? *Chest* 2003; **123**: 418–23.
5. Barnes TW, Morgenthaler TI, Olson EJ, *et al.* Sonographically guided thoracentesis and rate of pneumothorax. *J Clin Ultrasound* 2005; **33**: 442–6.
6. Runyon BA. Paracentesis of ascitic fluid: a safe procedure. *Arch Intern Med* 1986; **146**: 2259–61.
7. Bard C, Lafortune M, Breton G. Ascites: ultrasound guidance or blind paracentesis? *CMAJ* 1986; **135**: 209–10.
8. Nazeer SR, Dewbre H, Miller AH. Ultrasound-assisted paracentesis performed by emergency physicians vs the traditional technique: a prospective, randomized study. *Am J Emerg Med* 2005; **23**: 363–7.
9. Roy S, Dewitz A, Paul I. Ultrasound-assisted ankle arthrocentesis. *Am J Emerg Med* 1999; **17**: 300–1.
10. Smith SW. Emergency physician-performed ultrasonography-guided hip arthrocentesis. *Acad Emerg Med* 1999; **6**: 84–6.
11. Wiler JL, Costantino TG, Filippone L, Satz W. Comparison of ultrasound-guided and standard landmark techniques for knee arthrocentesis. *J Emerg Med* 2010; **39**: 76–82.
12. Hill R, Conron R, Greissinger P, Heller M. Ultrasound for the detection of foreign bodies in human tissue. *Ann Emerg Med* 1997; **29**: 353–6.
13. Orlinsky M, Knittel P, Feit T, Chan L, Mandavia D. The comparative accuracy of radiolucent foreign body detection using ultrasonography. *Am J Emerg Med* 2000; **18**: 401–3.
14. Nienaber A, Harvey M, Cave G. Accuracy of bedside ultrasound for the detection of soft tissue foreign bodies by emergency doctors. *Emerd Med Australas* 2010; **22**: 30–4.
15. Blankstein A, Cohen I, Heiman Z, *et al.* Localization, detection, and guided removal of soft tissue in the hands using sonography. *Arch Orthop Trauma Surg* 2000; **120**: 514–17.
16. Squire BT, Fox JC, Anderson C. ABSCESS: applied bedside sonography for convenient evaluation of superficial soft tissue infections. *Acad Emerg Med* 2005; **12**: 601–6.
17. Tayal VS, Hasan N, Norton HJ, Tomaszewski CA. The effect of soft-tissue ultrasound on the management of cellulitis in the emergency department. *Acad Emerg Med* 2006; **13**: 384–8.

18. Blaivas M, Theodoro D, Duggal S. Ultrasound-guided drainage of peritonsillar abscess by the emergency physician. *Am J Emerg Med* 2003; **21**: 155–8.
19. Grau T, Leipold RW, Conradi R, Martin E. Ultrasound control for presumed difficult epidural puncture. *Acta Anaesthesiol Scand* 2001; **45**: 766–71.
20. Peterson MA, Abele J. Bedside ultrasound for difficult lumbar puncture. *J Emerg Med* 2005; **28**: 197–200.
21. Abo A, Chen L, Johnston P, Santucci K. Positioning for lumbar puncture in children evaluated by bedside ultrasound. *Pediatrics*. 2010; **125**: e1149–53.
22. Stiffler KA, Jwayyed S, Wilber ST, Robinson A. The use of ultrasound to identify pertinent landmarks for lumbar puncture. *Am J Emerg Med*. 2007; **25**: 331–4.
23. Tsang TSM, El-Najdawi EK, Seward JB, *et al.* Percutaneous echocardiographically guided pericardiocentesis in pediatric patients: evaluation of safety and efficacy. *J Am Soc Echocardiogr* 1998; **11**: 1072–7.
24. Tsang TSM, Enriquez-Sarano M, Freeman WK, *et al.* Consecutive 1127 therapeutic echocardiographically guided pericardiocenteses: clinical profile, practice patterns, and outcomes spanning 21 years. *Mayo Clin Proc* 2002; **77**: 429–36.
25. Cho BC, Kang SM, Kim DH, *et al.* Clinical and echocardiographic characteristics of pericardial effusion in patients who underwent echocardiographically guided pericardiocentesis: Yonsei Cardiovascular Center experience, 1993–2003. *Yonsei Med J* 2004; **45**: 462–8.
26. Ettin D, Cook T. Using ultrasound to determine external pacer capture. *J Emerg Med* 1999; **17**: 1007–9.
27. Macedo W, Sturmann K, Kim LM, Kang L. Ultrasonographic guidance of transvenous pacemaker insertion in the emergency department: a report of three cases. *J Emerg Med* 1999; **17**: 491–6.
28. Baumann BM, McCans K, Stahmer SA, *et al.* Volumetric bladder ultrasound performed by trained nurses increases catheterization success in pediatric patients. *Am J Emerg Med* 2008; **26**: 18–23.
29. Aguilera PA, Choi T, Durham. Ultrasound-guided suprapubic cystostomy catheter placement in the emergency department. *J Emerg Med* 2004; **26**: 319–21.
30. Chen L, Hsiao AL, Moore CL, Dziura JD, Santucci KA. Utility of bedside bladder ultrasound before urethral catheterization in young children. *Pediatrics* 2005; **115**: 108–11.
31. Liebmann O, Price D, Mills C, *et al.* Feasibility of forearm ultrasonography-guided nerve blocks of the radial, ulnar, and median nerves for hand procedures in the emergency department. *Ann Emerg Med* 2006; **48**: 558–62.
32. Walker KJ, McGrattan K, Aas-Eng K, Smith AF. Ultrasound guidance for peripheral nerve blockade. *Cochrane Database Syst Rev* 2009; (**4**): CD006459.

33. Beaudoin FL, Nagdev A, Merchant RC, Becker BM. Ultrasound-guided femoral nerve blocks in elderly patients with hip fractures. *Am J Emerg Med* 2010; **28**: 76–81.
34. Stone MB, Wang R, Price DD. Ultrasound-guided supraclavicular brachial plexus nerve block vs procedural sedation for the treatment of upper extremity emergencies. *Am J Emerg Med* 2008; **26**: 706–10.

Index